MW01470206

Progress in Pain Research and Management
Volume 26

Pediatric Pain:
Biological and Social Context

Mission Statement of IASP Press®

The International Association for the Study of Pain (IASP) is a nonprofit, interdisciplinary organization devoted to understanding the mechanisms of pain and improving the care of patients with pain through research, education, and communication. The organization includes scientists and health care professionals dedicated to these goals. The IASP sponsors scientific meetings and publishes newsletters, technical bulletins, the journal *Pain*, and books.

The goal of IASP Press is to provide the IASP membership with timely, high-quality, attractive, low-cost publications relevant to the problem of pain. These publications are also intended to appeal to a wider audience of scientists and clinicians interested in the problem of pain.

Progress in Pain Research and Management
Volume 26

Pediatric Pain: Biological and Social Context

Editors

Patrick J. McGrath, PhD

*Departments of Psychology, Pediatrics, and Psychiatry,
Dalhousie University; Pediatric Pain Service,
IWK Health Centre, Halifax, Nova Scotia, Canada*

G. Allen Finley, MD, FRCPC

*Departments of Anesthesia and Psychology,
Dalhousie University; Pediatric Pain Service,
IWK Health Centre, Halifax, Nova Scotia, Canada*

IASP PRESS® • SEATTLE

© 2003 IASP Press®
International Association for the Study of Pain®

All rights reserved. No part of this publication may be reproduced, stored in a retrieval system, or transmitted, in any form or by any means, electronic, mechanical, photocopying, recording, or otherwise, without the prior written permission of the publisher.

Timely topics in pain research and treatment have been selected for publication, but the information provided and opinions expressed have not involved any verification of the findings, conclusions, and opinions by IASP®. Thus, opinions expressed in *Pediatric Pain: Biological and Social Context* do not necessarily reflect those of IASP or of the Officers and Councillors.

No responsibility is assumed by IASP for any injury and/or damage to persons or property as a matter of product liability, negligence, or from any use of any methods, products, instruction, or ideas contained in the material herein. Because of the rapid advances in the medical sciences, the publisher recommends that there should be independent verification of diagnoses and drug dosages.

Library of Congress Cataloging-in-Publication Data

Pediatric pain : biological and social context / editors, Patrick J. McGrath, G. Allen Finley.
     p. ; cm. -- (Progress in pain research and management ; v. 26)
  Includes bibliographical references and index.
  ISBN 0-931092-49-3 (alk. paper)
    1. Pain in children. 2. Pain in children--Social aspects. 3. Pediatrics. I. McGrath, Patrick J. II. Finley, G. Allen, 1954- III. Series.
  [DNLM: 1. Pain--Child. 2. Pain--Infant. WL 704 P3712 2003]
  RJ365.P433 2003
  618.92--dc21

                                                                2003051134

Published by:

IASP Press
International Association for the Study of Pain
909 NE 43rd Street, Suite 306
Seattle, WA 98105-6020 USA
Fax: 206-547-1703
www.iasp-pain.org
www.painbooks.org

Printed in the United States of America

Contents

List of Contributing Authors		vii
Preface		ix
1.	Long-Term Effects of Neonatal Pain: The Animal Literature *Sarita Garg, Umesh Narsinghani, Adnan T. Bhutta,* *Cynthia R. Rovnaghi, and K.J.S. Anand*	1
2.	Self-Regulation and Behavior in Preterm Children: Effects of Early Pain *Ruth Eckstein Grunau*	23
3.	Genetic Tools for the Study of Pain: Current Techniques and Findings *Shad B. Smith and Jeffrey S. Mogil*	57
4.	Social Development and Pain in Children *Carl L. von Baeyer and Lara J. Spagrud*	81
5.	The Role of Family Factors in Pediatric Pain *Christine T. Chambers*	99
6.	Chronic Illness and Pain in Children: A Review with Special Emphasis on Cancer *Gustaf Ljungman*	131
7.	Social Influences, Culture, and Ethnicity *Kenneth D. Craig and Rebecca R. Pillai Riddell*	159
8.	Health Center Policies and Accreditation *Ada K. Jacox and Carol D. Spengler*	183
9.	Availability of Opioid Analgesics for Cancer Pain Relief in Children *David E. Joranson, Aaron M. Gilson, Karen M. Ryan,* *and Martha A. Maurer*	201
Index		217

Contributing Authors

K.J.S. Anand, MBBS, DPhil *Departments of Pediatrics, Anesthesiology, Pharmacology, and Neurobiology, University of Arkansas for Medical Sciences, Little Rock, Arkansas, USA*

Adnan T. Bhutta, MBBS, FAAP *Department of Pediatrics, University of Arkansas for Medical Sciences, Little Rock, Arkansas, USA*

Christine T. Chambers, PhD *Department of Pediatrics, University of British Columbia; Centre for Community Child Health Research, British Columbia Research Institute for Children's and Women's Health; and Department of Psychology, British Columbia's Children's Hospital, Vancouver, British Columbia, Canada; currently Departments of Pediatrics and Psychology, Dalhousie University; and Pediatric Pain Research Laboratory, IWK Health Centre, Halifax, Nova Scotia, Canada*

Kenneth D. Craig, PhD *Department of Psychology, University of British Columbia, Vancouver, British Columbia, Canada*

Sarita Garg, PhD *Pain Neurobiology Laboratory, Arkansas Children's Hospital Research Institute, Little Rock, Arkansas, USA*

Aaron M. Gilson, PhD *Pain and Policy Studies Group, University of Wisconsin Comprehensive Cancer Center, World Health Organization Collaborating Center for Policy and Communications in Cancer Care, Madison, Wisconsin, USA*

Ruth Eckstein Grunau, PhD *Centre for Community Child Health Research, B.C. Research Institute for Children's and Women's Health, and Department of Pediatrics, University of British Columbia, Vancouver, British Columbia, Canada*

Ada K. Jacox, PhD, RN *School of Nursing, University of Virginia, Charlottesville, Virginia; and Clinical Practice Guidelines Program, American Pain Society, Glenview, Illinois, USA*

David E. Joranson, MSSW *Pain and Policy Studies Group, University of Wisconsin Comprehensive Cancer Center, World Health Organization Collaborating Center for Policy and Communications in Cancer Care, Madison, Wisconsin, USA*

Gustaf Ljungman, MD, PhD *Department of Children's and Women's Health, Uppsala University, and Unit for Pediatric Hematology and Oncology, University Children's Hospital, Uppsala, Sweden*

Martha A. Maurer, BS *Pain and Policy Studies Group, University of Wisconsin Comprehensive Cancer Center, World Health Organization Collaborating Center for Policy and Communications in Cancer Care, Madison, Wisconsin, USA*

Jeffrey S. Mogil, PhD *Department of Psychology, McGill University, Montreal, Quebec, Canada*

Umesh Narsinghani, MD, FAAP *Department of Pediatrics, Mercer University College of Medicine, Macon, Georgia, USA*

Rebecca R. Pillai Riddell, MA *Department of Psychology, University of British Columbia, Vancouver, British Columbia, Canada*

Cynthia R. Rovnaghi, MS *Pain Neurobiology Laboratory, Arkansas Children's Hospital Research Institute, Little Rock, Arkansas, USA*

Karen M. Ryan, MA *Pain and Policy Studies Group, University of Wisconsin Comprehensive Cancer Center, World Health Organization Collaborating Center for Policy and Communications in Cancer Care, Madison, Wisconsin, USA*

Shad B. Smith, BS *Department of Psychology, McGill University, Montreal, Quebec, Canada*

Lara J. Spagrud, BA (Hon) *Department of Psychology, University of Saskatchewan, Saskatoon, Saskatchewan, Canada*

Carol D. Spengler, PhD, RN *School of Nursing, University of Virginia, Charlottesville, Virginia; and Clinical Practice Guidelines Program, American Pain Society, Glenview, Illinois, USA*

Carl L. von Baeyer, PhD *Department of Psychology, University of Saskatchewan, Saskatoon, Saskatchewan, Canada*

Preface

Perhaps the most important thing we have learned about pain in the last 35 years is that context matters. Melzack and Wall set the stage in 1965 with their elegant theory that pain was not a simple straight-through system in which tissue damage occurring in the periphery propagates a signal that sets off an alarm in the brain in the form of the sensation of pain. Although Melzack and Wall did not explore how psychosocial and biological contexts interact to influence pain, their gate control theory broke the stranglehold that the specificity theory had previously held. Advances in neuroscience and in specific treatments for pain have moved forward our understanding of context by repeatedly demonstrating enormous variability in clinical pain situations. It is this variability that makes possible the study of context. Context includes all aspects of the internal or external environment independent of pain transmission itself. In this volume we present an overview of different contexts surrounding pediatric pain, beginning with the basic biological science data and then moving to psychological, social, and governmental contexts.

Early experience is a potent influence on the later experience of pain. While experimental human studies are not possible for ethical reasons, animal studies have begun to tell an interesting story. Rodent studies are contributing a great deal to the understanding of the possible effects of pain on development. Although direct generalization from rodents to humans is not possible, these studies provide clues as to where we should search for the effects of pain on humans. Anand and his colleagues have conducted some of the most intriguing studies in this area, and their chapter provokes us to take very seriously the long-term impact of pain on broad areas of human development.

Human studies of early experience are difficult to conduct rigorously and their interpretation is challenging because they rely exclusively on correlational methods or naturally occurring experiments that are almost always confounded. Grunau has done excellent work in this area, and her chapter draws on the widest range of literature to tell a coherent and challenging story.

Although pediatric pain research has increased dramatically in the last few years, some areas have lagged behind. For example, even though the genetics of pain is clearly important, very little animal work has focused on early development models that could correlate with pain-related pediatric conditions. It is clear that gene expression has a developmental course, at least in some disorders. For example, migraine is genetically transmitted, but only after puberty does it become evident in most migraineurs, and the condition appears to have differing heritability at different ages. Moreover, the ways in which development modifies the effects of gene expression on pediatric phenomena such as central sensitization and effects of sweet taste have not been investigated. Finally, infants and children may provide a particularly valuable resource for genetic research because of their relatively short learning history compared to adults. Smith and Mogil have provided an outstanding review of some of the most exciting work now occurring in pain genetics. Although the work has not used pediatric models, the information is generalizable to infants, children, and adolescents, and is of great importance to pediatric pain.

One of the least studied yet most important elements of context in pediatric pain is chronic illness. Many children with chronic illness suffer pain from their disease or from their treatment. Moreover, chronic illness may influence the ways in which these children and their family members react to pain. Unfortunately, most chronic illnesses and conditions occurring in the pediatric population have not been widely studied from a pain perspective, and most of the available research has focused on cancer. Ljungman, a pediatric oncologist, has reviewed the immediate and long-term impact of pain in children with cancer and other diseases.

We all know that children differ in their response to painful events. Some react very strongly whereas others seem to react very little, if at all. Many psychological factors may be involved. However, the scattered data on this topic have not been well integrated. Von Baeyer and Spagrud meet this challenge in bringing together the available information regarding attachment, temperament, socialization and social learning, and emotion regulation in the development of pain expression.

Most of the time we think of the pain experience as occurring within the boundaries of the skin of the individual. Indeed it does, but pain cannot be isolated within the individual. The social milieu profoundly affects the pain experience, and pain in turn influences the family and the larger social milieu. If the researcher's perspective is always restricted to the individual, only part of the story is told. If we fail to examine the environmental context, much will be lost, both in terms of understanding pain and in treating our patients.

The family is our genetic crucible. It nurtures our early experiences and our reactions to and understanding of pain. Too often families are not studied with scientific rigor, but Chambers has shown how families can be scientifically studied. In her chapter she thoroughly examines pain and the family while highlighting specific directions for further research.

Social influences of culture and ethnicity constitute the next level of analysis. This area has been plagued by stereotype and poor methodology. Much of the typically accepted "understanding" of social factors and culture is more a reflection of the prejudices of the authors than a true reflection of patients' behavior. Craig and Pillai disentangle the mythical from the real findings and present a clear path for future research.

Health services are designed to help children, but paradoxically often do not protect them from pain. Indeed, children often suffer pain from health care procedures. Hospital accreditation is a powerful tool to assist in modifying standard practice of such procedures in health centers in order to avoid unnecessary pain. Jacox and her colleagues are leaders in developing guidelines and practice standards for pain treatment and in promoting the recognition that effective pain treatment is an important outcome that must be accounted for in the accreditation process.

Government institutions probably form the least frequently studied context influencing pain, but their rules can have a major impact on its treatment. Government agencies enforce laws and regulations that control access to pain medications. Unfortunately, the most widely used and often the most effective class of drugs, the opioids, are the drugs most stringently restricted by governments worldwide. Legal restriction derives, of course, from their perceived potential for abuse, although this risk is greatly overstated. The risk of opioid diversion must be balanced against the real need for access to these drugs to relieve suffering. Joranson, a champion of sane drug laws and drug enforcement around opioids, details this story.

The biological and societal contexts of pain in infants, children, and youth play a critical role in the development and management of pain. By adopting a wider perspective that includes these contexts, clinicians and researchers can significantly improve their understanding, prevention, and treatment of pain.

This volume is based on the Fourth International Forum on Pediatric Pain, held at White Point Beach, Nova Scotia, Canada, September 19–22, 2002. We wish to thank McNeil Consumer Healthcare, Canada, who provided an educational grant for this meeting, all the participants who contributed to the discussion, and our patients, who provide the inspiration.

PATRICK J. MCGRATH
G. ALLEN FINLEY

1

Long-Term Effects of Neonatal Pain: The Animal Literature

Sarita Garg,[a] Umesh Narsinghani,[b] Adnan T. Bhutta,[a,c] Cynthia R. Rovnaghi,[a] and K.J.S. Anand[a,c]

[a]*Pain Neurobiology Laboratory, Arkansas Children's Hospital Research Institute, Little Rock, Arkansas, USA;* [b]*Department of Pediatrics, Mercer University College of Medicine, Macon, Georgia, USA;* [c]*Departments of Pediatrics, Anesthesiology, Pharmacology, and Neurobiology, University of Arkansas for Medical Sciences, Little Rock, Arkansas, USA*

NEONATAL PAIN AS A CLINICAL PROBLEM

Pain, whether or not it involves tissue injury, activates widely distributed and highly variable elements in the peripheral and central nervous systems, depending on features of the noxious stimulus, the context in which it occurs, and characteristics of the subject such as age, species, gender, and previous experiences of pain. Different types of pain (physiological, inflammatory, visceral, and neuropathic) are transmitted by distinct molecular mechanisms and increase pain sensitivity via the activation, modulation, or modification of different elements within the pain system (Woolf and Salter 2000).

Newborn infants admitted to the hospital frequently undergo painful and invasive procedures. Pain in infancy is also a developmental issue, because the immaturity of spinal cord sensory processing in the newborn leads to lower thresholds for excitation and sensitization, thus maximizing the central effects of noxious inputs. Furthermore, the plasticity of both peripheral and central sensory connections in the neonatal period means that early damage in infancy can lead to prolonged structural and functional alterations in pain pathways that last into adult life (Lidow 2002).

Our thinking about infant pain has changed dramatically in the past 20 years. Researchers thought that young children did not experience pain, due to their assumption that the immature nervous system offered protection against the experience of acute pain. Also, they considered that newborn infants would not remember early experiences and that exposure to neonatal pain would thus have no lasting effects on behavior or development (Swafford and Allen 1968). Recent research, however, has highlighted the need for prevention and management of pain in neonates (Anand 2001; Banos et al. 2001), because even the most premature neonates possess the basic neuronal circuitry needed for the processing of nociceptive information (Fitzgerald and Beggs 2001). They are capable of mounting the behavioral distress and physiological stress responses elicited by noxious stimulation in older age groups (Anand 1998; Guinsburg et al. 1998). Furthermore, preterm neonates exhibit lower pain thresholds compared to older infants, and these thresholds decrease even further following exposure to repeated painful stimuli (Andrews and Fitzgerald 1999, 2002; Narsinghani and Anand 2000).

Clinical and basic scientific research focusing on the long-term effects of neonatal pain is important because large numbers of both preterm and full-term neonates routinely experience repetitive acute or prolonged inflammatory pain during their exposure to neonatal intensive care. These experiences occur at a time when the infants' sensitivity to pain, vulnerability to neuronal cell death, and mechanisms of neuroplasticity (synaptogenesis, dendritic morphogenesis) are developmentally accentuated. Several clinical studies show that early exposure to repetitive pain is subsequently correlated with altered pain processing, poor cognitive development, and atypical behaviors during childhood. Therefore, a deeper understanding of the mechanisms leading to these long-term changes may allow the development of novel therapeutic approaches to prevent the long-term effects of pain in the developing brain.

The objectives of this chapter are to critically appraise the findings and issues related to animal studies on the long-term consequences of repetitive neonatal pain, to scrutinize the mechanistic insights on the function and development of the immature pain system obtained from these studies, and wherever possible, to examine the relevance of these animal models for reproducing the clinical situations in critically ill or preterm neonates. It is well documented that neonates and infants in neonatal intensive care units (NICUs) experience repeated painful events (Barker and Rutter 1995; Johnston et al. 1997; Porter and Anand 1998). Research on the long-term consequences of repeated pain in preterm and full-term neonates is described by Grunau (this volume). Repetitive neonatal pain or stress can produce permanent alterations in various sensory systems (Berardi et al. 2000), and their long-term effects often depend on the stage of maturation at which the adverse experience or noxious stimulation occurs. Thus, windows of vulnerability for long-term modification depend on the maturational stage of the nociceptive circuitry in preterm and newborn babies (Anand and Carr 1989). For both ethical and practical reasons, it is difficult to study the long-term effects of repetitive pain in human infants. Clinical, demographic, genetic, social, and environmental factors often confound the interpretation of findings from long-term follow-up studies, requiring inordinately large sample sizes to control for these factors. Therefore, animal models have greatly contributed to our understanding of neonatal processing and the long-term consequences of pain.

MODELS EXAMINING THE LONG-TERM EFFECTS OF NEONATAL PAIN

Although animal models may never match the complexity of the human condition, they provide a unique opportunity to investigate a number of basic mechanisms that are conserved across mammalian evolution. Animal models give an insight into basic mechanisms underlying the long-term consequences of pain and also provide sufficient data to generate hypotheses that can be tested in human infants (Johnston et al. 2002; Lidow 2002). Many confounding variables can be controlled by the experimental setting and study design, which helps in clarifying the direct effects of the applied manipulations. Experiments using specific strains of rodents, for example, with littermates subjected to different experimental paradigms, allow us to reduce the genetic variability between experimental groups. Animals are kept in well-controlled environments with less variability than a NICU, which decreases the sample size required for studying a given effect. Because the lifespan of many animal species is shorter than that of humans, experiments on the long-term effects of pain can be concluded within a relatively short time. Amongst the mammalian species, rodents have been used most commonly for pain and neurodevelopmental research, because of their short lifespan, easy availability, low cost, simple requirements for housing, diet, and animal husbandry, and previous standardization and validation of behavioral tests. A few models have used nonhuman primates because of their evolutionary or social relevance, although these studies require the scientific justification for a primate model, are subject to greater costs of procurement and limited availability, and require complex laboratory maintenance and higher security.

RODENT MODELS

Human infants and neonatal rat pups display a variety of behavioral and physiological responses in response to acute pain. These responses have highly conserved developmental or age-specific patterns (Guy and Abbott 1992; Johnston et al. 1993). Similarities in the pain system of newborn rodents and humans include exaggerated cutaneous reflexes (Fitzgerald et al. 1988), functional polymodal nociceptors (Fitzgerald 1987), sensitization caused by repeated noxious stimulation (Fitzgerald et al. 1989; Taddio et al. 2002), relatively large receptive fields of dorsal horn cells (Yi and Barr 1995), and immaturity of the descending inhibitory systems (Fitzgerald and Koltzenburg 1986). Pain-related neurotransmitters in the spinal cord including substance P, galanin, met-enkephalin, somatostatin, calcitonin gene-related peptide (CGRP), vasoactive intestinal polypeptide (VIP), and other ligands appear to follow similar developmental patterns of expression in newborn rats and human neonates (Marti et al. 1987). Previous studies have assumed that the neurological maturity of neonatal rat pups at birth (P0) or at 7 days (P7) is similar to that of 24-week preterm or term neonates, respectively (Dobbing 1981; Fitzgerald and Anand 1993; Alvares et al. 2000; Lidow 2002). However, recent data suggest that rat pups are even less mature than previously thought (Mattson and Rychlik 1991; Clancy et al. 2001; Sugiura et al. 2001) (see Fig. 1).

Rodent models addressing the long-term consequences of neonatal pain can be divided into four groups, designed to examine the effects of inflammatory pain, physiological pain, visceral pain, and neuropathic pain (Woolf and Salter 2000).

Inflammatory pain. A model for the long-term effects of neonatal pain was based on intraplantar injections of complete Freund's adjuvant (CFA) into the hindpaw of neonatal rat pups (Ruda et al. 2000; Tachibana et al. 2001). A single CFA injection at P0 or P3 caused inflammation of the hindpaw lasting for 5–7 days, associated with abnormal sprouting of sciatic primary afferents on the ipsilateral side, which encroached on spinal segments of the dorsal horn (L6, S1) that do not normally receive sensory input from the sciatic nerve. In the adult rats, dorsal horn neurons (in laminae I/II) receiving input from these thinly myelinated or unmyelinated nerve fibers were hyperexcitable, demonstrating increased activity at rest and in response to tactile or noxious stimuli (Ruda et al. 2000). Behavioral testing of these adult rats showed no abnormality in their paw-withdrawal latencies to thermal stimulation. However, when the hindpaw was re-inflamed by CFA injections in adulthood, the rats exhibited high thermal hyperalgesia associated with a significantly higher density of fos-immunoreactive dorsal horn

Developmental Time across Species

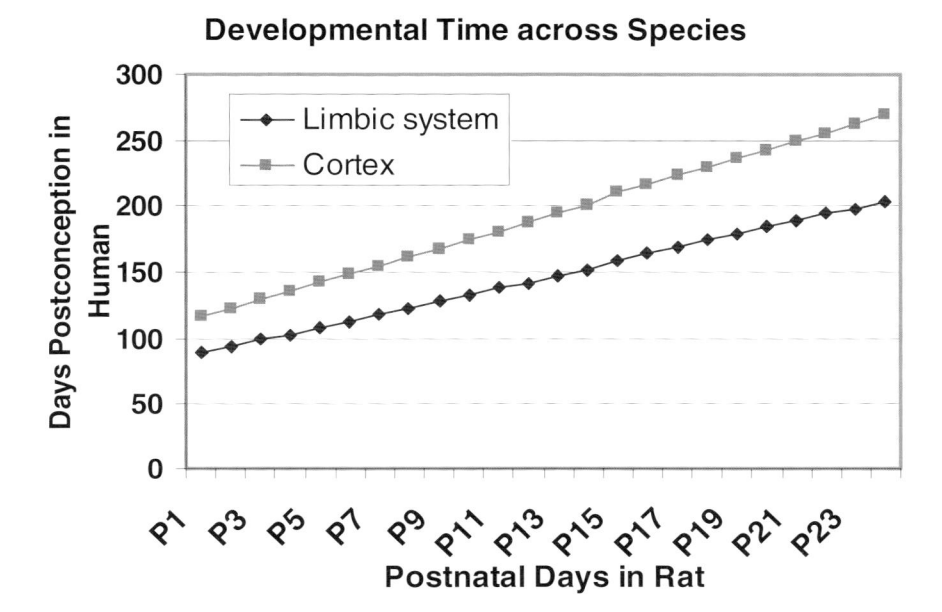

Fig. 1. Comparison of developmental events in the rat brain during the postnatal period with prenatal development of the human brain. Data are based on Clancy et al. (2000, 2001).

neurons on the ipsilateral as compared to the contralateral side. Vulnerability to these changes was limited to the early newborn period, because animals injected with CFA at P14 failed to manifest any of these long-term effects (Ruda et al. 2000; Tachibana et al. 2001). In evaluating the clinical relevance of these findings, we must take into account the developmental differences between newborn rats and humans, as well as the considerable differences in brain complexity and adaptability. In addition, the localized fibrosis, limb deformities, and other trophic changes caused by localized inflammation lasting for 5–7 days in newborn rat pups and a systemic inflammatory response leading to CFA-induced arthritis may have contributed to these findings (Anand 2000).

Models of inflammatory pain are induced by injections of formalin (Bhutta et al. 2001), bee venom (Lariviere and Melzack 1996), carrageenan (Rahman et al. 1997), injection or topical application of capsaicin (Marsh et al. 1999b; Liu et al. 2003). Formalin injections produce behavioral signs of inflammatory pain that last for about 30 minutes in infant rats and an hour in adult rats (Guy and Abbott 1992; Abbott and Guy 1995; Teng and Abbott 1998), although hyperalgesia and inflammatory changes may persist for 6–8 hours after injection (Bhutta et al. 2001). Repeated formalin injections in the early neonatal period were associated with thermal hyposensitivity in adult male and female rats; this long-term effect was partially ameliorated by morphine pretreatment in the male rats, but not in the females (Bhutta et al. 2001). Repetitive neonatal inflammatory pain decreased ethanol preference and locomotor activity during adulthood, to a greater extent in the males than in females (Bhutta et al. 2001).

Carrageenan injections produce inflammation lasting for up to 48 hours (Alvares et al. 2000), although a single carrageenan injection can be calibrated to produce edema of the injected paw and increased nocifensive behaviors lasting for 24 hours (Lidow et al. 2001). Infant rats injected with carrageenan at P0 or P1 showed alterations in the phenotype of primary sensory neurons (Beland and Fitzgerald 2001), decreases of 33% in the receptive field of dorsal horn neurons (Rahman et al. 1997), and mechanical and thermal hyposensitivity of the neonatally injected paw (but accentuated hyperalgesia following CFA-induced re-inflammation) during adulthood (Cleland et al. 1999; Lidow et al. 2001). Many of these long-term effects were absent in rats injected with carrageenan at P14, suggesting that even brief local inflammation can lead to long-term changes in nociception, as long as this insult takes place during a critical developmental window in neonatal rats.

Physiological pain (tissue injury). The most commonly performed invasive procedure in preterm and full-term neonates is the heel stick for blood sampling (Barker and Rutter 1995; Porter and Anand 1998). To model the long-term effects of repeated heel sticks in human neonates, rat pups were subjected to four daily needle sticks (one to each paw, applied at hourly intervals) from P1 to P7. Similar to the data from human neonates (Fitzgerald et al. 1989; Taddio et al. 2002), the results showed that repetitive needle sticks were associated with a thermal hypersensitivity during subsequent development (at P16 and P22), but this effect was not maintained into adulthood (Anand et al. 1999). Behavioral changes during adulthood in these rats, however, showed increased preference for alcohol, greater anxiety and defensive withdrawal, and prolonged memory for chemosensory cues, associated with diminished neuronal activation in the somatosensory cortex following thermal pain (Anand et al. 1999). Another preliminary report suggests that the long-term effects of repeated needle sticks in neonatal rats may be blunted by maternal grooming (Johnston and Walker 2000). Other models have reported thermal hyposensitivity and enhanced effects of morphine analgesia in adult rats that were exposed to repeated foot shocks from birth to P21 (Shimada et al. 1990), although the clinical relevance of this model has been questioned (Lidow 2002).

To model the surgical incisions performed in human neonates during procedures such as circumcision or chest tube insertion, Reynolds and Fitzgerald (1995) removed a small piece of skin from the hindpaw of neonatal rat pups at P0, P7, and P14. Neonatal skin wounds resulted in the exuberant sprouting of cutaneous nerve fibers supplying the area of injured skin, originating from C fibers, Aδ fibers, and sympathetic nerve fibers. The younger the age at the time of injury, the more profound was this hyperinnervation response, which was associated with significant and long-term decreases in localized sensory thresholds. Hyperinnervation of neonatal wounds involved not only local collaterals from nearby damaged nerve branches but also sprouting of sensory fibers drawn from deep tissue and noncutaneous nerve bundles (Alvares et al. 2000). Blockade of nerve impulses from the injured area (local anesthetic sciatic nerve block) or spinal anesthesia did not block the nerve sprouting, suggesting that axonal transport of growth factors from the dorsal root ganglia (DRG) or efferent impulses from the spinal cord do not influence the peripheral nerve sprouting (De Lima et al. 1999). Cutaneous nerve sprouting was inhibited by anti-nerve growth factor antibodies in adult rats but not in neonatal rat pups, suggesting a role for other growth factors released locally in the area of tissue injury (Reynolds et al. 1997a,b).

Visceral pain. Animal models for early visceral pain were not investigated until recently because the lack of clinical data suggested that visceral pain or hyperalgesia may occur rarely, or perhaps not at all, during infancy or early childhood. Recent data have challenged this concept, showing significant reductions in the abdominal skin reflex following surgical operations in neonates and small infants, as well as visceral hyperalgesia resulting from hydronephrosis and dilatation of the renal pelvis (Andrews and Fitzgerald 2002; Andrews et al. 2002).

To develop an adult animal model for irritable bowel syndrome, Al-Chaer and colleagues (2000) applied colorectal distension (mechanical stimulation) or intracolonic injection of mustard oil (chemical stimulation) daily to developing rats from P8 to P21. These animals developed visceral hyperalgesia during adolescence and adulthood, determined by an increased activity of spinal viscerosensitive neurons both at baseline and following colorectal distension, which is associated with increased sensitivity for abdominal withdrawal reflexes. Following repetitive neonatal stress, in the form of daily maternal separation from P2 to P14, adult animals developed signs of visceral hyperalgesia, stress-induced colonic motility, somatic hypoalgesia, and stress-induced increased fecal output, thus mimicking the cardinal features of irritable bowel syndrome (Coutinho et al. 2002). Thus, it is likely that repetitive noxious and stressful stimuli in the neonatal period lead to abnormal processing of visceral pain in later life. In this regard, it is intriguing that gastric suction in healthy, full-term human infants at birth was associated with a threefold increased risk for developing irritable bowel syndrome in later life (K.J.S. Anand et al., unpublished manuscript).

Neuropathic pain (nerve injury). Studies on the long-term consequences of neonatal sciatic nerve sectioning or ligation have shown that rat pups lose up to 75% of axotomized neurons as compared to only 30% of neurons lost in adult animals (Himes and Tessler 1989; Lewis et al. 1999). The resulting cortical reorganization, however, is restricted in newborn rats as compared to adult rats (Cusick 1996). Active loss of immature neurons results in the sprouting of central dorsal root terminals of nearby intact nerves in the spinal cord to occupy areas that are normally the exclusive territory of the sectioned sciatic nerve (Fitzgerald 1985; Fitzgerald and Shortland 1988; Shortland and Fitzgerald 1994). These newly sprouted nerve fibers form inappropriate functional connections with dorsal horn cells in areas outside of their normal termination, leading to a permanent distortion of the nervous system with disproportionately increased cutaneous inputs from areas surrounding the denervated skin (Shortland and Molander 2000; Sugimoto et al. 2000). Rats subjected to chronic constriction injury of the sciatic nerve showed spontaneous pain behaviors for more than 12 weeks, associated with increased activity in anterior dorsal thalamus, habenular complex, cingulate cortex, and retrosplenial cortex. Thermal hyperalgesia in these rats was correlated with activity in the somatosensory cortex, hypothalamic paraventricular nucleus, and basolateral amygdala, but mechanical allodynia was associated with changes in the ventrolateral and ventroposterolateral thalamus. Thus, peripheral nerve damage leads to persistent abnormalities in the sensory thalamocortical axis (Paulson et al. 2002).

PRIMATE MODELS

Both rodent and primate models have reported that early adverse experiences can alter behavioral and neuroendocrine responsiveness, brain morphology, gene expression and neurochemical markers regulating their developmental processes (Sanchez et al. 2001; Gorman et al. 2002). Relatively few reports, however, have assessed the long-term effects of neonatal pain exposure in primates. Experiments involving early life stress in nonhuman primates suggest that many of the behavioral and biochemical changes resemble those of rodents undergoing early pain. Hence, we will focus on the behavioral and neurobiological sequelae of exposure to early adverse events in nonhuman primates.

One of the most important environmental regulatory factors in early development is parental care (Hofer 1994). The rhesus monkey (*Macaca mulatta*) is the primate species most frequently used to study the developmental effects of the early social environment. Apart from the relative physical maturity of the rhesus infant at birth, a difference between the early development of infant humans and rhesus monkeys is the amount of physical contact between mother and neonate (Seay and Gottfried 1975). The macaque infant remains closely attached to the mother's ventral surface for several weeks and sleeps in close ventral contact with the mother for nearly a year, at which time weaning occurs. Any spontaneous or experimental deviation of care may result in infant stress responses. Hyperactivity of immature stress systems such as the limbic-hypothalamic-pituitary-adrenal (HPA) axis and the limbic-sympatho-adrenomedullary axis can alter their subsequent reactivity across the lifespan (Pryce et al. 2002). Monkey and human infants exhibit similarities in their behavioral reactions to maternal separation. The rhesus infant's initial reaction to maternal separation consists of a "protest phase" with increased activity and vocalization, physiological reactions such as defecation (Harlow et al. 1971), and increased HPA function (Bayart et al. 1990). Pigtail macaques respond even more intensely to maternal separation than do rhesus monkeys (Kaufman and Rosenblum 1967).

In addition, early maternal and social deprivation interferes with the normal cognitive development of primates (Beauchamp and Gluck 1988; Beauchamp et al. 1991; Sanchez et al. 1998). It produces altered stress physiology with high basal adrenocorticotropic hormone (ACTH) and glucocorticoid levels and accentuated HPA responsiveness to stress (Clarke et al. 1994; Coplan et al. 1996). The mothers of bonnet macaque monkeys that have unpredictable foraging demands in their environment are more aggressive toward and less nurturing of their infants. As adults, offspring raised by such macaque mothers exhibited persistently elevated cerebrospinal fluid (CSF) concentrations of corticotropin-releasing factor (CRF) (Coplan et al. 1996), consistent with the evidence for increased CRF levels in adult rats exposed to maternal separation as infants (Plotsky and Meaney 1993). Because the hyperactivity of CRF-releasing neurons has been implicated in the pathophysiology of human affective and anxiety disorders, this finding provides a neurobiological mechanism by which early-life stressors may contribute to adult psychopathology. This vulnerability may also be, at least in part, heritable. Studies in squirrel monkeys demonstrated that paternal half-siblings that exhibit prolonged adrenocortical and vocalization responses to maternal separation are the ones that spend more time near the mother in the undisturbed groups (Lyons et al. 1999), thus indicating an individual variability in "coping" and "recovering" from adverse experiences that has both genetic and experiential components in agreement with human twin studies (Silove et al. 1995; Kendler and Karkowski-Shuman 1997). Prenatal models of maternal stress in rhesus monkeys during mid-to-late gestation (E90–E145) or early gestation (E45–E90) have many similar long-term effects.

Dysregulation of monoaminergic systems has been reported in isolated or peer-reared primates. Either excessive or insufficient dopamine neurotransmission can impair prefrontal cognitive functions involving working memory, as well as behavioral inhibition (Arnsten and Goldman-Rakic 1998; Collins et al. 1998). Recent evidence suggests that disruptions in forebrain dopamine neurotransmission induced by excessive exposure to cortisol may lead to prefrontal cognitive deficits (Lyons et al. 2000).

In summary, multiple rodent and primate models have examined the long-term behavioral outcomes of exposure to neonatal pain or early adverse experiences such as maternal separation, but the neurobiological bases for these behavioral changes are not completely understood. Further investigation of the mechanisms leading to changes in pain-related and other behaviors will allow the development of novel therapeutic and preventive approaches to diminish the persistent effects of neonatal pain and stress. These mechanisms must be investigated in the spinal cord as well as in supraspinal areas.

LONG-TERM CHANGES IN SPINAL PAIN MECHANISMS

Investigation of the neurochemistry, electrophysiological properties, and connectivity of sensory neurons in the developing DRG and dorsal horn of spinal cord in rats has shed light on the way in which the newborn central nervous system is altered by exposure to noxious stimuli. Long-term changes in spinal pain processing are developmentally regulated and depend on the maturation of spinal pain system at the time that postnatal exposure to noxious stimulation occurs.

EXCITATORY MECHANISMS

Acute pain or inflammation produces robust and specific pain behaviors and induces neuronal *Fos* expression in the dorsal horn (Yi and Barr 1995), leading to A-fiber-mediated sensitization and C-fiber-mediated windup (the mechanisms underlying primary and secondary hyperalgesia) (Fitzgerald et al. 1989; Jennings and Fitzgerald 1998; Woolf and Salter 2000). Zhou and colleagues have demonstrated that neurotrophins from DRG cells are responsible for generating the long-term hyperalgesia and allodynia following peripheral nerve injury, and are also involved in the survival of neurons in the dorsal horn and sympathetic ganglia (Theodosiou et al. 1999; Huang et al. 2000; Zhou et al. 2000). These data provided the first evidence that DRG-derived neurotrophins mediate the prolonged neuropathic pain after peripheral nerve injury, but their inhibition may lead to neurodegenerative changes in the dorsal horn (Zhou et al. 1998; Deng et al. 2000). Prostaglandin E_2 (PGE_2) and its receptor are key factors contributing to the generation of hyperalgesia caused by inflammation. Spinal plasticity resulting from carrageenan-induced inflammation was associated with time-dependent increases in prostaglandin E_2 concentrations, activation of its receptors, and increase in calcium in the spinal dorsal horn neurons (Nakayama et al. 2002). Downstream from these mediators, the regulatory Iβ subunit of protein kinase A probably plays an important role in hyperalgesia, because mice with a null mutation for this factor were protected from inflammatory and tissue-injury-related nociception (Malmberg et al. 1997).

Glutamate is the primary excitatory neurotransmitter in the spinal cord and brain, whereas its receptors, N-methyl D-aspartate (NMDA), α-amino-3-hydroxy-5-methyl-4-isoxazole propionate (AMPA)/kainate, and metabotropic glutamate receptor 1 (mGluR1), play a central role in the activity-dependent changes of dendritic length or spine density, synaptic stability, long-term potentiation (LTP) or depression (LTD), and other processes that mediate a heightened plasticity in the neonatal brain and spinal cord. Numerous reports show that NMDA-dependent mechanisms are implicated not only in spinal transmission of pain but also in the long-term effects of pain (Dubner and Ruda 1992; Chiang et al. 1997; Sakurada et al. 1998; Svendsen et al. 1998; Zhuo 1998; Baba et al. 2000).

Neonatal rats exposed to repeated needle sticks from P0 to P7 developed a prolonged thermal hyperalgesia noted at 16 and 22 days of age (Anand et al. 1999). Prolonged localized inflammation caused by CFA injections in neonatal rat pups led to increased sprouting of primary sensory fibers and abnormal extension into caudal segments of the spinal cord (L6, S1). These events were associated with hyperexcitability in the dorsal horn neurons connected with these fibers and were correlated with increased pain behaviors in adult rats (Ruda et al. 2000). Significant increases in Fos-like immunoreactivity in the lumbar spinal cord of these rats suggested that neonatal peripheral inflammation results in increased responses of spinal cord neurons to peripheral inflammation in adult rats (Tachibana et al. 2001). Localized inflammation for 48 hours, caused by injecting carrageenan into the hindpaws of P1 rats, led to a marked reduction of 33% in the receptive field size of dorsal neurons to subsequent noxious stimulation (Rahman et al. 1997). Peripheral inflammation induced by 0.25% carrageenan in rat pups at birth (P0) led to significant increases in the withdrawal latency to thermal and mechanical stimulation in the absence of ongoing inflammation, with significant decreases in these parameters in the presence of CFA-induced inflammation during adulthood (Lidow et al. 2001).

In contrast to acute tissue injury, which leads to hyper-responsiveness to pain, long-term effects of early inflammatory pain may lead to decreased responsiveness (Bhutta et al. 2001; Lidow et al. 2001), no change (Alvares et al. 2000), or an increased sensitivity to pain (Ruda et al. 2000; Tachibana et al. 2001). The conflicting findings of these studies may be attributed to the use of different inflammatory agents and paradigms; Bhutta et al. used daily formalin injections, Alvares et al. used a single dose of carrageenan, and Ruda et al. used CFA. Thus, the persistent changes from neonatal pain depend on the type and timing of stimulation, the age and species of rat pups (Mogil et al. 1999a,b; Lariviere et al. 2002), and other factors such as concurrent treatments with opioids (Bhutta et al. 2001).

MODULATORY MECHANISMS

The development of diffuse noxious inhibitory controls (DNICs) from the periaqueductal gray, pontine reticular nuclei, locus ceruleus, and other foci in the brainstem is functionally mature by P21, but not yet effective at P12 (Boucher et al. 1998). This development follows a rostrocaudal pattern, associated with higher pain thresholds in the forelimbs as compared to the hindlimbs of 10-day-old rats (Ren et al. 1997). Due to immature gating mechanisms, newborns are incapable of filtering peripheral sensory stimulation, with exaggerated behavioral responses and the potential for widespread and long-term alteration of the supraspinal microcircuitry involved in pain processing.

Endogenous analgesic mechanisms in the postnatal period are mediated via pathways requiring orogustatory, orotactile, and generalized tactile inputs (Blass et al. 1995; Barr et al. 1999; Blass and Watt 1999). Opioid receptors mediate many of the inhibitory mechanisms in the dorsal horn, but other physiological roles also affect the regulation of dendritic growth and spine formation in developing neurons (Hauser et al. 1989).

In summary, neonatal interventions lead to permanent alterations in the structure and function of the adult pain system, with hyperinnervation in areas of wounded skin (Reynolds and Fitzgerald 1995), an increased sprouting of primary afferent fibers, and hyperexcitability of dorsal horn neurons (Ruda et al. 2000), leading to adaptive changes within the dorsal horn that decrease the receptive field size of these afferent neurons (Rahman et al. 1997). Putative mechanisms for such adaptive changes include reduced dendritic arborization of dorsal horn neurons, increased inhibitory interneurons, upregulation of inhibitory receptors or ion channels, or enhanced activity of the DNICs from supraspinal centers. Behavioral studies demonstrate lower pain thresholds in neonatal and infant rats, mediated by immature mechanisms at several levels of the pain system (Anand et al. 1999). Normal development of the spinal pain system occurs in the absence or near-absence of noxious stimulation, and multiple studies suggest that acute, repetitive, or prolonged pain in the neonatal period permanently alters the structure and function of the developing pain system.

LONG-TERM CHANGES IN SUPRASPINAL PROCESSING

Pain has been described as an unpleasant experience that includes discriminative, affective, and cognitive components to produce a unified sensory experience, each component mediated via separate and interactive forebrain mechanisms (Casey 1999). Recent years have seen an increased focus on understanding the supraspinal processing of pain, both in animal models and in humans. The introduction of imaging techniques such as positron emission tomography (PET) and autoradiography has led to the elucidation of specific brain regions involved in supraspinal pain processing. Autoradiography-measured regional cerebral blood flow (rCBF) during formalin injections in Sprague-Dawley rats showed increased flow in the somatosensory cortex, parts of the limbic system, medial thalamus, and ventral posterior (VPL) thalamus. In humans, the ability to localize a somatic stimulus and grade its intensity are functions of the primary somatosensory cortex (S1) and VPL thalamus (Derbyshire et al. 1997; Derbyshire and Jones 1998). Lesions in these areas, however, do not produce analgesia. In contrast, lesions in the anterior cingulate cortex (ACC) and insular cortex have no effect on pain localization, but they do affect the perceived unpleasantness of noxious stimuli (Derbyshire and Jones 1998, Casey 1999). Human PET scans measuring cerebral activity before and after hypnotic suggestions found that modulation of pain intensity produced significant changes in pain-evoked activity in the S1 cortex, while modulation of the perceived unpleasantness produced significant changes in the ACC (Rainville et al. 1997; Hofbauer et al. 2001). Patients with chronic facial pain had increased blood flow in the ACC and decreased blood flow in the prefrontal cortex, structures that are closely related to the "medial pain system" (Derbyshire et al. 1994). The anatomical connections between these regions and with caudal structures like the thalamus are illustrated in Fig. 2, showing the putative supraspinal processing of pain.

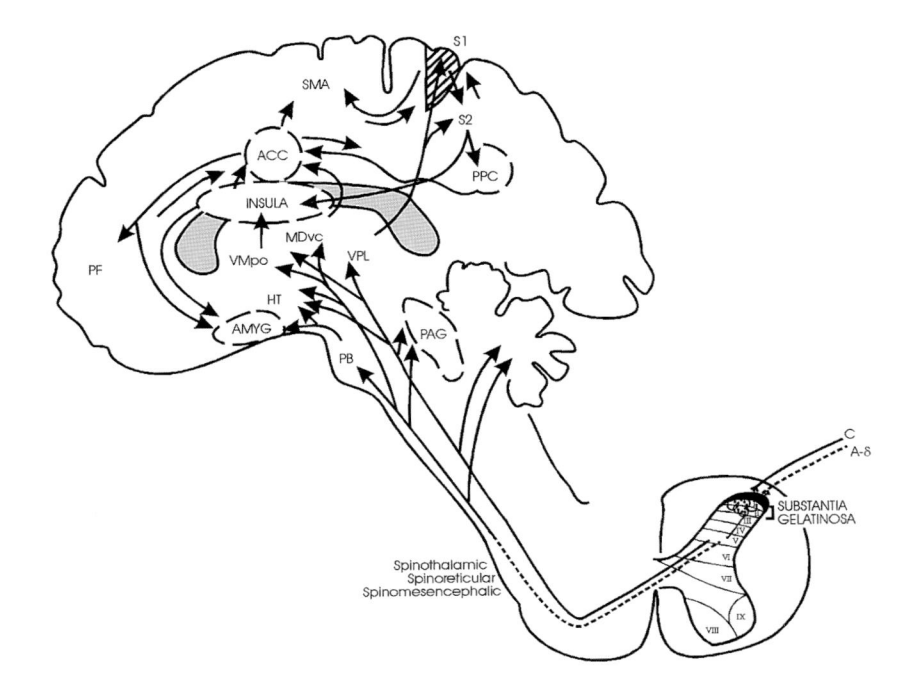

Fig. 2. Spinal and supraspinal structures involved in pain processing and the long-term effects of pain. ACC = anterior cingulate cortex; AMYG = amygdala; HT = hypothalamus; MDvc = medial dorsal nucleus, ventrocaudal part; PAG = periaqueductal gray matter; PB = parabrachial nucleus; PF = prefrontal cortex; PPC = posterior parietal cortex; S1 and S2 = primary and secondary somatosensory cortical areas; SMA = supplementary motor area; VMpo = ventromedial nucleus, posterior part; VPL = ventroposterior lateral nucleus of the thalamus.

Despite growing awareness of the role of various supraspinal regions in pain processing, the long-term effects of pain on these regions is not well understood. For 24 to 41 days after intraspinal injection of quisqualic acid (an AMPA/mGluR1 agonist) in Long-Evans rats, rCBF was increased in the arcuate nucleus, the hindlimb area of the S1 cortex, the parietal cortex, and the posterior ventral thalamic nuclei (VPL and ventroposteromedial [VPM]) (Morrow et al. 2000). Following chronic constriction injury of the sciatic nerve, persistent spontaneous pain behaviors were correlated with activation of limbic system structures (the anterior dorsal thalamus, habenular complex, and cingulate and retrosplenial cortices). Thermal hyperalgesia was correlated with the activation of the somatosensory cortex, hypothalamic paraventricular nucleus, and basolateral amygdala, and mechanical allodynia was correlated with changes in ventrolateral and VPL thalamic activity, indicating that persistent changes in pain behavior were associated with functional derangements of the limbic-thalamo-cortical axis (Paulson et al. 2002). Forebrain-targeted overexpression of the NMDA-receptor subunit NR2B (in the ACC and insular cortex, but not in the spinal cord) was associated with enhanced responsiveness to formalin- and CFA-induced inflammatory pain (Wei et al. 2001). Double knockouts of the calmodulin-stimulated adenylyl cyclases (AC1 and AC8), which couple NMDA-receptor activation to cyclic adenosine monophosphate (cAMP) signaling in the ACC and forebrain areas, were indistinguishable from normal rats in tests of acute pain but showed vastly reduced behavioral allodynia following inflammatory pain (Wei et al. 2002). More recently, we have found that capsaicin-induced hyperalgesia in P21 rats was associated with upregulation of neuronal adenylyl cyclase and uncoupling of opioid receptors in the forebrain. Opioid receptor desensitization in the forebrain may reduce opioidergic inputs to the descending inhibitory controls, associated with persistent hyperalgesia and reduced responses to morphine analgesia in capsaicin-injected young rats (Liu et al. 2003).

Behavioral changes in adult rats following exposure to repetitive noxious stimuli as neonates also reflect long-term supraspinal changes, although the specific mechanisms remain undefined. Adult rats exhibited an increased preference for alcohol, greater anxiety and defensive withdrawal behavior, prolonged chemosensory memory, and diminished activation of the somatosensory cortex by thermal pain following exposure to repeated needle sticks in the neonatal period (Anand et al. 1999). Neonatal rat pups exposed to repeated formalin injections (P1–P7) exhibited prolonged latencies on hot-plate testing as adults, suggesting delayed supraspinal pain processing (Bhutta et al. 2001). These rats also exhibited decreased alcohol preference and reduced locomotor activity, suggesting that plasticity of the neonatal brain allows permanent changes in brain development secondary to noxious stimuli. The underlying mechanisms may include, among other explanations, increases in the rate of naturally occurring neuronal cell death in the cortical areas associated with nociceptive processing (Newton et al. 2000; Bhutta and Anand 2001). We have proposed that enhanced neuronal death in the immature neonatal period may occur due to two primary mechanisms: (1) NMDA-mediated excitotoxicity and (2) enhanced naturally occurring neuronal apoptosis during early development (Anand and Scalzo 2000; Bhutta and Anand 2001). Repetitive or prolonged pain, especially in the vulnerable neonatal period when neuronal plasticity is at its peak, thus can lead to long-term anatomical and behavioral changes. The neurobiological mechanisms underlying these changes remain the focus of intense research activity.

DIRECTIONS FOR FURTHER RESEARCH ON NEONATAL PAIN

A large body of scientific and clinical data supports the development of animal models of neonatal pain to study the long-term changes resulting from acute, repetitive, prolonged, or chronic pain. Although numerous models have been reported, very little information is currently available to identify the precise mechanisms leading to these long-term changes. Across the different laboratory models used and the mechanisms investigated, it is increasingly clear that neonatal experiences of pain will be recorded in the hard-wiring of the immature brain and may persist, perhaps for the entire life of the individual. The pattern and magnitude of these cellular, ultrastructural, or architectural abnormalities will depend on genetic variability as well as the timing, intensity, and duration of pain and adverse experiences. These early experiences may establish an increased or decreased vulnerability to subsequent pain and stress during infancy and childhood. Cumulative brain damage during infancy may lead to reductions in brain volume, poor cognitive outcomes, abnormal behaviors, and neuroendocrine dysregulation during adolescence and adult life. The importance of preventing or ameliorating the subtle brain damage caused by neonatal pain and stress cannot be overestimated. Thus, concerted efforts by clinicians and neuroscientists should investigate the mechanisms underlying early neuronal injury, minimize the impact of early adverse experiences in neonates, and investigate novel therapeutic strategies for treating neonatal pain and stress.

ACKNOWLEDGMENTS

Supported by Arkansas Children's Hospital Foundation and the National Institute for Child Health and Human Development (HD36484 to K.J.S. Anand).

REFERENCES

Abbott FV, Guy ER. Effects of morphine, pentobarbital and amphetamine on formalin-induced behaviours in infant rats: sedation versus specific suppression of pain. *Pain* 1995; 62:303–312.

Al-Chaer ED, Kawasaki M, Pasricha PJ. A new model of chronic visceral hypersensitivity in adult rats induced by colon irritation during postnatal development. *Gastroenterology* 2000; 119:1276–1285.

Alvares D, Torsney C, Beland B, et al. Modelling the prolonged effects of neonatal pain. *Prog Brain Res* 2000; 129:365–373.

Anand KJS. Clinical importance of pain and stress in preterm neonates. *Biol Neonate* 1998; 73:1–9.

Anand KJS. Pain, plasticity, and premature birth: a prescription for permanent suffering? *Nat Med* 2000; 6:971–973.

Anand KJS. International Evidence-Based Group for Neonatal Pain. Consensus statement for the prevention and management of pain in the newborn. *Arch Pediatr Adolesc Med* 2001; 155:173–180.

Anand KJS, Carr DB. The neuroanatomy, neurophysiology, and neurochemistry of pain, stress, and analgesia in newborns and children. *Pediatr Clin N Am* 1989; 36:795–822.

Anand KJS, Scalzo FM. Can adverse neonatal experiences alter brain development and subsequent behavior? *Biol Neonate* 2000; 77:69–82.

Anand KJS, Coskun V, Thrivikraman KV, Nemeroff CB, Plotsky PM. Long-term behavioral effects of repetitive pain in neonatal rat pups. *Physiol Behav* 1999; 66:627–637.

Andrews K, Fitzgerald M. Cutaneous flexion reflex in human neonates: a quantitative study of threshold and stimulus-response characteristics after single and repeated stimuli. *Dev Med Child Neurol* 1999; 41:696–703.

Andrews K, Fitzgerald M. Wound sensitivity as a measure of analgesic effects following surgery in human neonates and infants. *Pain* 2002; 99:185–95.

Andrews KA, Desai D, Dhillon HK, Wilcox DT, Fitzgerald M. Abdominal sensitivity in the first year of life: comparison of infants with and without prenatally diagnosed unilateral hydronephrosis. *Pain* 2002; 100:35–46.

Arnsten AF, Goldman-Rakic PS. Noise stress impairs prefrontal cortical cognitive function in monkeys: evidence for a hyperdopaminergic mechanism. *Arch Gen Psychiatry* 1998; 55:362–368.

Baba H, Doubell TP, Moore KA, Woolf CJ. Silent NMDA receptor-mediated synapses are developmentally regulated in the dorsal horn of the rat spinal cord. *J Neurophysiol* 2000; 83:955–962.

Banos JE, Ruiz G, Guardiola E. An analysis of articles on neonatal pain published from 1965 to 1999. *Pain Res Manage* 2001; 6:45–50.

Barker DP, Rutter N. Exposure to invasive procedures in neonatal intensive care unit admissions. *Arch Dis Child Fetal Neonatal Ed* 1995; 72:F47–F48.

Barr RG, Pantel MS, Young SN, et al. The response of crying newborns to sucrose: is it a "sweetness" effect? *Physiol Behav* 1999; 66:409–417.

Bayart F, Hayashi KT, Faull KF, Barchas JD, Levine S. Influence of maternal proximity on behavioral and physiological responses to separation in infant rhesus monkeys (*Macaca mulatta*). *Behav Neurosci* 1990; 104:98–107.

Beauchamp AJ, Gluck JP. Associative processes in differentially reared monkeys (*Macaca mulatta*): sensory preconditioning. *Dev Psychobiol* 1988; 21:355–364.

Beauchamp AJ, Gluck JP, Fouty HE, Lewis MH. Associative processes in differentially reared rhesus monkeys (*Macaca mulatta*): blocking. *Dev Psychobiol* 1991; 24:175–189.

Beland B, Fitzgerald M. Influence of peripheral inflammation on the postnatal maturation of primary sensory neuron phenotype in rats. *J Pain* 2001; 2:36–45.

Berardi N, Pizzorusso T, Maffei L. Critical periods during sensory development. *Curr Opin Neurobiol* 2000; 10:138–145.

Bhutta AT, Anand KJS. Abnormal cognition and behavior in preterm neonates linked to smaller brain volumes. *Trends Neurosci* 2001; 24:129–130; 131–132.

Bhutta AT, Rovnaghi CR, Simpson PM, et al. Interactions of inflammatory pain and morphine treatment in infant rats: long-term behavioral effects. *Physiol Behav* 2001; 73:51–58.

Blass EM, Watt LB. Suckling- and sucrose-induced analgesia in human newborns. *Pain* 1999; 83:611–623.

Blass EM, Shide DJ, Zaw-Mon C, Sorrentino J. Mother as shield: differential effects of contact and nursing on pain responsivity in infant rats—evidence for nonopioid mediation. *Behav Neurosci* 1995; 109:342–353.

Boucher T, Jennings E, Fitzgerald M. The onset of diffuse noxious inhibitory controls in postnatal rat pups: a C-Fos study. *Neurosci Lett* 1998; 257:9–12.

Casey KL. Forebrain mechanisms of nociception and pain: analysis through imaging. *Proc Natl Acad Sci USA* 1999; 96:7668–7674.
Chiang CY, Hu JW, Sessle BJ. NMDA receptor involvement in neuroplastic changes induced by neonatal capsaicin treatment in trigeminal nociceptive neurons. *J Neurophysiol* 1997; 78:2799–2803.
Clancy B, Darlington RB, Finlay BL. The course of human events: predicting the timing of primate neural development. *Dev Sci* 2000; 3(1):57–66.
Clancy B, Darlington RB, Finlay BL. Translating developmental time across mammalian species. *Neuroscience* 2001; 105:7–17.
Clarke AS, Wittwer DJ, Abbott DH, Schneider ML. Long-term effects of prenatal stress on HPA axis activity in juvenile rhesus monkeys. *Dev Psychobiol* 1994; 27:257–269.
Cleland CL, Ritter SM, Hawkins AR, Broghammer AM, Gebhart GF. Neonatal inflammation causes permanent, dose-dependent changes in thermal pain sensitivity in rats. *Abstracts: 9th World Congress on Pain.* Seattle: IASP Press, 1999, p 413.
Collins P, Roberts AC, Dias R, Everitt BJ, Robbins TW. Perseveration and strategy in a novel spatial self-ordered sequencing task for nonhuman primates: effects of excitotoxic lesions and dopamine depletions of the prefrontal cortex. *J Cogn Neurosci* 1998; 10:332–354.
Coplan JD, Andrews MW, Rosenblum LA, et al. Persistent elevations of cerebrospinal fluid concentrations of corticotropin-releasing factor in adult nonhuman primates exposed to early-life stressors: implications for the pathophysiology of mood and anxiety disorders. *Proc Natl Acad Sci USA* 1996; 93:1619–1623.
Coutinho SV, Plotsky PM, Sablad M, Miller, et al. Neonatal maternal separation alters stress-induced responses to viscerosomatic nociceptive stimuli in rat. *Am J Phys Gastro Liver Physiol* 2002; 282:G307–G316.
Cusick CG. Extensive cortical reorganization following sciatic nerve injury in adult rats versus restricted reorganization after neonatal injury: implications for spatial and temporal limits on somatosensory plasticity. *Prog Brain Res* 1996; 108:379–390.
De Lima J, Alvares D, Hatch DJ, Fitzgerald M. Sensory hyperinnervation after neonatal skin wounding: effect of bupivacaine sciatic nerve block. *Br J Anaesth* 1999; 83:662–664.
Deng YS, Zhong JH, Zhou XF. Effects of endogenous neurotrophins on sympathetic sprouting in the dorsal root ganglia and allodynia following spinal nerve injury. *Exp Neurol* 2000; 164:344–350.
Derbyshire SW, Jones AK. Cerebral responses to a continual tonic pain stimulus measured using positron emission tomography. *Pain* 1998; 76:127–135.
Derbyshire SW, Jones AK, Devani P, et al. Cerebral responses to pain in patients with atypical facial pain measured by positron emission tomography. *J Neurol Neurosurg Psychiatry* 1994; 57:1166–1172.
Derbyshire SW, Jones AK, Gyulai F, et al. Pain processing during three levels of noxious stimulation produces differential patterns of central activity. *Pain* 1997; 73:431–445.
Dobbing J. Nutritional growth restriction and the nervous system. In: Davison AN, Thompson RHS (Eds). *The Molecular Basis of Neuropathology.* London: Edward Arnold, 1981.
Dubner R, Ruda MA. Activity-dependent neuronal plasticity following tissue injury and inflammation. *Trends Neurosci* 1992; 15:96–103.
Fitzgerald M. The sprouting of saphenous nerve terminals in the spinal cord following early postnatal sciatic nerve section in the rat. *J Comp Neurol* 1985; 240:407–413.
Fitzgerald M. Cutaneous primary afferent properties in the hind limb of the neonatal rat. *J Physiol* 1987; 383:79–92.
Fitzgerald M, Anand KJS. The developmental neuroanatomy and neurophysiology of pain. In: Schechter N, Berde C, Yaster M (Eds). *Pain Management in Infants, Children and Adolescents.* Baltimore: Williams & Williams, 1993, pp 11–32.
Fitzgerald M, Beggs S. The neurobiology of pain: developmental aspects. *Neuroscientist* 2001; 7:246–257.

Fitzgerald M, Koltzenburg M. The functional development of descending inhibitory pathways in the dorsolateral funiculus of the newborn rat spinal cord. *Brain Res* 1986; 389:261–270.

Fitzgerald M, Shortland P. The effect of neonatal peripheral nerve section on the somadendritic growth of sensory projection cells in the rat spinal cord. *Brain Res* 1988; 470:129–136.

Fitzgerald M, Shaw A, MacIntosh N. The postnatal development of the cutaneous flexor reflex: a comparative study in premature infants and newborn rat pups. *Dev Med Child Neurol* 1988; 30:520–526.

Fitzgerald M, Millard C, McIntosh N. Cutaneous hypersensitivity following peripheral tissue damage in newborn infants and its reversal with topical anaesthesia. *Pain* 1989; 39:31–36.

Gorman JM, Mathew S, Coplan J. Neurobiology of early life stress: nonhuman primate models. *Semin Clin Neuropsychiatry* 2002; 7:96–103.

Guinsburg R, Kopelman BI, Anand KJS, et al. Physiological, hormonal, and behavioral responses to a single fentanyl dose in intubated and ventilated preterm neonates. *J Pediatr* 1998; 132:954–959.

Guy ER, Abbott FV. The behavioral response to formalin in preweanling rats. *Pain* 1992; 51:81–90.

Harlow HF, Harlow MK, Suomi SJ. From thought to therapy: lessons from a primate laboratory. *Am Scientist* 1971; 59:538–549.

Hauser KF, McLaughlin PJ, Zagon IS. Endogenous opioid systems and the regulation of dendritic growth and spine formation. *J Comp Neurol* 1989; 281:13–22.

Himes BT, Tessler A. Death of some dorsal root ganglion neurons and plasticity of others following sciatic nerve section in adult and neonatal rats. *J Comp Neurol* 1989; 284:215–230.

Hofbauer RK, Rainville P, Duncan GH, Bushnell MC. Cortical representation of the sensory dimension of pain. *J Neurophysiol* 2001; 86:402–411.

Hofer MA. Early relationships as regulators of infant physiology and behavior. *Acta Paediatr* 1994; 397(Suppl):9–18.

Huang BR, Gu JJ, Ming H, Lai DB, Zhou XF. Differential actions of neurotrophins on apoptosis mediated by the low affinity neurotrophin receptor p75NTR in immortalised neuronal cell lines. *Neurochem Int* 2000; 36:55–65.

Jennings E, Fitzgerald M. Postnatal changes in responses of rat dorsal horn cells to afferent stimulation: a fibre-induced sensitization. *J Physiol* 1998; 509:859–868.

Johnston CC, Walker CD. The effects of exposure to repeated minor pain during the neonatal period on long-term inflammatory and thermal pain response. Canadian Pain Society Meeting, Banff, Alberta, Canada, 2000.

Johnston CC, Stevens B, Craig KD, Grunau RV. Developmental changes in pain expression in premature, full-term, two- and four-month-old infants. *Pain* 1993; 52:201–208.

Johnston CC, Collinge JM, Henderson SJ, Anand KJS. A cross-sectional survey of pain and pharmacological analgesia in Canadian neonatal intensive care units. *Clin J Pain* 1997; 13:308–312.

Johnston CC, Filion F, Snider L, et al. Routine sucrose analgesia during the first week of life in neonates younger than 31 weeks' postconceptional age. *Pediatrics* 2002; 110:523–528.

Kaufman IC, Rosenblum LA. Depression in infant monkeys separated from their mothers. *Science* 1967; 155:1030–1031.

Kendler KS, Karkowski-Shuman L. Stressful life events and genetic liability to major depression: genetic control of exposure to the environment? *Psychol Med* 1997; 27:539–547.

Lariviere WR, Melzack R. The bee venom test: a new tonic-pain test. *Pain* 1996; 66:271–277.

Lariviere WR, Wilson SG, Laughlin TM, et al. Heritability of nociception. III. Genetic relationships among commonly used assays of nociception and hypersensitivity. *Pain* 2002; 97:75–86.

Lewis SE, Mannion RJ, White FA, et al. A role for HSP27 in sensory neuron survival. *J Neurosci* 1999; 19:8945–8953.

Lidow MS. Long-term effects of neonatal pain on nociceptive systems. *Pain* 2002; 99:377–383.

Lidow MS, Song Z-M, Ren K. Long-term effects of short-lasting early local inflammatory insult. *Neuroreport* 2001; 12:399–403.

Liu JG, Rovnaghi CR, Garg S, Anand KJS. Hyperalgesia in young rats associated with opioid receptor desensitization in the forebrain. *J Pharmacol Exp Ther* 2003; in press.

Lyons DM, Martel FL, Levine S, Risch NJ, Schatzberg AF. Postnatal experiences and genetic effects on squirrel monkey social affinities and emotional distress. *Horm Behav* 1999; 36:266–275.

Lyons DM, Lopez JM, Yang C, Schatzberg AF. Stress-level cortisol treatment impairs inhibitory control of behavior in monkeys. *J Neurosci* 2000; 20:7816–7821.

Malmberg AB, Brandon EP, Idzerda RL, et al. Diminished inflammation and nociceptive pain with preservation of neuropathic pain in mice with a targeted mutation of the type I regulatory subunit of cAMP-dependent protein kinase. *J Neurosci* 1997; 17:7462–7470.

Marsh D, Dickenson A, Hatch D, Fitzgerald M. Epidural opioid analgesia in infant rats II: responses to carrageenan and capsaicin. *Pain* 1999b; 82:33–38.

Marti E, Gibson SJ, Polak JM, et al. Ontogeny of peptide and amino-containing neurons in motor, sensory, and autonomic regions of rat and human spinal cord. *J Comp Neurol* 1987; 266:332–359.

Mattson MP, Rychlik B. Comparison of rates of neuronal development and survival in human and rat cerebral cortical cell cultures. *Mech Ageing Dev* 1991; 60:171–187.

Mogil JS, Wilson SG, Bon K, et al. Heritability of nociception I: responses of 11 inbred mouse strains on 12 measures of nociception. *Pain* 1999a; 80:67–82.

Mogil JS, Wilson SG, Bon K, et al. Heritability of nociception II. 'Types' of nociception revealed by genetic correlation analysis. *Pain* 1999b; 80:83–93.

Morrow TJ, Paulson PE, Brewer KL, Yezierski RP, Casey KL. Chronic, selective forebrain responses to excitotoxic dorsal horn injury. *Exp Neurol* 2000; 161:220–226.

Nakayama Y, Omote K, Namiki A. Role of prostaglandin receptor EP1 in the spinal dorsal horn in carrageenan-induced inflammatory pain. *Anesthesiology* 2002; 97:1254–1262.

Narsinghani U, Anand KJS. Developmental neurobiology of pain in neonatal rats. *Lab Anim* 2000; 29:27–39.

Newton BW, Rovnaghi CR, Narsinghani U, et al. Supraspinal fos expression may have neuroprotective effects in inflammation-induced neuronal cell death: a FluoroJade-B and C-fos study. *Soc Neurosci Abstracts* 2000; 26:435.

Paulson PE, Casey KL, Morrow TJ. Long-term changes in behavior and regional cerebral blood flow associated with painful peripheral mononeuropathy in the rat. *Pain* 2002; 95:1–40.

Plotsky PM, Meaney MJ. Early postnatal experience alters hypothalamic corticotropin-releasing factor (CRF) mRNA, median eminence CRF content and stress-induced release in adult rats. *Mol Brain Res* 1993; 18:195–200.

Porter FL, Anand KJS. Epidemiology of pain in neonates. *Res Clin Forums* 1998; 20:9–16.

Pryce CR, Ruedi-Bettschen D, Dettling AC, Feldon J. Early life stress: long-term physiological impact in rodents and primates. *News Physiol Sci* 2002; 17:150–155.

Rahman W, Fitzgerald M, Aynsley-Green A, Dickenson AH. The effects of neonatal exposure to inflammation and/or morphine on neuronal responses and morphine analgesia in adult rats. In: Jensen TS, Turner JA, Wiesenfeld-Hallin Z (Eds). *Proceedings of the 8th World Congress on Pain,* Progress in Pain Research and Management, Vol. 8. Seattle: IASP Press, 1997, pp 783–794.

Rainville P, Duncan GH, Price DD, Carrier B, Bushnell MC. Pain affect encoded in human anterior cingulate but not somatosensory cortex. *Science* 1997; 277:968–971.

Ren K, Blass EM, Zhou Q, Dubner R. Suckling and sucrose ingestion suppress persistent hyperalgesia and spinal Fos expression after forepaw inflammation in infant rats. *Proc Natl Acad Sci USA* 1997; 94:1471–1475.

Reynolds ML, Fitzgerald M. Long-term sensory hyperinnervation following neonatal skin wounds. *J Comp Neurol* 1995; 358:487–498.

Reynolds M, Alvares D, Middleton J, Fitzgerald M. Neonatally wounded skin induces NGF-independent sensory neurite outgrowth in vitro. *Brain Res Dev Brain Res* 1997a; 102:275–283.

Reynolds ML, Ward A, Graham CF, Coggeshall R, Fitzgerald M. Decreased skin sensory innervation in transgenic mice overexpressing insulin-like growth factor-II. *Neuroscience* 1997b; 79:789–97.

Ruda MA, Ling Q-D, Hohmann AG, Peng YB, Tachibana T. Altered nociceptive neuronal circuits after neonatal peripheral inflammation. *Science* 2000; 289:628–631.

Sakurada T, Wako K, Sugiyama A, et al. Involvement of spinal NMDA receptors in capsaicin-induced nociception. *Pharmacol Biochem Behav* 1998; 59:339–345.

Sanchez MM, Hearn EF, Do D, Rilling JK, Herndon JG. Differential rearing affects corpus callosum size and cognitive function of rhesus monkeys. *Brain Res* 1998; 812:38–49.

Sanchez MM, Ladd CO, Plotsky PM. Early adverse experience as a developmental risk factor for later psychopathology: evidence from rodent and primate models. *Dev Psychopathol* 2001; 13:419–449.

Seay B, Gottfried NW. A phylogenetic perspective for social behavior in primates. *J Gen Psychol* 1975; 92:5–17.

Shimada C, Kurumiya S, Noguchi Y, Umemoto M. The effect of neonatal exposure to chronic footshock on pain-responsiveness and sensitivity to morphine after maturation in the rat. *Behav Brain Res* 1990; 36:105–111.

Shortland P, Fitzgerald M. Neonatal sciatic nerve section results in a rearrangement of the central terminals of saphenous and axotomized sciatic nerve afferents in the dorsal horn of the spinal cord of the adult rat. *Eur J Neurosci* 1994; 6:75–86.

Shortland P, Molander C. Alterations in the distribution of stimulus-evoked c-fos in the spinal cord after neonatal peripheral nerve injury in the rat. *Brain Res Dev Brain Res* 2000; 119:243–250.

Silove D, Manicavasagar V, O'Connell D, Morris-Yates A. Genetic factors in early separation anxiety: implications for the genesis of adult anxiety disorders. *Acta Psychiatr Scand* 1995; 92:17–24.

Sugimoto T, Li YL, Kishimoto H, Fujita M, Ichikawa H. Compensatory projection of primary nociceptors and c-fos induction in the spinal dorsal horn following neonatal sciatic nerve lesion. *Exp Neurol* 2000; 164:407–414.

Sugiura N, Patel RG, Corriveau RA. N-methyl-D-aspartate receptors regulate a group of transiently expressed genes in the developing brain. *J Biol Chem* 2001; 276:14257–14263.

Svendsen F, Tjolsen A, Hole K. AMPA and NMDA receptor-dependent spinal LTP after nociceptive tetanic stimulation, *Neuroreport* 1998; 9:1185–1190.

Swafford L, Allen D. Pain relief in the pediatric patient. *Med Clin N Am* 1968; 52:131–136.

Tachibana T, Ling QD, Ruda MA. Increased Fos induction in adult rats that experienced neonatal peripheral inflammation. *Neuroreport* 2001; 12:925–927.

Taddio A, Shah V, Gilbert-MacLeod C, Katz J. Conditioning and hyperalgesia in newborns exposed to repeated heel lances. *JAMA* 2002; 288:857–861.

Teng CJ, Abbott FV. The formalin test: a dose-response analysis at three development stages. *Pain* 1998; 76:337–347.

Theodosiou M, Rush RA, Zhou XF. et al. Hyperalgesia due to nerve damage: role of nerve growth factor. *Pain* 1999; 81:245–255.

Wei F, Wang GD, Kerchner GA, et al. Genetic enhancement of inflammatory pain by forebrain NR2B overexpression. *Nat Neurosci* 2001; 4:164–169.

Wei F, Qiu CS, Kim SJ, et al. Genetic elimination of behavioral sensitization in mice lacking calmodulin-stimulated adenylyl cyclases. *Neuron* 2002; 36:713–726.

Woolf CJ, Salter MW. Neuronal plasticity: increasing the gain in pain. *Science* 2000; 288:1765–1768.

Yi DK, Barr GA. The induction of Fos-like immunoreactivity by noxious thermal, mechanical and chemical stimuli in the lumbar spinal cord of infant rats. *Pain* 1995; 60:257–265.

Zhou XF, Cameron D, Rush RA. Endogenous neurotrophin-3 supports the survival of a subpopulation of sensory neurons in neonatal rat. *Neuroscience* 1998; 86:1155–1164.

Zhou XF, Deng YS, Xian CJ, Zhong JH. Neurotrophins from dorsal root ganglia trigger allodynia after spinal nerve injury in rats. *Eur J Neurosci* 2000; 12:100–105.

Zhuo M. NMDA receptor-dependent long term hyperalgesia after tail amputation in mice. *Eur J Pharmacol* 1998; 349:211–220.

Correspondence to: K.J.S. Anand, MBBS, DPhil, Arkansas Children's Hospital, S-431, 800 Marshall Street, Little Rock, AR 72202, USA. Tel: 501-364-1008; Fax: 501-364-3188; email: anandsunny@exchange.uams.edu.

2

Self-Regulation and Behavior in Preterm Children: Effects of Early Pain

Ruth Eckstein Grunau

Centre for Community Child Health Research, B.C. Research Institute for Children's and Women's Health, and Department of Pediatrics, University of British Columbia, Vancouver, British Columbia, Canada

Early repetitive pain has been viewed as affecting two broad aspects of infant and child functioning in premature infants, namely pain systems and cognitive and social-emotional development (Anand 2000; Grunau 2000). While it appears reasonable to expect differential effects on the neurobiology of these systems, this distinction between effects on *pain* as separate from effects on other aspects of *development* has been primarily for the convenience of researchers grappling conceptually with the issues in this emerging field of investigation (Grunau 2002). Yet adaptation to external stimulation may be affected broadly in preterm infants, cutting across different types of stimuli encompassing physical "threat" as well as novel, inherently nonaversive stimulation. It is postulated that dysregulation initiated by early stress may affect an infant's threshold to reactivity and recovery across various stimulus situations. These effects may be most pronounced under conditions of novelty, threat, or uncertainty, which are central to the construct of arousal. However, despite extensive exposure to nociceptive stimulation early in life, preterm infants are by no means a homogeneous population, and the determinants of relative resilience and risk in this group are poorly understood. Genetic factors, intrinsic traits, and environmental context (prenatal, neonatal, parenting, and cultural factors) all are likely to play dynamic interactive roles for infants born prematurely, as they do in the development of term-born infants.

This chapter will first consider the construct of arousal, with a focus on disruptive effects of early pain. Then the importance of caregiver interaction in the development of self-regulatory behaviors will be highlighted. Evidence that parenting style can moderate the developing behaviors of the very young child, thereby ameliorating some of the potential negative effects of early pain exposure, will be examined. New data from our center that bear on parental (mainly maternal) factors as moderators of young children's behavior will be presented. Relationships of maternal behavior during mother-child interaction with child temperament and child behaviors during cognitive assessment will be examined in former preterm children of normal intelligence born with extremely low birth weight (up to 1 kg) and low gestational age (up to 28 weeks), as compared with children born with normal birth weight at term. Child pain sensitivity, as rated by parents, will also be examined in relation to task behaviors in both groups. The aims of this chapter are to integrate these findings into the emerging literature, which suggests the developmental importance of early pain; to illustrate the plasticity of the developing nervous system in the emergence of self-regulatory behaviors; and to emphasize that pain reactivity in young preterm children is related to a continuum of adaptability to environmental demands.

AROUSAL

The concept of arousal as a state of central nervous system (CNS) regulation is key to theories of sensory processing and attention (Rothbart and Goldsmith 1985). Arousal regulation is assessed through physiological and behavioral responses that are assumed to reflect changes in CNS activation. Arousal varies with context conditions: a novel stimulus can be positively or negatively exciting; it may or may not be frightening. The capacity to regulate arousal varies among individuals depending on their temperamental traits, and it also changes across the developmental lifespan, although there appears to be continuity at the extremes (Kagan et al. 1988; Kagan 1997). Currently there are no comprehensive theories of child development that attempt to account for multiple dimensions of functioning, and that are applicable to the continuum of typical children as well as those with developmental disabilities or psychopathology. However, there is consensus that regulation of arousal is central to understanding early development. Some theoretical formulations or models have been proposed that specifically relate to the development of arousal regulation (e.g., Mayes 2000; Posner 2002); others are conceptualized within the construct of temperament (Rothbart et al. 1992) or development of emotion (e.g., Gray 1991). Arousal regulation is an organizing construct for integrating relationships among sensory stimulation, stress, cortical activity, and performance (e.g., Rothbart and Goldsmith 1985; Mayes 2000).

Even the relatively short-term impact of prior pain on subsequent pain response in human preterm infants is complex. Recent pain exposure is associated with decreased pain threshold (Andrews and Fitzgerald 1994; Porter et al. 1998) and with increased response to intrusive procedures (Grunau et al. 2000a). Conversely, greater exposure to early pain over longer time periods of several weeks is associated with decreased behavioral reactivity to pain (Johnston and Stevens 1996; Grunau et al. 2001b). Dampening to (faster recovery from) subsequent pain also has been observed many months after hospital discharge following finger lancing (Grunau et al. 2001b), especially in the smallest and sickest babies (Oberlander et al. 2000). In another study overall dampening was reported by parents of former preterm infants at a corrected chronological age (CCA) of 18 months, adjusted for prematurity (Grunau 1994a). However, this picture is further complicated by differences in immediate reactivity versus dampening following acute pain. At 8 months' CCA, immediate pain reactivity was greater in extremely low birth-weight (ELBW[1]) infants (weighing up to 800 g) than in term-born full-birth-weight infants (suggesting greater sensitivity), but recovery (dampening) was significantly faster in the ELBW infants, suggesting less persistence of pain (Grunau et al. 2001a).

Based on multiple lines of physiological, behavioral, and neurobiological evidence, it is clear that interactive multilevel excitatory and inhibitory gating systems not only protect the cortex from excessive stimulation but also facilitate coordination between sensory, attentional, and executive cortical systems (Mayes 2000). Emphasizing the different CNS origins of behavioral response is necessary in order to reconcile apparent contradictions in the effects of early pain on subsequent pain response in the neonatal intensive care unit (NICU). Landmark research by Fitzgerald and her colleagues has consistently shown, in both human and animal studies, that pain threshold was lower at very low gestational ages, and dropped further with repetitive tactile stimulation (Fitzgerald et al. 1988; Fitzgerald and Beggs 2001). In contrast, others have consistently found that facial reactivity to pain was lowest at early gestational ages, and increased to its maximum in term-born infants (Craig et al. 1993; Stevens and Johnston 1996). Furthermore, greater early exposure to pain was associated with lower pain threshold, i.e., increased behavioral response (Fitzgerald and Beggs 2001), but decreased facial reactivity (Stevens and Johnston 1996; Grunau et al. 2001b). Pain threshold was measured using reflex leg extension to von Frey hairs

---

[1] The standard definition of ELBW is ≤1 kg. Some studies have included infants with specific birth weight ranges that may be lower to examine the highest risk infants.

(Andrews and Fitzgerald 1994), while behavioral reactivity to acute pain was determined using facial response. In the first study to examine both of these behaviors concurrently, Morison et al. (2001) confirmed both the earlier findings, namely that greater early exposure to pain was associated with subsequently *more* leg extension but *less* facial reactivity. These apparently contradictory findings can be explained by considering the level of the CNS system generating the response. Leg extension is viewed as a spinal-level reflex response (Fitzgerald and Andrews 1998), whereas facial reactivity may be mediated at the supraspinal level of the CNS (K.J.S. Anand, personal communication).

The classical model of the relationship between arousal and performance is the inverted "U shaped curve" (Hebb 1955). Low and high states of arousal are associated with poor performance, with optimum performance occurring when the individual is in a "medium" state of arousal. Recently Mayes (2000) proposed that current evidence suggests a double curve model—one curve reflecting more prefrontal functions, and a second reflecting increasing dominance of more subcortical and automatic posterior functions with increasing arousal (Fig. 1). This formulation is potentially powerful in accounting for apparently contradictory reactivity in increasingly stressful situations, wherein the individual switches from more executive to more automatic functions. For example, after discharge from the NICU, at 8 months' post-term CCA, Grunau and colleagues (2001a) found that the immediate facial reactivity to blood collection was *greater* for preterm compared to term-born infants, then switched to *less* response in the recovery phase (i.e.,

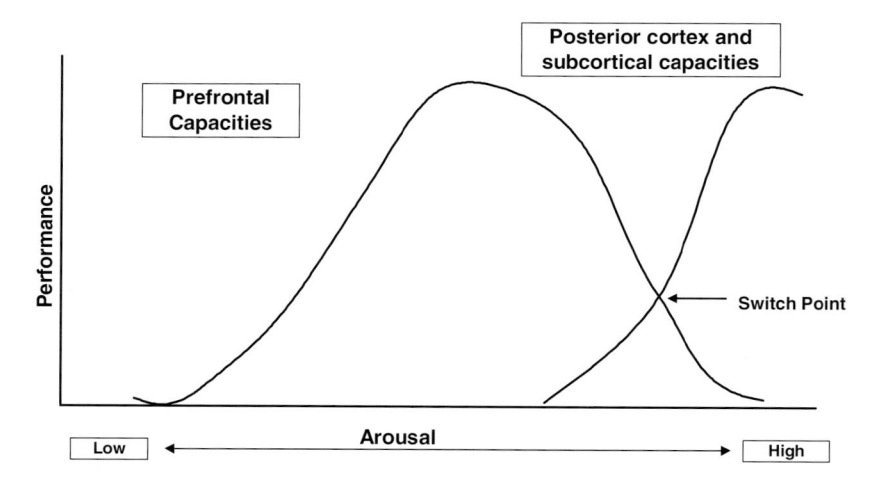

Fig. 1. Interactive arousal systems and performance. Reprinted from Mayes (2000), with permission.

faster dampening). One interpretation is that the initial heightened reactivity might reflect a startle response, followed by relatively faster "shutdown." However, Mayes' model suggests another interpretation. Multiple studies of preterm and full-term infants have shown that the most aversive phase of blood collection by heel lance is the squeezing that follows the lance, rather than the lance itself (e.g., Grunau and Craig 1987; Grunau 1998, 2001b). If we assume that this is also true of finger lance, then the initial lance stimulus may be only moderately arousing, and the higher initial response may be cortically mediated (as in the left side of Fig. 1). Subsequently, as the infant shifts into a higher arousal state during the squeezing phase (as in the right side of Fig. 1), the response shifts to a brain-stem-mediated "shutdown" response evident earlier in development in the NICU after weeks of exposure to pain (see Grunau 2001b). The second explanation is appealing, because it is more likely that increased facial response on the Neonatal Facial Coding System (Grunau and Craig 1987) would reflect heightened pain, rather than startle. Increased heart rate is ambiguous, because it is consistent with either startle or pain. Furthermore, the initial heightened response may demonstrate memory for pain in the preterm group. Mayes' formulation is also appealing due to the power of the model for generating testable hypotheses. This model will help move the area of pain in preterm infants beyond the current phase of mainly descriptive studies.

In terms of broader aspects of arousal, infants born at extremely low birth weight (up to 800 g) or extremely low gestational age (up to 25 weeks), and thereby exposed to repeated early pain in the NICU, showed signs of stress when exposed to novel tasks during cognitive assessment at 18 months' CCA. The Bayley Behavior Rating Scale was completed by the examiner as part of standardized assessment using the Mental Scale of the Bayley Scales of Infant Development. The percentile scores on the dimensions of orientation/engagement and emotional regulation were compared (see Fig. 2). These high-risk toddlers displayed adequate engagement during unfamiliar cognitive tasks, but problematic regulatory capacity. These findings are consistent with the premise that early pain exposure may be associated with disruption of the development of self-regulation of stress arousal.

LEARNING AND MEMORY OF PAIN

Denial of the capacity of infants to "remember" pain is due to a misconception that cognition is a prerequisite for memory. Chapman and Nakamura (1999) have even proposed that conscious experience is a prerequisite for pain perception. This is clearly not the case. Consciousness may or may not

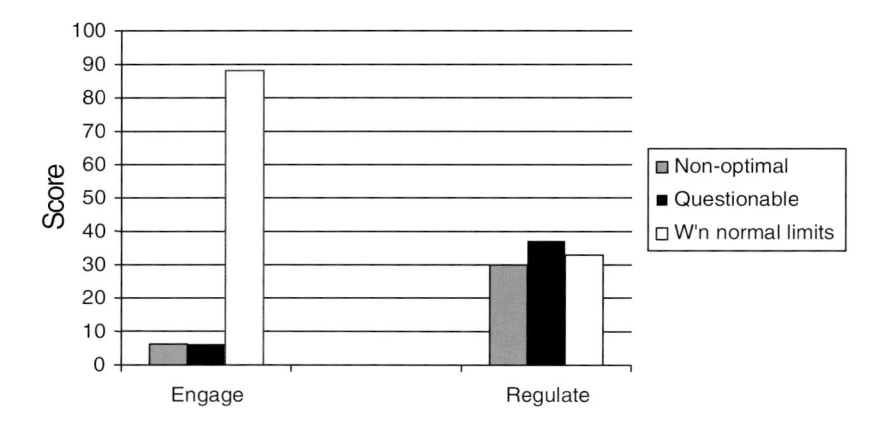

Fig. 2. Behavior rating during standardized testing at age 18 months on the mental scale of the Bayley Test of Infant Development. Engage refers to Orientation/Engagement; Regulate refers to Emotional Regulation.

be present at any level of animal phylogeny, but this is extremely difficult to determine objectively. Perception of pain is fundamental to survival in allowing an organism to perceive and respond to threat (Anand and Craig 1996).

A massive body of literature exists on conditioning in animals, and conditioning implies memory. For example, pigeons learn (remember) to peck a lever to acquire food pellets following a number of learning trials (Neuringer 1969). Conditioning to physically aversive stimulation is extremely rapid, and fear conditioning is very easily acquired in mammals. For example, "one-trial learning" can occur in studies of rats conditioned to avoid electric shock (Kopp et al. 1968). The significantly greater behavioral response to the initial pain seen at 8 months' CCA in the preterm infants (Grunau et al. 2001a) could reflect a generalized hyper-reactivity due to immature neurobehavioral modulation. However, an equally, if not more, plausible explanation is that this behavior indicates a learned response acquired in the NICU and reflects early "biological memory" for pain in these infants. Conditioned memory for pain in the NICU is consistent with other evidence. In a study of pain response to blood collection at 32 weeks' postconceptional age (PCA), infants were grouped according to the number of prior skin-breaking procedures to which they had been exposed since birth. Infants who had undergone 20 or fewer skin-breaking procedures in the NICU displayed a pattern of facial responses consistent with term-born infants never exposed to pain (Grunau 2001b), namely a slight increase in facial activity to first contact by the laboratory technician, a further increase to swabbing to cleanse the heel, then a significant increase to lance, a further increase to squeezing, and then a rapid drop during recovery. In contrast, infants exposed to more than 20 prior invasive procedures, and particularly those exposed to more than 180 procedures, showed a *drop* in facial response to first contact. The increase shown to first contact in the relatively pain-naive group (20 or fewer prior procedures) is consistent with "orienting" to tactile contact, whereas the decrease to the same stimulus in the remaining groups suggests "withdrawal" consistent with aversive conditioning. This interpretation is consistent with the results of a recent study demonstrating that preterm infants between 28 and 32 weeks' gestational age demonstrated anticipatory increase in heart rate prior to heel lance for blood collection (Goubet et al. 2001).

Alternatively, greater prior pain exposure is associated with higher early illness severity, and might suggest that compromise to the CNS is mediating altered pain response at 32 weeks. However, this option is unlikely, given that we recently found no differences in behavioral or cardiac reactivity to pain between infants with and without intraparenchymal brain injury (on cranial ultrasound) in the neonatal period (Oberlander et al. 2002). In that study, pain responses were examined at 32 weeks' PCA, and the two groups were matched for gestational age at birth and gender.

CAREGIVER INFLUENCES

Mother-infant interaction has long been viewed not only as a critical determinant of the development of the individual, but also as a "regulator" of social and emotional interaction and competence (Lewis and Ramsay 1999). A transactional model of development proposes that child outcomes are the product of dynamic interactions between the child and others, including the family and social context across time (Sameroff and Chandler 1975). Numerous studies have shown that positive caregiving promotes cognitive and social development (see Bornstein 1995), both in term-born infants and in those biologically at risk due to prematurity (Greenberg and Crnic 1988). It is well established that markers of socioeconomic status (SES), such as mother's education, become increasingly associated with child intelligence over time, in children born preterm (Resnick et al. 1990). For example, in a recent study designed to evaluate the combined influence of medical and SES background factors on cognitive outcome at 5.5 years of age (Bohm et al. 2002), parental education was the single best predictor of intelligence quotient (IQ). However, as has been found previously (Grunau et al. 1990; Taylor et al. 1998), neonatal factors such as birth weight contributed more to prediction of visually based abilities reflected in performance IQ, as compared to verbal IQ, which is typically more closely related to environmental circumstances. In general, as the number of biological and environmental risks increase, cognitive outcome declines (e.g., Liaw and Brooks-Gunn 1994; Sameroff et al. 1998). Although neonatal factors are related to some extent to later cognition in extremely premature children, SES becomes increasingly important over time (Jefferis et al. 2002). Most of the relevant studies have addressed SES rather than specific caregiver factors.

Recently, Grunau and colleagues examined the role of maternal factors in cognitive functioning in high-risk survivors of neonatal intensive care. Maternal sensitivity to child cues (measured during mother-child interaction) and maternal organization and responsivity (from the Home Screening Questionnaire, described in Grunau 2002) were significant predictors of subsequent IQ at age 4.5 years (Grunau et al. 2000b).

Among extremely premature infants (<801 g birth weight or <26 weeks gestation), maternal style of interaction was significantly associated with behavior in very young children (18 months' CCA) *after controlling for cognitive development* (Grunau et al. 2002). Higher maternal gratification from interaction was significantly associated with greater child enjoyment, organization, responsiveness, and involvement during a structured teaching task. Child involvement was also promoted by better maternal organization and greater maternal sensitivity to child cues. Conversely, child activity level was independent of all the maternal factors measured. Activity during novel tasks may reflect the altered capacity for self-regulation of arousal that could be induced by NICU experiences such as pain, and may be less prone to amelioration by caregiver style. However, the relative plasticity of different aspects of self-regulation over time and relative influences of caregiver characteristics on specific child behaviors require far more study. The extent to which amelioration or exacerbation of effects is possible probably varies widely across individuals.

Plasticity can be viewed as stages of development in which options are available for alternative developmental pathways (Johnson 2001). Therefore, while early exposure to repeated pain may set in motion alterations to behavioral trajectories, it is expected that developmental plasticity in human infancy and early childhood may allow considerable opportunity for environmental moderation of early adverse effects of NICU care.

DEVELOPMENT OF SELF-REGULATION

In developmental cognitive psychology, the mechanisms thought to be involved in self-regulation are collectively viewed as "attention" (Posner and Rothbart 2000). In the first year of life, landmark periods have been described with regard to orienting to objects and control of distress (Ruff and Rothbart 1996), and in the second year and beyond, in children's abilities to plan and to regulate their growing cognitive skills (Posner and Rothbart 1998). Multiple studies have shown that preterm infants are more easily stressed, less alert, less responsive, and less able to provide clear signals of distress, and that they display more interactional difficulties compared to healthy term-born infants in the first few months of life (e.g., Als 1982; Greenberg and Crnic 1988; Eckerman et al. 1999). Furthermore, quality of parent-infant interaction at 6 months post-term mediated the relationship between neonatal risk status and cognitive development at 12 months (Poehlmann and Fiese 2001). Differences in preterm infants' orientation and interaction with objects have been identified (Ruff 1986), but the mechanisms of altered attention and self-regulation, particularly the potential links with early pain exposure, are still a matter of conjecture (Grunau 2000). In the early months of life, control of distress is a major focus of the infant and caregiver, and attention plays an important role in this process (Rainville et al. 1997). In addition to holding and rocking the infant, following the first few months of life, caregivers increasingly use visual orienting (distraction) to redirect the infant's attention and reduce distress.

Posner and Rothbart (2000) reviewed converging evidence in adults from neuroimaging studies that suggests that specific midline frontal cortical areas are engaged in emotional response to tasks, for example, before the start of a task that subjects expect to be difficult (Murtha et al. 1996). These brain areas are also involved in awareness of emotion in evaluating pain (Rainville et al. 1997). From this basis, Posner and Rothbart (2000) proposed that early interactions between infant and caregiver during distress may promote the infant's own control of distress and lead to the development of more general control systems for negative emotion (probably in the midfrontal cortical areas). Further, these authors suggested that later in development, when *cognitive* challenges arise, a system for regulating brain areas may already be under way. Infants who effectively utilize attention control strategies to regulate their arousal are thereby thought to be more likely to interact effectively with their environment. Caution must be used regarding the importance of single constructs such as infant capacity to regulate arousal outside of the bigger picture of infant history and developmental context. For example, the substantial majority of healthy term-born infants with "colic" (early excessive crying) later show totally normal capacities to be responsive in interactive contexts with parents (Barr 1998). These differing findings suggest that the etiology of arousal difficulties must be considered. For example, colic is a common, short-term, time-limited condition in otherwise healthy, normally developing infants, who appear to be at no greater risk of later interactional difficulties than other term-born children, assuming an appropriate caregiver environment. Furthermore, effects of temperament are bidirectional, in that the infant's interactive style affects responses from others in the social environment. Thus child temperament may affect learning by influencing the nature and quality of interaction with others, particularly with the caregiver, at early ages (Halpern et al. 2001). However, the etiology of normal individual differences is very different from the etiology of regulatory difficulties in biologically at-risk infants. In vulnerable infants who have undergone lengthy hospitalization in the NICU, it is likely that "rewiring" of circuits in the brain has taken place, such that certain functions come under the control of cortical regions that were not designed to carry them out. While this rewiring may allow for considerable compensation and recovery to occur, processing is likely to be affected in subtle ways. While a positive caregiving environment contributes to improved cognitive outcome in the development of biologically at-risk children (e.g., Greenberg and Crnic 1988; Halpern et al. 2001), there may be less potential for amelioration of NICU effects in the infants at the lower end of the gestational age range of survivors (Taylor et al. 1998). However, very little is known about the particular caregiver factors, or their interaction with characteristics of the child, that may contribute to altered outcome in specific areas of development and behavior.

ETIOLOGY OF ALTERED SELF-REGULATION

In very young infants, capacity to regulate arousal is initially seen in the development of cyclical sleep and waking states. In preterm infants in the NICU, regulation of sleep and waking states is altered in response to procedures (Sell et al. 1992; Stevens et al. 1996; Grunau et al. 1998). Disruption of sleep/wake cycles is one potential mechanism linking early repetitive pain to subsequent development of behavioral dysregulation. Higher-order executive functioning in childhood may be related initially to capacity to modulate arousal, attention, and self-regulation in infancy. Development of these critical functions, which are essential for learning and memory, may initially depend on appropriate maturation of sleep and waking state regulation.

The role of sleep in attention, cognitive tasks, and memory consolidation has been recognized for many years (Rotenberg 1992). Neurophysiological studies using EEG during sleep suggest that even healthy preterm neonates display altered functional brain maturation compared to term-born infants (Scher 1997a,b). Altered characteristics of sleep in preterm, compared to term-born, infants appear to be predictive of later neurodevelopment. Sleep cycle length and the active sleep component of the cycle measured in the neonatal period predicted mental development at 6 months (Borghese et al. 1995). In a sample of healthy preterm and term-born infants, lower spectral beta EEG energies were associated with lower mental and motor development at 12 months' CCA (Scher et al. 1996), and with lower SES. While these are correlational findings indicating association rather than causation, they suggest that disruption of the development of normal sleep cycles, which is known to occur in relation to NICU procedures, may be one mechanism of altered neurodevelopment, even in apparently normal preterm infants. Serial EEG studies during infancy are needed to check whether former preterm infants display continued differences in sleep measures. Persistently lower spectral beta EEG energies during infancy might be more closely related to lower developmental outcome, and therefore different patterns may emerge in infants whose EEG during sleep differed in only the neonatal period to those who continue to display dysmaturity (Scher et al. 1996). Episodic pain potentially disrupts development of sleep/waking state regulation during the weeks when organized states emerge (Fajardo et al. 1992). These alterations in the sleep and waking state may affect critical aspects of functional development.

Organization of sleep and waking states reflects the neurobiological integrity and competence of the CNS, and sleep-wake arousal patterns do not mature in the same way in preterm and term infants (Davis and Thoman 1987). Multiple functions have been proposed as important roles for active sleep, including physiological restoration, brain maturation, behavioral adaptation, and cognitive functioning; however, very little is known about the neonatal period (Blumberg and Lucas 1996). The developmental psychobiology of sleep-waking state regulation has close links to control of arousal, affect, and attention (Dahl 1996). Early pain and stress are thus likely to directly affect the development of systems related to regulation of attention, arousal, emotion, and executive control functions. Gating and coordination of changes in sleep-waking state include involvement of the prefrontal cortex in interaction with other cortical and subcortical systems (Horne 1993). Emotional regulation also involves a complex interplay of cortical and subcortical systems, including the limbic system and the amygdala, with the prefrontal cortex playing a central role of integration and modulation; stress responses overlap with these systems (Valentino et al. 1992). The nature of these effects probably changes at each developmental stage, resurfacing in some new expression of function as cognitive demands are reorganized and increase during the childhood years.

Arousal regulation is an organizing construct for relating behavioral, physiological, and hormonal responses to stimulation and stress, presumably reflecting changes in CNS activation, and the capacity to modulate excitability, leading to altered performance (Mayes 2000). The development of self-regulation and coping is proposed as key to understanding effects of repeated stressors, potentially affecting pain systems as well as cognitive, emotional, and social development.

Self-regulation is a central concept in organizing and integrating biobehavioral reactivity in infancy. The dynamic, transactional nature of maternal care and infant reciprocity, shaping the mutual behavioral sequences of early interaction, is viewed as intrinsically important to human development, and continues over a relatively prolonged time period compared to other mammals (Spangler et al. 1994). Stress and pain both activate neuroendocrine systems, and the continuum of tactile and invasive stimuli can have cumulative and potentially permanent effects. Responses of the hypothalamic-pituitary-adrenal (HPA) axis in adult animals appear to be shaped by experiences very early in life (Meaney et al. 1991). Johnson (2001) emphasized the importance of activity-dependent processes in prenatal and postnatal life in contributing to aspects of specialization of the cerebral cortex. Over the course of human infant development, appropriate interactive social experience is likely to contribute further to the specialization of later-developing systems of the cerebral cortex.

TEMPERAMENT AND EFFORTFUL CONTROL

Increasingly in early childhood, voluntary attention mechanisms and executive processes have important implications for the development of behavioral and emotional control. Temperament has been described as a psychobiological mediator of stress reactivity (Boyce et al. 1992; Lewis 1992). While often referred to as a single construct, temperament is conceived as a set of factors whose dimensions vary somewhat depending on the model under consideration. However, numerous temperament theorists include a construct that taps threshold or reactivity to external stimulation (e.g., Carey and McDevitt 1978; Rothbart and Derryberry 1981; Buss and Plomin 1984; Goldsmith et al. 1987). Rothbart and Bates (1997) defined temperament as individual differences in motor and emotional reactivity and self-regulation. Posner and Rothbart (2000) point out that traditionally the major theories of temperament have primarily focused on the child's arousal to stimulation and his or her reactivity to positive and negative situations and affect. An additional construct of "effortful control," related to self-regulatory executive attention, has recently been proposed (Shoda et al. 1990; Kochanska et al. 1995; Posner and Rothbart 2000). The dimension of effortful control taps the development of executive attention in early childhood.

Response to novelty is viewed as a potential stressor. For preterm infants, the combination of effortful control, in a context of responding to novelty task demands, appears to be noticeably challenging (Whitfield et al. 1997). It is proposed here that these difficulties may reflect problems integrating executive control functions with self-regulatory mechanisms relating to external stress.

Temperamental individual propensity for behavioral approach and inhibition has important implications for understanding coping, because it implies that certain individuals are predisposed to respond to situations as stressful, making them more likely to withdraw (Tobin 1989; Rothbart 1991; Kagan et al. 1995). Temperament has been viewed by some investigators in this area as biologically based and genetically determined (Buss and Plomin 1984); however, adverse early experience may itself alter early temperament.

Ethically acceptable paradigms for studying experimentally induced stress in human infants and children are very limited. In our center we have examined child behaviors during the novel, and potentially stressful, demands of structured cognitive assessment in order to address these questions. At 18 months' CCA, infants born at extremely low birth weight (up to 800 g) or extremely low gestational age (up to 25 weeks) displayed adequate engagement during unfamiliar cognitive tasks, but problematic regulatory capacity (as shown in Fig. 2). At age 9 years, preterm children who escaped major sensory, motor, or cognitive impairment displayed difficulties maintaining engagement when tasks were challenging during cognitive assessment, compared to term-born socially comparable peers, even after controlling for IQ (Whitfield et al. 1997).

A STUDY ASSESSING THE ETIOLOGY OF CHILD BEHAVIORS

This section presents data from a study conducted at the Neonatal Follow-up Programme at the Children's and Women's Health Centre of British Columbia to explore relationships between perinatal experience, parenting influences, and development of behaviors related to effortful control during novel task demands. The primary focus of this study was to investigate behaviors during unfamiliar cognitive tasks during standardized testing of intelligence in preterm preschoolers, with an emphasis on whether child temperament and parent interaction might affect these behaviors. A second goal was to examine whether temperament was associated with neonatal factors, and in addition, whether parental ratings of pain and touch reactivity were related to neonatal factors. A third aim was to explore whether, in addition to temperament characteristics rated by a parent, pain reactivity might be a further index of environmental response linked to other behavioral systems.

PURPOSE OF THE STUDY

Data are presented here with the aim of examining whether maternal factors may moderate child behaviors during novel tasks at age 3 years, above and beyond perinatal factors. In addition, we examined parent ratings of child sensitivity to pain to test the hypothesis that in very young children, pain reactivity is an indicator of more general capacity to modulate arousal, rather than an independent characteristic.

This work focused on preterm children of extremely low birth weight with normal intelligence. The study included a control group of term-born peers. Children born small for their gestational age (i.e., whose growth was retarded in utero) were excluded because their outcomes presumably reflect influences of insufficient placental delivery, whereas our focus was the influences of postnatal environment. Other exclusion criteria was periventricular leukomalacia and grade IV intraventricular hemorrhage on neonatal ultrasound. Number of days in the level III NICU was used as a marker of exposure to the NICU environment. We did not obtain detailed data on pain and medication exposure for these children.

PARTICIPANTS

The study sample comprised 103 ELBW infants (46 boys, 57 girls) of very low gestational age (VLGA), born at a weight of no more than 1 kg at 28 weeks' gestation or less. These infants were seen for psychometric assessment in the Neonatal Follow-up Programme at the Children's and Women's Health Centre of British Columbia at 3 years' CCA and again at age 4.5 years. Mean birth weight of the VLGA group was 814.7 g (SD = 116.7) with a range of 560–1000 g, mean gestational age at birth was 26.0 weeks (SD = 1.3) with a range of 23–28 weeks, and mean time spent in the level III NICU was 100 days (SD = 70.6) with a range of 24–500 days. We included only infants whose birth weight was appropriate for gestational age (i.e., above the 10th percentile on intrauterine growth curves), and who displayed intelligence in the normal range at age 3 years, with a composite IQ score on the Stanford Binet Intelligence Scale of at least 85. We included a control group of 38 healthy term-born children (20 boys, 18 girls) for comparison at age 3 years, all with normal IQ, as described previously (Grunau et al. 1994b).

MEASURES

Age 3 years' CCA. Child behaviors during standardized cognitive assessment on the Stanford-Binet Intelligence Scale (Thorndike et al. 1986) were rated by the psychology examiner (a psychometrician or psychologist), using the Stanford-Binet Behavior Rating Scale (SBR; Thorndike et al. 1986). The SBR is comprised of 14 behaviors, each rated on a five-point scale. A rating of speech articulation is also part of this scale, but we excluded it in order to focus exclusively on child behavior. Parent behavior was evaluated during observations of parent-child dyadic interaction during teaching tasks (Greenberg and Crnic 1988), in which three global dimensions (parent gratification, sensitivity, and affect) were rated on five-point scales. We have previously reported good reliability with this scale in the clinic setting (Grunau et al. 1994b). In the VLGA group, 84% of caregivers were mothers, 13% fathers, and 3% another caregiver, usually a grandmother or aunt. In the control group all caregivers were mothers. The caregiver completed the temperament questionnaire (Buss and Plomin 1984), which provides measures of shyness, activity, sociability, and emotionality. In addition, we included caregiver ratings of child pain sensitivity and response to touch, as used previously (Grunau et al. 1994a,b). Parent-child dyadic interaction at age 3 years was evaluated, using the methods of Greenberg and Crnic (1988) in "real time" during structured teaching tasks, which we have described previously (Grunau 2000a). The examiner, who rated the child's behavior during cognitive assessment and the parent behavior during parent-child interaction, was blinded to perinatal medical data and to all parent questionnaire data, but was aware of group status (i.e., VLGA or control), which is a limitation of this clinically based work.

Age 4.5 years' CCA. The Personality Inventory for Children (PIC; Lachar and Gdowski 1979), a questionnaire that has been widely used to measure child behaviors, was completed by a parent, usually the mother. We examined four factors scales from the PIC (undisciplined/poor self control, social incompetence, internalization/somatic symptoms, and cognitive development). We completed a PIC for 83 of the 103 VLGA children seen at both age 3 years and age 4.5 years.

DATA ANALYSIS AND RESULTS

Age 3 years' CCA. We compared the 14 behaviors on the SBR between the two groups (VLGA and controls), using two-way (Group × Gender) multivariate analysis of variance (MANOVA). The overall effect for Group was highly significant ($F_{14,122} = 5.99$, $P = 0.0001$). Surprisingly, there was no significant overall main effect of Gender ($F_{14,122} = 0.55$, $P = 0.90$), and no Gender × Group interaction ($F_{14,122} = 0.76$, $P = 0.71$). Univariate ANOVA tests showed that at age 3 years the VLGA children had statistically significantly poorer scores, compared to controls, on 12 of the 14 behaviors: easily distracted ($P = 0.0001$), abnormal activity ($P = 0.003$), waits to be told ($P = 0.41$), urging needed ($P = 0.009$), insecure ($P = 0.001$), distrusts own ability ($P = 0.0001$), ill-at-ease ($P = 0.02$), anxious ($P = 0.0001$), gives up easily ($P = 0.0001$), reacts to failure unrealistically ($P = 0.0001$), seeks to terminate the task ($P = 0.001$), prefers only easy tasks ($P = 0.0001$), needs constant praise and encouragement ($P = 0.0001$), and shows difficulty establishing

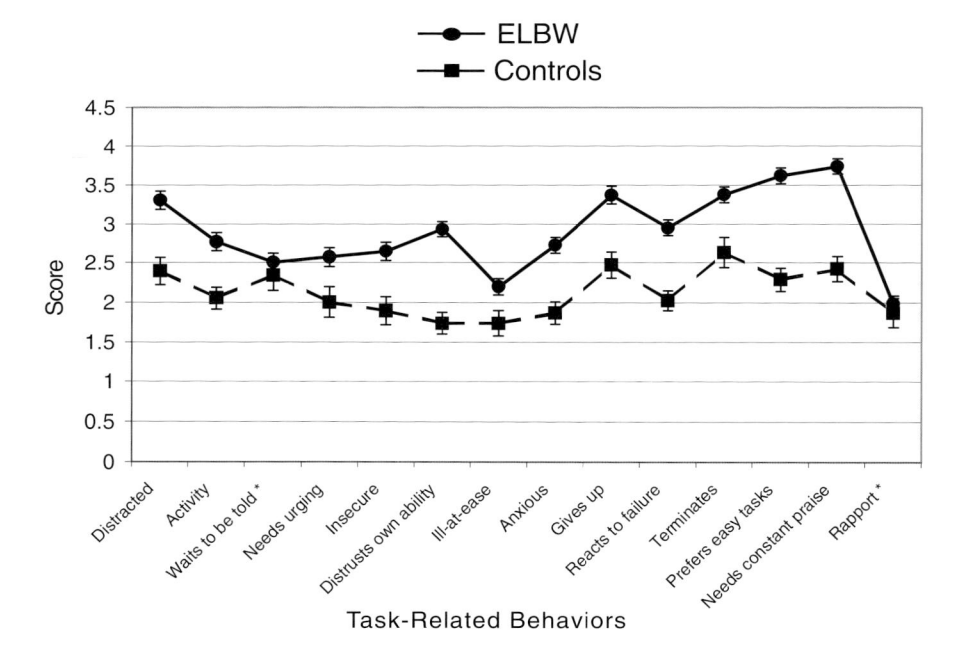

Fig. 3. Behaviors during psychological assessment at age 3 years in preterm children with extremely low birth weight and term-born controls. Task-related behaviors were rated using the Stanford Binet Behavior Rating Scale (Thorndike et al. 1986). Differences between groups were statistically significant at $P < 0.0001$, except where marked with an asterisk (*) to denote nonsignificance.

Table I
Pearson correlations of temperament at 3 years' CCA and parent
ratings of child sensitivity to pain and touch

	Emotionality	Sociability	Activity	Pain Sensitivity	Touch Sensitivity
VLGA					
Shyness	0.18	−0.37**	−0.31	0.05	0.37***
Emotionality		−0.01	−0.09	0.46***	0.27**
Sociability			0.53***	0.12	−0.23
Activity				−0.06	−0.24
Pain sensitivity					0.10
Control					
Shyness	−0.03	−0.20	−0.48**	−0.10	0.14
Emotionality		0.320	0.22	0.321*	0.12
Sociability			0.35*	0.22	−0.10
Activity				0.05	−0.19
Pain sensitivity					−0.09

Abbreviations: CCA = corrected chronological age; VLGA = very low gestational age. *$P < 0.05$; **$P < 0.01$; ***$P < 0.001$.

rapport ($P = 0.50$). These results, showing poorer self-regulatory behaviors in the VLGA group at age 3 years, are displayed graphically in Fig. 3.

Second, to reduce the behavioral outcome data, we summed the 14 individual SBR ratings to produce a single overall score of behavior during cognitive assessment for each child at 3 years' CCA. For the VLGA group, we conducted Pearson correlations to evaluate the relationships of neonatal factors and the summed SBR behavior score. The summary SBR behavior score during cognitive testing at age 3 years was significantly correlated with the number of days in the level III NICU ($r = 0.25$, $P = 0.01$), but not with gestational age at birth ($r = −0.02$, $P = 0.84$) or birth weight ($r = −0.02$, $P = 0.85$). In addition, we examined intercorrelations between child temperament scores and parent ratings of child sensitivity to pain and to touch at 3 years' CCA (see Table I). In order to compare the relative magnitude of association in correlation coefficients between the VLGA and control children, given the differences in sample size for each group, $P < 0.01$ was used as the cutoff for statistical significance in the VLGA group, and $P < 0.05$ in the control group. The relationships among the temperament variables were similar in each group, with high activity level associated with low shyness and high sociability, and high pain sensitivity with high emotionality. In the VLGA group, but not the controls, high sensitivity to touch was related to high shyness and high emotionality.

Table II
Pearson correlations between neonatal variables and temperament,
pain, and touch sensitivity at 3 years' CCA for the VLGA group

	Time in Level III NICU (Days)	Gestational Age at Birth	Birth Weight
Shyness	0.02	–0.05	0.12
Emotionality	–0.07	–0.12	–0.05
Sociability	0.13	0.05	–0.01
Activity	0.05	0.07	–0.03
Pain sensitivity	–0.13	0.09	0.13
Touch sensitivity	0.27**	–0.23*	–0.13

Abbreviations: See Table I footnote; NICU = neonatal intensive care unit. $*P < 0.05$; $**P < 0.01$.

We then examined the intercorrelations of the neonatal variables with child temperament, and with sensitivity to pain and to touch (see Table II). The temperament variables were not associated with any perinatal variable. Pain sensitivity at age 3 years was not associated with neonatal factors; however, sensitivity to touch was related to longer time spent in the level III NICU and to lower gestational age at birth. No correlation among predictor variables was above 0.60, indicating that these measures were sufficiently independent to be used as predictors in regression analyses without concerns of multicollinearity.

When we examined the intercorrelations among the NICU variables, we found that a higher number of days in the level III NICU was associated with lower gestational age ($r = -0.22$, $P = 0.03$) and lower birth weight ($r = -0.30$, $P = 0.002$). Higher gestational age at birth was significantly associated with higher birth weight ($r = 0.71$); however, we retained both measures for regression analysis.

Age 4.5 years' CCA. Scores on the four factor scales on the PIC were compared between the two groups (VLGA, controls), using two-way (Group × Gender) MANOVA. The overall effect for Group was highly significant ($F_{4,114} = 6.26$, $P = 0.0001$). There was no significant overall main effect of Gender ($F_{4,114} = 0.66$, $P = 0.62$), and no Gender × Group interaction ($F_{4,114} = 0.75$, $P = 0.56$). Univariate ANOVA tests showed that the differences mainly reflected parent ratings of cognitive development being lower in the VLGA group ($F_{1,117} = 21.64$, $P = 0.0001$); internalization/somatic symptoms also contributed to the overall difference ($F_{1,117} = 3.22$, $P = 0.075$).

Table III
Summary of regression analyses of the summed
Stanford Behavior Rating Scale scores
at 3 years' CCA for VLGA boys

	R	R^2	β*	P
Parent affect	0.46	0.22	0.48	0.002
Avoidance of touch	0.56	0.31	−0.31	0.03

*Standardized beta coefficient.

PREDICTION OF CHILD BEHAVIOR DURING NOVEL TASKS AT AGE 3 YEARS

We performed hierarchical multiple regression analysis separately for each group. The outcome measure was the summary SBR score of child behavior during cognitive assessment at 3 years' CCA. Furthermore, for the VLGA group, the analyses were completed separately for boys and girls. In the VLGA group the predictor variables were perinatal variables (birth weight, gestation, and number of days in the level III NICU), entered at Step 1; parent behaviors during parent-child interaction (gratification, sensitivity, and affect) at age 3 years, entered at Step 2; and child variables including temperament (shyness, emotionality, sociability, and activity), pain sensitivity, and touch at age 3 years, entered at Step 3. For the control group the predictor variables were the same, except that the neonatal variables were excluded; the number of subjects was too low to carry out separate analyses by gender.

Among the VLGA boys (see Table III), higher positive parent affect during interaction in teaching tasks was associated with better overall child behavior during novel tasks. In addition, greater child avoidance of touch at 3 years' CCA was associated with more problem behavior. No perinatal factors predicted child behavior at 3 years' CCA. For VLGA girls (see Table IV), a higher number of days in the level III NICU, greater child shyness, and greater pain insensitivity were associated with more problem behavior at age 3 years.

Table IV
Summary of regression analyses of the summed Stanford
Behavior Rating Scale scores at 3 years' CCA for VLGA girls

	R	R^2	β*	P
Time in level III NICU (days)	0.38	0.15	0.36	0.007
Shyness	0.58	0.33	0.46	0.0001
Pain sensitivity	0.63	0.39	−0.25	0.04

*Standardized beta coefficient.

Table V
Summary of regression analyses of the summed Stanford Behavior Rating Scale scores at 3 years' CCA for the control group

	R	R^2	β*	P
Parent gratification	0.38	0.15	−0.44	0.003
Shyness	0.53	0.28	0.40	0.007
Pain sensitivity	0.61	0.37	0.31	0.03

Note: There were nine predictor variables (three for parent interaction, four for child temperament [shyness, emotionality, sociability, activity], one for child pain sensitivity, and one for child touch). We had 38 control subjects. Exploratory regression analysis requires five cases per predictor, so analyses could not be conducted separately by gender, and these results are highly tentative.
*Standardized beta coefficient.

Among the controls (see Table V), higher parent gratification during interaction and lower child shyness were associated with better behavior during novel tasks. Higher pain sensitivity was related to more problem behavior in the control group, which was opposite to the relationships found with the VLGA children (i.e., touch and pain sensitivity).

In order to examine whether temperament was itself affected by prematurity, we used MANOVA to compare shyness, activity, sociability, and emotionality ratings between the VLGA and term-born control groups. We

Table VI
Summary of regression analyses of the VLGA group on the Personality Inventory for Children factor scales at age 4.5 years

	R	R^2	β*	P†
Undisciplined/Poor Self-Control				
Child emotionality (temperament)	0.33	0.11	0.45	0.0001
Child sensitivity to pain	0.42	0.17	−0.28	−0.02
Social Incompetence				
Parent affect during interaction	0.43	0.18	−0.42	0.0001
Child sensitivity to pain	0.52	0.27	0.26	0.01
Temperament/shyness	0.56	0.31	0.21	0.05
Internalization/Somatic Symptoms				
Parent gratification during interaction	0.27	0.07	−0.22	0.056
Child emotionality (temperament)	0.35	0.12	0.23	0.046
Cognitive Development				
Gestational age at birth	0.35	0.12	−0.35	0.003

*Standardized beta coefficient.
†P values for predictors at the final step.

Table VII
Summary of regression analyses of the control group on the Personality
Inventory for Children factor scales at age 4.5 years

	R	R^2	β*	P†
Undisciplined/Poor Self-Control				
Parent affect during interaction	0.38	0.15	−0.38	0.01
Child activity (temperament)	0.51	0.26	0.34	0.03
Social Incompetence				
Child activity (temperament)	0.50	0.25	−0.57	0.0001
Child emotionality (temperament)	0.59	0.34	0.31	0.04
Internalization/Somatic Symptoms				
Child emotionality (temperament)	0.41	0.17	0.41	0.01

*Standardized beta coefficient.
†P values for predictors at the final step.

found no statistically significant differences between the VLGA and control children ($F < 1$, P = n.s.). Furthermore, there were no statistically significant associations between temperament and neonatal variables, as shown in Table II.

PREDICTION OF PERSONALITY INVENTORY FOR CHILDREN AT AGE 4.5 YEARS

We conducted hierarchical regression analyses for the VLGA (see Table VI) and control (see Table VII) groups separately; we did not address gender due to an insufficient sample size. The outcome measures were the four factor scales of the PIC outlined above. The predictor variables were the same as used at 3 years.

Factor 1: Undisciplined/poor self-control. In the VLGA group, greater child emotionality and insensitivity to pain (both at 3 years' CCA) predicted poorer self-control at age 4.5 years; no parent or perinatal factors were significant. In contrast, for the controls, lower parent affect and higher child activity (both at 3 years) predicted poorer self-control at age 4.5 years.

Factor 2: Social incompetence. In the VLGA group, poorer parent affect, higher child shyness, and great sensitivity to pain (all at 3 years' CCA) predicted greater social incompetence at age 4.5 years. For the controls, lower child activity and greater emotionality (both at 3 years' CCA) predicted greater social incompetence at age 4.5 years.

Factor 3: Internalization/somatic symptoms. In the VLGA group, lower parent gratification, higher child emotionality (at 3 years' CCA) predicted more internalization/somatic symptoms at age 4.5 years. For the controls, greater emotionality (at 3 years' CCA) predicted more internalization/somatic symptoms at age 4.5 years.

Factor 4: Cognitive development. In the VLGA group, low gestational age at birth predicted more problems with cognitive development. There were no significant predictors for the control group.

CONCLUSIONS OF THE STUDY

Reactions to novelty are viewed in the arousal literature as mild stressors. Our study showed that VLGA children with normal intelligence displayed poorer self-regulatory behaviors during novel tasks carried out during standardized cognitive assessment, compared to term-born control children. These behaviors generally reflected poorer executive planning and control; for example, the VLGA children were more easily distracted, needed urging to attempt or complete unfamiliar tasks, distrusted their ability, gave up easily, sought to terminate activities, preferred easy tasks, and required constant praise and encouragement. Another aim was to examine whether parent interaction measured independently during teaching interactions with the child might influence the child's competence in novel problem solving (in interaction with a psychology examiner). We also explored associations of child temperament with child behavior and examined child pain and touch reactivity (rated by parents at age 3 years) as further indices of arousal response to the external environment, which might relate to child capacity to self-regulate.

The VLGA children showed problems with *effortful control* during problem solving at 3 years' CCA, as reflected in poorer attention and self-regulation, especially as tasks became more cognitively challenging. Overall, these behavior problems were related to longer time spent in the NICU, rather than to gestation or birth weight. As expected from the developmental literature, for term-born controls, positive parenting during teaching tasks was associated with better problem-solving behavior. However, in the VLGA group, parenting was associated with behavior for boys but not for girls. Child temperament was related to behavior for controls and for VLGA girls, but not for VLGA boys. *Parent* ratings of pain or touch sensitivity was associated with behavior rated by the *examiner,* above and beyond temperament. However, among the controls, children who were more sensitive to pain showed worse task-related behavior, whereas among the VLGA children, those who were more sensitive to touch or pain demonstrated better task-related behavior.

These findings suggest, first, that pain and touch sensitivity may be an important individual differences factor that is not tapped by traditional temperament measures. Second, the differing history of tactile experiences in early infancy may have altered the relationships between tactile sensitivity and other aspects of child functioning. Further, pain sensitivity may be altered by factors other than early pain exposure. For example, in rodents, early maternal presence can buffer pain response (Blass et al. 1995). Furthermore, in another study, early maternal separation altered adult pain sensitivity, and this effect could be prevented with prophylactic treatment strategies (Stephan et al. 2002). These findings may bear on why pain sensitivity was related to other child behaviors in the term-born controls, as well as in the preterm children at age 3 years.

Parent ratings of child behaviors at age 4.5 years using four factors of the PIC scale revealed that lower gestational age was associated with greater parental concern regarding cognitive development among the VLGA children, whereas for controls there were no associations with this factor. More positive parenting at 3 years' CCA was associated with better social competence and less internalization/somatic complaints among VLGA children, and less lack of discipline/poor self-control among the term-born controls at age 4.5. Temperament factors at 3 years' CCA were significant predictors of all the behavior factors at age 4.5 years, for both groups. For the VLGA children, 31% of the variance in social incompetence was accounted for by the combined contributions of parent affect during interaction (18%), child sensitivity to pain (additional 9%), and temperamental shyness (additional 4%). In contrast, for controls, social incompetence was explained only by temperament factors (34%). In predicting behaviors at 4.5 years, parent rating of pain sensitivity at age 3 years was a significant predictor of lack of discipline/poor self-control and social incompetence, but only for the VLGA children. These associations between pain sensitivity and other behaviors are intriguing, but any relations with pain exposure in the NICU are highly speculative, and the data presented here are tentative.

We have previously found that the child-rearing environment can modify effects of pain exposure in the NICU, either positively or negatively. Poor family relations and low maternal sensitivity to child cues significantly exacerbated the relationship between prematurity and increased somatization (Grunau et al. 1994a). In another data set, maternal factors were associated with altered pain response reported by parents of ELBW preterm infants (Grunau 2002). At 8 months' CCA, greater facial reactivity to pain was associated with a lower number of pain procedures and higher exposure to morphine in the NICU, and with positive maternal responsivity (Grunau 2002). Increased heart rate reactivity to lance was significantly associated with less exposure to pain and more morphine in the NICU; however, we only found a trend with maternal responsivity (Grunau 2002).

Caregiver factors are likely to moderate effects of early exposure to pain and stress. However, relationships among specific aspects of NICU experience, child, parent, and family factors, and social context in the development of high-risk children are clearly complex. These questions need to be explored using large samples so that effects can be examined longitudinally, and separately for girls and boys.

LONG-TERM EFFECTS OF EARLY PAIN: THE HUMAN DATA

PAIN

While multiple lines of evidence compel concern for potential long-lasting effects of early pain experience (Grunau 2000; also see Garg et al., this volume), we lack human studies directly related to long-term effects of pain in preterm infants that examine outcomes following discharge from the NICU. To my knowledge, almost all the empirical studies later in infancy and childhood are from our center. Initially, we established through questionnaires that parents of children born at extremely low birth weight rated their toddlers as significantly less sensitive to pain at 18 months' CCA, compared to the ratings of parents of children born at heavier low birth weight or at full term (Grunau et al. 1994a). At 4.5 years, parents rated somatization as significantly more prevalent in former ELBW children than in term-born peers, and this finding was confirmed independently elsewhere (Sommerfelt et al. 1996). Furthermore, there were differences in child ratings at 8–10 years of pictures of children in pain situations (Grunau et al. 1998). Recently we carried out biobehavioral studies that confirmed that former ELBW infants display differences in pain response at 4 (Oberlander et al. 2000) and 8 (Grunau et al. 2001b) months' CCA, in studies of blood collection by finger lance, a "pain-naive" site that had not been used previously.

DEVELOPMENT

The main evidence directly linking early pain to subsequent development comes from studies in which infants have been randomized to receive morphine versus placebo during initial acute care in the NICU (MacGregor 1998; Anand et al. 1999). However, these studies utilized small samples and have not provided conclusive evidence of improved outcomes attributable to early pharmacological pain management. Furthermore, little is known about longer-term or repeated exposure to analgesic agents. For example, even repeated sucrose exposure may not be innocuous (Johnston 2002). Recently Gormally and colleagues (2001) suggested that we pay more attention to evolutionary or environmental adaptations to manage pain, rather than rely too heavily on pharmacology. Positioning and containment (Fearon et al.

1997), music (Butt and Kisilevsky 2000), sucking (Stevens and Johnston 1993), and suckling (Blass and Watt 1999), for example, may facilitate early coping with stressful interventions. However, with infants at very low gestational age, these efforts at environmental soothing will most likely be complimentary to the use of pharmacological agents such as morphine.

A further challenge to evaluating the contribution of early pain experience to all aspects of development is the fact that exposure to prenatal stress has long-term effects on offspring (e.g., Lehman et al. 2000). However, what is more surprising is that prenatal stress also alters pain responses subsequently. For example, prenatal stress altered the timing and intensity of inflammatory pain responses in juvenile rats (Butkevich and Vershinina 2001). The importance of prenatal stress is particularly important in studying the development of preterm infants, because in most cases the causal factors initiating the preterm delivery are unknown. Prenatal stressors may themselves cumulatively contribute to preterm labor (Whitehead et al. 2002).

ONTOGENETIC ADAPTATION

Adaptation is viewed as a modification of structure and function to "fit" the environment. Premature infants, especially at extremely low gestational age, may "shut down" during periods of sensory "overload" (Tronick et al. 1990; Als 1995). The infant's incapacity to modulate arousal and to recover is often only evident some time after the acute procedures are over, and thus may not be noticed unless the infant's coping is carefully evaluated (Als 1982, 1995). These withdrawal periods may be adaptive to the organism in the short run, conserving energy for maintaining physiological stability. However, the cost may be high when repeated challenges are encountered, with the potential for altered arousal over time (Grunau et al. 2001a). Furthermore, shutting down responses to invasive stimulation may be an appropriate adaptation to intrusive aspects of the NICU in the short run to maintain energy. This adaptation may be a rudimentary form of protective response due to the unnatural NICU environment (Tronick et al. 1990). Expectancy formation contributes to the infant's ability to organize responses to recurring stimuli in the environment over time. Experimental evidence indicates that preterm infants in the NICU can be successfully conditioned, provided that a low-energy response is chosen. Ingersoll and Thoman (1994) demonstrated that infants at 33 weeks' PCA learned to approach and achieve contact with a "breathing" teddy bear placed in the isolette. Recently, Goubet et al. (2001) showed that preterm infants between 28 and 32 weeks' gestational age learn to predict painful stimulation. Thus a conditioning paradigm appears operative in relation to procedures in the NICU. Given the primacy of negative conditioning in animal models, it is conceptually likely that a conditioned response may be learned, even in very young neonates experiencing repetitive pain. However, it is also possible that "shutting down" alters pain perception itself, which also would be protective in the short run.

Preterm infants may display either hyposensitivity or hypersensitivity to novel stimuli. In early infancy, persisting alteration in face-to-face interaction with caregivers may be one of a number of unwanted sequelae affecting long-term development of social interaction. Whereas in the NICU this protective response may have been adaptive in response to early sensory overload, if it persisted later, it could be maladaptive. Increased prevalence of withdrawal, social difficulties, anxiety, and depression amongst children of very low birth weight warrants concern that, as adults, they might be at increased risk for specific types of later psychopathology. However, these links are only conjectural at this point. Even within the emotional domain, the relative contributions of birth weight and psychosocial variables can vary, with adolescent depression relatively more related to family environment, and anxiety more related to birth weight (Levy-Shiff et al. 1994). Tonic negative affect over a prolonged period could set a background for ongoing nonspecific anxiety. Conversely, progression to depression may be triggered or precipitated by the additional presence of nonoptimal family relationships.

Traditionally, stress has been viewed as resulting in disturbance of an organism's physiological homeostasis (Selye 1975). However, mild stress is not considered inherently damaging; rather, in mature organisms some degree of stress can be motivating. The key issue is that stress is not necessarily inherent to a given stimulus, but is relative to the organism and situation; the stressor must be appropriate developmentally. In other words, a stimulus or situation easily regulated by a healthy term-born infant may be highly stressful for a sick baby or a VLGA baby. For example, bathing is demonstrably stressful for a VLGA infant in the NICU and potentially disruptive for some term-born neonates, but is generally positive for healthy infants a short time later. Furthermore, confronting novelty can be either invigorating or stressful, depending on inherent temperamental traits and environmental history. In young children, security of attachment to the primary caregiver can affect the degree of distress caused by novel stimuli. Gunnar (1994) has shown that inhibited children with poor attachments show cortisol elevations when placed in arousing, unfamiliar situations, whereas those who are securely attached do not.

Relationships between stress, outcomes, and coping are complex (Compas et al. 1999), especially in preterm infants, who are more sensitive to environmental context at all stages of development. For example, stressful maternal life events, but not emotional distress, moderated the effect of an intervention program on child cognitive scores (Klebanov et al. 2001). The same study, when data were adjusted for maternal education and family income, showed that former preterm children whose mothers experienced more stressful life events were less able to benefit from intervention to promote their development.

Interestingly, even in much more simple mammals such as the rat, physical and emotional stressors are fundamentally different; for example, effects of cues differ depending on the nature of the stressor. Recently, Pijlman and colleagues (2002) examined long-term behavioral effects of cues to physical versus emotional stressors in adult rats. Presenting a cue prior to an unavoidable stressor can influence the response. After repeated pairing of a cue with a stressor, the cue becomes a predictor of the stressor. Over time, behavioral stress effects appeared to be reduced when a warning, such as a light, was always presented as a warning signal (cue) prior to foot shock (Pijlman et al. 2002). Thus predictable stress was viewed as less severe than unpredictable stress. However, the opposite was also observed in this study. Cueing stress had greater effects on physical than emotional stressors, and the results were in the opposite direction. Animals cued prior to physical stress became inactive, whereas emotional stress led to increased activity regardless of cueing. Cueing prior to physical stress may be analogous to wiping the foot prior to heel lance in preterm infants; the infants learn over time that heel swab predicts pain (Goubet et al. 2001). Furthermore, the reduction in facial response that characteristically follows long-term pain exposure (Johnston and Stevens 1996; Grunau 2001b) may also reflect behavioral inhibition comparable to the animals' response to cued physical pain mentioned above.

CONCLUSION

In very early human development, mechanisms of attention, social-emotional regulation, temperament, and cognitive functioning are interwoven. At the outset of this chapter I proposed that early repetitive pain in preterm neonates is likely to affect arousal and interaction with the environment, particularly in unfamiliar situations or in approaching novel tasks. Rather than considering pain reactivity and cognitive approach or avoidance as separate domains, under this view we would see them both as different aspects of underlying difficulties in arousal regulation. The specific responses would depend on the level of the CNS involved, from automatic conditioned reactivity to higher or executive and attention capabilities. This chapter has presented multiple lines of evidence that converge to support the proposed schema. However, a great deal of work is needed to understand the mechanisms involved in these developmental processes.

ACKNOWLEDGMENTS

The author's research program is primarily supported by grant HO39783 from the National Institute for Child Health and Human Development (USA) and by grant MOP42469 from the Canadian Institutes for Health Research. The author is a Senior Scholar with the Michael Smith Foundation for Health Research.

REFERENCES

Als H. The unfolding of behavioral organization in the face of biological violation. In: Tronick EZ (Ed). *Social Interchange In Infancy: Affect, Cognition, and Communication.* Baltimore: University Park Press, 1982.

Als H. The preterm infant: a model for the study of fetal brain expectation. In: Lecanuet JP, Fifer WP, Krasnegor NA, Smotherman WP (Eds). *Fetal Development: A Psychobiological Perspective.* Hillsdale, NJ: Erlbaum, 1995, pp 439–471.

Anand KJS. Effects of perinatal pain and stress. In: Mayer EA, Saper CB (Eds). *Progress in Brain Research.* Amsterdam: Elsevier Science, 2000, pp 117–129.

Anand KJS, Craig KD. New perspectives on the definition of pain. *Pain* 1996; 67:3–6.

Anand KJ, Barton BA, McIntosh N, et al. Analgesia and sedation in preterm neonates who require ventilatory support: results from the NOPAIN trial. Neonatal Outcome and Prolonged Analgesia in Neonates. *Arch Pediatr Adolesc Med* 1999; 153:331–338.

Andrews K, Fitzgerald M. The cutaneous withdrawal reflex in human neonates: sensitization, receptive fields, and the effects of contralateral stimulation. *Pain* 1994; 56:95–101.

Barr RG. Crying in the first year of life: good news in the midst of distress. *Child Care Health Dev* 1998; 24:425–439.

Blass EM, Watt LB. Suckling- and sucrose-induced analgesia in human newborns. *Pain* 1999; 83:611–623.

Blass EM, Shide DJ, Zaw-Mon C, Sorrentino J. Mother as a shield: differential effects of contact and nursing on pain reactivity in infant rats—evidence for nonopioid mediation. *Behav Neurosci* 1995; 109(2):342–353.

Blumberg MS, Lucas DE. A developmental and component analysis of active sleep. *Dev Psychobiol* 1996; 29:1–22.

Bohm B, Katz-Salamon M, Institute K, et al. Developmental risks and protective factors for influencing cognitive outcome at 5 1/2 years of age in very-low-birthweight children. *Dev Med Child Neurol* 2002; 44:508–516.

Borghese IF, Minard KL, Thoman EB. Sleep rhythmicity in premature infants: implications for development status. *Sleep* 1995; 18:523–530.

Bornstein MH. *Handbook of Parenting.* Mahwah, NJ: Lawrence Erlbaum, 1995.

Boyce WT, Barr RG, Zeltzer LK. Temperament and the psychobiology of childhood stress. *Pediatrics* 1992; 90:483–486.

Buss AH, Plomin R. *Temperament: Early Developing Personality Traits.* Hillsdale, NJ: Erlbaum, 1984.
Butkevich IP, Vershinina EA. Prenatal stress alters time characteristics and intensity of formalin-induced pain responses in juvenile rats. *Brain Res* 2001; 915:88–93.
Butt ML, Kisilevsky BS. Music modulates behavior of premature infants following heel lance. *Can J Nurs Res* 2000; 31:17–39.
Carey WB, McDevitt SC. Revision of the infant temperament questionnaire. *Pediatrics* 1978; 61:735–739.
Chapman CR, Nakamura Y. A passion of the soul: an introduction to pain for consciousness researchers. *Conscious Cogn* 1999; 8:391–422.
Compas B, Connor J, Saltzman H, Harding Thomsen A, Wadsworth M. Getting specific about coping: effortful and involuntary responses to stress in development. In: Lewis M, Ramsay DS (Eds). *Soothing and Stress.* Mahwah, NJ: Lawrence Erlbaum, 1999, pp 229–256.
Craig KD, Whitfield MF, Grunau RV, Linton J, Hadjistavropoulos HD. Pain in the preterm neonate: behavioural and physiological indices. *Pain* 1993; 52:287–299.
Dahl RE. The impact of inadequate sleep on children's daytime cognitive function. *Semin Pediatr Neurol* 1996; 3:44–50.
Davis DH, Thoman EB. Behavioral states of premature infants: implications for neural and behavioral development. *Dev Psychobiol* 1987; 20:25–38.
Eckerman CO, Hsu HC, Molitor A, Leung EH, Goldstein RF. Infant arousal in an en-face exchange with a new partner: effects of prematurity and perinatal biological risk. *Dev Psychol* 1999; 35:282–293.
Fajardo B, Browning M, Fisher D, Paton J. Early state organization and follow-up over one year. *J Dev Behav Pediatr* 1992; 13:83–88.
Fearon I, Kisilevsky BS, Hains SM, Muir DW, Tranmer J. Swaddling after heel lance: age-specific effects on behavioral recovery in preterm infants. *J Dev Behav Pediatr* 1997; 18:222–232.
Fitzgerald M, Andrews K. Flexion reflex properties in the human infant: a measure of spinal sensory processing in the newborn. In: Finley GA, McGrath PJ (Eds). *Measurement of Pain in Infants and Children,* Progress in Pain Research and Management, Vol. 10. Seattle: IASP Press, 1998, pp 47–57.
Fitzgerald M, Beggs S. The neurobiology of pain: developmental aspects. *Neuroscientist* 2001; 7:246–257.
Fitzgerald M, Shaw A, MacIntosh N. Postnatal development of the cutaneous flexor reflex: comparative study of preterm infants and newborn rat pups. *Dev Med Child Neurol* 1988; 30:520–526.
Goldsmith HH, Buss AH, Plomin R, et al. Roundtable: what is temperament? Four approaches. *Child Dev* 1987; 58:505–529.
Gormally S, Barr RG, Wertheim L, et al. Contact and nutrient caregiving effects on newborn infant pain responses. *Dev Med Child Neurol* 2001; 43:28–38.
Goubet N, Clifton RK, Shah B. Learning about pain in preterm newborns. *J Dev Behav Pediatr* 2001; 22:418–424.
Gray L. The neuropsychology of temperament. In: Strelau J, Angleitner A (Eds). *Explorations in Temperament: International Perspectives on Theory and Measurement.* New York: Plenum, 1991, pp 105–128.
Greenberg MT, Crnic KA. Longitudinal predictors of developmental status and social interaction in premature and full-term infants at age two. *Child Dev* 1988; 59:554–570.
Grunau R. Long-term consequences of pain in human neonates. In: McGrath PJ, Stevens BJ, Anand KJS (Eds). *Pain in Neonates: Pain Research and Clinical Management.* Amsterdam: Elsevier Science, 2000, pp 55–76.
Grunau RE. Early pain in preterm infants: a model of long term effects. *Clin Perinatol* 2002; 29:373–394.

Grunau RE, Kearney SM, Whitfield MF. Language development at 3 years in pre-term children of birth weight below 1000 g. *Br J Disord Commun* 1990; 25:173–182.

Grunau RE, Oberlander T, Holsti L, Whitfield MF. Bedside application of the Neonatal Facial Coding System in pain assessment of premature neonates. *Pain* 1998; 76:277–286.

Grunau RE, Holsti L, Whitfield MF, Ling E. Are twitches, startles, and body movements pain indicators in extremely low birth weight infants? *Clin J Pain* 2000a; 16:37–45.

Grunau RE, Whitfield MF, Petrie J. Predicting IQ of biologically "at risk" children from age 3 to school entry: sensitivity and specificity of the Stanford-Binet Intelligence Scale IV. *J Dev Behav Pediatr* 2000b; 21:401–407.

Grunau RE, Oberlander T, Whitfield MF, et al. Pain reactivity in former extremely low birth weight infants at corrected age 8 months compared with term born controls. *Infant Behav Dev* 2001a; 24:41–55.

Grunau RE, Oberlander TF, Whitfield MF, Fitzgerald C, Lee SK. Demographic and therapeutic determinants of pain reactivity in very low birth weight neonates at 32 weeks' post-conceptional age. *Pediatrics* 2001b; 107:105–112.

Grunau RE, Whitfield MF, Petrie JH, Morison SJ, Davis CG. Mother-child dyadic interaction in extremely high risk premature toddlers. *Pediatr Res* 2002; 49(4):336A.

Grunau RV, Craig KD. Pain expression in neonates: facial action and cry. *Pain* 1987; 28:395–410.

Grunau RV, Whitfield MF, Petrie JH. Pain sensitivity and temperament in extremely low-birth-weight premature toddlers and preterm and full-term controls. *Pain* 1994a; 58:341–346.

Grunau RV, Whitfield MF, Petrie JH, Fryer EL. Early pain experience, child and family factors, as precursors of somatization: a prospective study of extremely premature and fullterm children. *Pain* 1994b; 56:353–359.

Gunnar MR. Psychoendocrine studies of temperament and stress in early childhood: expanding current models. In: Bates JE, Wachs TD (Eds). *Temperament: Individual Differences at the Interface of Biology and Behavior*. Washington, DC: American Psychological Association, 1994; pp 25–38.

Halpern LF, Garcia Coll CT, Meyer EC, Bendersky K. The contributions of temperament and maternal responsiveness to the mental development of small-for-gestational-age and appropriate-for-gestational-age infants. *Appl Dev Psychol* 2001; 22:199–224.

Hebb DO. Drives and the CNS (conceptual nervous system). *Psychol Rev* 1955; 62:243–254.

Horne JA. Human sleep, sleep loss and behavior: implications for the prefrontal cortex and psychiatric disorder. *Br J Psychiatry* 1993; 162:413–419.

Ingersoll EW, Thoman EB. The breathing bear: effects on respiration in premature infants. *Physiol Behav* 1994; 56:855–859.

Jefferis BJ, Power C, Hertzman C. Birth weight, childhood socioeconomic environment, and cognitive development in the 1958 British birth cohort study. *BMJ* 2002; 325:305.

Johnson M. Functional brain development during infancy. In: Bremner G, Fosel A (Eds). *Handbook of Infant Development*. Malden, MA: Blackwell, 2001.

Johnston CC, Stevens BJ. Experience in a neonatal intensive care unit affects pain response. *Pediatrics* 1996; 98:925–930.

Johnston CC, Stevens B, Craig KD, Grunau RV. Developmental changes in pain expression in premature, full-term, two- and four-month-old infants. *Pain* 1993; 52:201–208.

Johnston CC, Stevens BJ, Yang F, Horton LJ. Differential response to pain by very premature neonates. *Pain* 1995; 61:471–479.

Johnston CC, Stremler RL, Stevens BJ, Horton LJ. Effectiveness of oral sucrose and simulated rocking on pain response in preterm neonates. *Pain* 1997; 72:193–199.

Johnston CC, Stremler R, Horton L, Friedman A. Effect of repeated doses of sucrose during heel stick procedure in preterm neonates. *Biol Neonate* 1999; 75:160–166.

Johnston CC, Filion F, Snider L, et al. Routine sucrose analgesia during first week of life in neonates less than 31 weeks' post-conceptual age. *Pediatrics* 2002; 110:523–528.

Kagan J. Temperament and the reactions to unfamiliarity. *Child Dev* 1997; 68:139–143.

Kagan J, Reznick JS, Snidman N. Temperamental influences on reactions to unfamiliarity and challenge. *Adv Exp Med Biol* 1988; 245:319–339.

Kagan J, Snidman N, Arcus D. The role of temperament in social development. *Ann NY Acad Sci* 1995; 771:485–490.

Klebanov PK, Brooks-Gunn J, McCormick MC. Maternal coping strategies and emotional distress: results of an early intervention program for low birth weight young children. *Dev Psychol* 2001; 37:654–667.

Kochanska G, Aksan N, Koenig AL. A longitudinal study of the roots of preschoolers' conscience: committed compliance and emerging internalization. *Child Dev* 1995; 66:1752–1769.

Kopp R, Bohdanecky Z, Jarvik ME. Proactive effect of a single electroconvulsive shock (ECS) on one-trial learning in mice. *J Comp Physiol Psychol* 1968; 65:514–517.

Lachar D, Gdowski CL. Problem-behavior factor correlates of Personality Inventory for Children profile scales. *J Consult Clin Psychol* 1979; 47:39–48.

Lehman J, Stohr T, Feldon J. Long-term effects of prenatal stress experiences and postnatal maternal separation on emotionality and attentional processes. *Behav Brain Res* 2000; 107:133–144.

Levy-Shiff R, Einat G, Mogilner MB, Lerman M, Krikler R. Biological and environmental correlates of developmental outcome of prematurely born infants in early adolescence. *J Pediatr Psychol* 1994; 19:63–78.

Lewis M. Individual differences in response to stress. *Pediatrics* 1992; 90:487–490.

Lewis M, Ramsay DS. Effect of maternal soothing on infant stress response. *Child Dev* 1999; 70:11–20.

Liaw F, Brooks-Gunn J. Cumulative familial risks and low-birthweight children's cognitive and behavioral development. *J Clin Child Psychol* 1994; 23:360–372.

MacGregor R, Evans D, Sugden D, Gaussen T, Levene M. Outcome at 5–6 years of prematurely born children who received morphine as neonates. *Arch Dis Child Fetal Neonatal Ed* 1998; 79:F40–F43.

Mayes LC. A developmental perspective on the regulation of arousal states. *Semin Perinatol* 2000; 24:267–279.

Meaney MJ, Mitchell JB, Aitken DH, et al. The effects of neonatal handling on the development of the adrenocortical response to stress: implications for neuropathology and cognitive deficits in later life. *Psychoneuroendocrinology* 1991; 16:85–103.

Merskey H. On the development of pain. *Headache* 1970; 10:116–123.

Morison SJ, Grunau RE, Oberlander TF, Whitfield MF. Relations between behavioral and cardiac autonomic reactivity to acute pain in preterm neonates. *Clin J Pain* 2001; 17:350–358.

Murtha AP, Chertkow H, Beauregard M, Dixon R, Evans A. Anticipation causes increased blood flow to the anterior cingulate cortex. *Hum Brain Mapp* 1996; 4:103–112.

Neuringer AJ. Animals respond for food in the presence of free food. *Science* 1969; 166:399–401.

Oberlander TF, Grunau RE, Whitfield MF, et al. Biobehavioral pain responses in former extremely low birth weight infants at four months' corrected age. *Pediatrics* 2000; 105:e6.

Oberlander TF, Grunau RE, Fitzgerald C, Whitfield MF. Does parenchymal brain injury affect biobehavioral pain responses in very low birth weight infants at 32 weeks' postconceptional age? *Pediatrics* 2002; 110:570–576.

Pijlman F, Wolterink G, van Ree J. Cueing unavoidable physical but not emotional stress increases long-term behavioral effects in rats. *Behav Brain Res* 2002; 134:393.

Poehlmann J, Fiese BH. Parent-infant interaction as a mediator of the relation between neonatal risk status and 12-month cognitive development. *Infant Behav Dev* 2001; 24:171–188.

Porter FL, Wolf CM, Miller JP. The effect of handling and immobilization on the response to acute pain in newborn infants. *Pediatrics* 1998; 102:1383–1389.

Posner MI. Convergence of psychological and biological development. *Dev Psychobiol* 2002; 40(3):339–343.

Posner MI, Rothbart MK. Attention, self-regulation and consciousness. *Philos Trans R Soc Lond B Biol Sci* 1998; 353:1915–1927.

Posner MI, Rothbart MK. Developing mechanisms of self-regulation. *Dev Psychopathol* 2000; 12:427–441.

Rainville P, Duncan GH, Price DD, Carrier B, Bushnell MC. Pain affect encoded in human anterior cingulate but not somatosensory cortex. *Science* 1997; 277:968–971.

Resnick MB, Stralka K, Carter RL, et al. Effects of birth weight and sociodemographic variables on mental development of neonatal intensive care unit survivors. *Am J Obstet Gynecol* 1990; 162:374–378.

Rotenberg VS. Sleep and memory. I: The influence of different sleep stages on memory. *Neurosci Biobehav Rev* 1992; 16:497–502.

Rothbart MK. Temperament: a developmental framework. In: Strelau J, Angleitner A (Eds). *Explorations in Temperament: International Perspectives on Theory and Measurement.* New York: Plenum Press, 1991, pp 61–74.

Rothbart MK, Derryberry JE. Development of individual differences in temperament. In: Lamb ME, Brown AL (Eds). *Advances in Developmental Psychology.* Hillsdale, NJ: Lawrence Erlbaum, 1981, pp 37–86.

Rothbart MK, Goldsmith HH. Three approaches to the study of infant temperament. *Dev Rev* 1985; 5:237–260.

Rothbart MK, Ziaie H, O'Boyle CG. Self-regulation and emotion in infancy. *New Dir Child Dev* 1992; 7–23.

Rothbart MK, Bates JE. Temperament. In: Eisenberg N (Ed). *Social, Emotional, and Personality Development,* Handbook of Child Psychology, Vol. 3. New York: Wiley, 1997; pp 105–175.

Ruff HA. Attention and organization of behavior in high-risk infants. *J Dev Behav Pediatr* 1986; 7:298–301.

Ruff HA, Rothbart MK. *Attention in Early Development: Themes and Variations.* New York: Oxford University Press, 1996.

Sameroff AJ. Environmental risk factors in infancy. *Pediatrics* 1998; 5(Suppl E)102:1287–1292.

Sameroff AJ, Chandler MJ. Reproductive risk and the continuum of caretaking casualty. In: Horowitz FD, Hetherington M, Scarr-Salapatek S, Siegel EG (Eds). *Review of Child Development Research,* Vol. 4. Chicago: University of Chicago Press, 1975, pp 187–244.

Scher MS. Neurophysiological assessment of brain function and maturation: I. A measure of brain adaptation in high risk infants. *Pediatr Neurol* 1997a; 16:191–198.

Scher MS. Neurophysiological assessment of brain function and maturation. II. A measure of brain dysmaturity in healthy preterm neonates. *Pediatr Neurol* 1997b; 16:287–295.

Scher MS, Steppe DA, Banks DL. Prediction of lower developmental performances of healthy neonates by neonatal EEG-sleep measures. *Pediatr Neurol* 1996; 14:137–144.

Sell EJ, Hill-Mangan S, Holberg CJ. Natural course of behavioral organization in premature infants. *Infant Behav Develop* 1992; 15:461–478.

Selye H. Confusion and controversy in the stress field. *J Hum Stress* 1975; 1:37–44.

Shoda Y, Mischel W, Peake PK. Predicting adolescent cognitive and self-regulatory competencies from preschool delay of gratification: identifying diagnostic conditions. *Dev Psychol* 1990; 26:978–986.

Sommerfelt K, Troland K, Ellertsen B, Markestad T. Behavioral problems in low-birthweight preschoolers. *Dev Med Child Neurol* 1996; 38(10):927–940.

Spangler G, Schieche M, Ilg U, Maier U, Ackermann C. Maternal sensitivity as an external organizer for biobehavioral regulation in infancy. *Dev Psychobiol* 1994; 27:425–437.

Stephan M, Helfritz F, Pabst R, von Horsten S. Postnatally induced differences in adult pain sensitivity depend on genetics, gender and specific experiences: reversal of maternal deprivation effects by additional postnatal tactile stimulation or chronic imipramine treatment. *Behav Brain Res* 2002; 133:149–158.

Stevens BJ, Johnston CC. Pain in the infant: theoretical and conceptual issues. *Maternal Child Nurs J* 1993; 21:3–14.

Stevens BJ, Johnston CC, Horton L. Factors that influence the behavioral pain responses of premature infants. *Pain* 1994; 59:101–109.

Stevens B, Johnston C, Petryshen P, Taddio A. Premature Infant Pain Profile: development and initial validation. *Clin J Pain* 1996; 12:13–22.

Taylor HG, Klein N, Schattschneider C, Hack M. Predictors of early school age outcomes in very low birth weight children. *J Dev Behav Pediatr* 1998; 19:235–243.

Thorndike RL, Hagen EP, Sattler JM. *The Stanford-Binet Intelligence Scale,* 4th ed. Chicago: Riverside, 1986.

Tobin MJ. Constraints upon parenting: experience of a psychologist. *Child Care Health Dev* 1989; 15:37–43.

Tronick EZ, Scanlon KB, Scanlon JW. Protective apathy, a hypothesis about the behavioral organization and its relation to clinical and physiologic status of the preterm infant during the newborn period. *Clin Perinatol* 1990; 17:125–154.

Valentino RJ, Page M, Van Bockstaele E, Aston-Jones G. Corticotropin-releasing factor innervation of the locus coeruleus region: distribution of fibers and sources of input. *Neuroscience* 1992; 48:689–705.

Weinberg J. Recent studies on the effects of fetal alcohol exposure on the endocrine and immune systems. *Alcohol Alcohol Suppl* 1994; 2:401–409.

Weinberg J, Kim CK, Yu W. Early handling can attenuate adverse effects of fetal ethanol exposure. *Alcohol* 1995; 12:317–327.

Whitehead N, Hill H, Brogan D, Blackmore-Prince C. Exploration of threshold analysis in the relation between stressful life events and preterm delivery. *Am J Epidemiol* 2002; 155:117–124.

Whitfield MF, Grunau RV, Holsti L. Extremely premature (≤ 800 g) schoolchildren: multiple areas of hidden disability. *Arch Dis Child Fetal Neonatal Ed* 1997; 77(2):F85–90.

Correspondence to: Ruth E. Grunau, PhD, Centre for Community Child Health Research, Room L408, 4480 Oak Street, Vancouver, BC, Canada V6H 3V4. Email: rgrunau@cw.bc.ca.

3

Genetic Tools for the Study of Pain: Current Techniques and Findings

Shad B. Smith and Jeffrey S. Mogil

Department of Psychology, McGill University, Montreal, Quebec, Canada

Pain sensitivity is a complex trait whose variability among individuals can prove frustrating to clinicians and researchers alike. The source of this variation is, of course, some combination of nature (inherited genetic factors) and nurture (environmental and experiential factors), but until recently little has been known about the latter and nothing at all about the former. Researchers and clinicians have long observed that the objective intensity of a noxious stimulus (or, in clinical situations, the severity of an injury) often does not correspond with the degree of pain perceived. We have come to appreciate pain as a highly subjective sensory and emotional experience (IASP Subcommittee on Taxonomy 1979), one that can depend as much on current and past environmental circumstances as on physiological nociceptive processes.

Despite a number of challenges, sophisticated anatomical, electrophysiological, pharmacological, and behavioral techniques have facilitated great advances in our understanding of basic nociceptive mechanisms. Researchers have begun to explain pain phenomena on the cellular level. Pain-related neurotransmitters, receptors, ion channels, transducers, and enzymes have been identified. Most recently, advances in molecular biological technology, such as the polymerase chain reaction and DNA sequencing, have allowed us to probe pain on the most basic level of biological reductionism, the gene itself. Some genetic studies have capitalized on the natural differences among individuals to elucidate the causes of variability. This chapter describes the methodologies being used to isolate, identify, and manipulate the actions of individual genes responsible for the variability observed in pain and analgesia sensitivities. The reader is directed also to published comprehensive reviews on this subject (Mogil et al. 1996b, 2000; Mogil and Grisel 1998;

Mogil 1999; Mogil and McCarson 2000). The latter portion of this chapter explores the known genetic bases of pain-related human pathological conditions featuring pediatric onset.

INTERINDIVIDUAL VARIABILITY IN PAIN AND ANALGESIA

HUMAN STUDIES

Libman (1934) reported that he could divide his patients into high, normal, and zero sensitivity categories based on pain response when he surreptitiously applied pressure to the mastoid bone in the direction of the styloid process. Later, more quantitative research established that this variability could be observed across a range of painful stimuli, including noxious pressure (Sherman 1943; Chapman and Jones 1944), noxious heat (Clark and Bindra 1956; Wolff and Jarvik 1963, 1964), and electrical current (Lanier 1943; Clark and Bindra 1956). Differences in baseline pain threshold as well as tolerance to pain were observed in these early experiments, and in more recent studies (Brennum et al. 1989; Chen et al. 1989; Jacobs et al. 1995; Isselee et al. 1997). Variability in responses to clinical pain remains much less well studied, although it is appreciated that neuropathic pain after traumatic injury is highly variable (Richards 1967; Jensen et al. 1985; Bonica 1990).

The efficacy of analgesic drugs also shows a high level of variability among individuals. Opioids that presumably act at the same receptor sites can have widely ranging analgesic potencies and side-effect profiles in different patients (Buchsbaum et al. 1981; Levine et al. 1981; Chapman et al. 1990; Galer et al. 1992; Maier et al. 2002). Lasagna and Beecher (1954) found in a classic study that the standard clinical dose of morphine, 10 mg, successfully alleviated pain in only about 65% of their patients. Almost 10% of Caucasians do not respond to the opiate codeine, being unable (by virtue of inheriting certain allelic variants of the *CYP2D6* gene) to convert the drug into its active metabolite, morphine (Gonzales et al. 1988; see Sindrup and Brosen 1995). Interestingly, this gene has also been implicated in nociceptive sensitivity on the cold pressor test (Sindrup et al. 1993). Individual differences in response to nonsteroidal anti-inflammatory drugs also have been thoroughly documented (e.g., Wolff et al. 1965; Bellamy 1985; Day 1993; Walker et al. 1994, 1997).

A few heritable, pain-related conditions can now be attributed to specific genetic determinants, and many more are thought to have significant genetic components. Congenital insensitivity to pain with anhidrosis (CIPA, also classified as hereditary sensory neuropathy, type IV), a rare condition involving the total loss of pain sensation unaccompanied by loss of other sensory modalities (Thrush 1973), was the first such condition to garner research attention, due to its extreme nature. The subject of one early case report (Dearborn 1932) made his living as a carnival side show, "The Human Pincushion." A recent study by Indo and colleagues (1996) revealed that any one of a number of mutations of the *NTRK1* gene, which codes for the high-affinity receptor (TRKA) for nerve growth factor, is responsible for virtually all cases of CIPA. Without the TRKA receptor, nociceptors do not develop in such individuals. Another example of a heritable pain pathology with an elucidated genetic basis is familial hemiplegic migraine, distinguished from the more common migraine with aura by the co-occurrence of some degree of motor weakness in at least one side of the body. It has an autosomal dominant pattern of inheritance, and linkage analysis has implicated chromosome 19p13 in the disease (Joutel et al. 1993). Ophoff and colleagues (1996) demonstrated that mutations in the *CACNA1A* gene on chromosome 19 were responsible. This gene codes for a calcium channel subunit; the missense mutations causing the pathology affect the kinetic properties and voltage dependence of activation of the α_{1A} calcium channel (Kraus et al. 1998).

Much more commonly, however, genetic factors merely predispose individuals to express high or low sensitivity to a pain-related trait, or to be susceptible or resistant to developing a pain-associated disease. The extent of such susceptibility can be expressed as "heritability," or the proportion of overall phenotypic variance explained by genetic factors. Using twin studies (see Martin et al. 1997), researchers have estimated the heritability of many common painful maladies: 39–58% for migraine (Honkasalo et al. 1995; Larsson et al. 1995; Ziegler et al. 1998), 55% for menstrual pain (Treloar et al. 1998), 50% for back pain (Bengtsson and Thorson 1991), 46% for carpal tunnel syndrome (Hakim et al. 2002), and 21% for sciatica (Heikkila et al. 1989). Fibromyalgia runs in families (e.g., Buskila et al. 1996), but myofascial temporomandibular disorder apparently does not (Raphael et al. 1999; Michalowicz et al. 2000).

ANIMAL STUDIES

In human studies, environmental and psychosocial factors generally contribute more to the variability of pain-related traits than do genetic factors. However, using identically housed and reared laboratory mice, we have estimated the heritabilities for various nociceptive and analgesic sensitivity traits as ranging from 28% to 76% (Belknap et al. 1983; Kest et al. 1999; Mogil et al. 1999a,b). The mouse is the animal model of choice for genetic studies for reasons beyond simply the practical; the genetics community has also benefited from the extensive pedigree records maintained for most commercially available strains. The usefulness of the mouse is reflected in the fact that it will be the first mammal (after humans) to have its genome fully mapped, and a draft sequence with 96% coverage is already publicly available (www.ensembl.org/Mus_musculus/). The relevance of research conducted on nonhuman species is always in question, but the extensive linkage homology between mice and humans (Copeland et al. 1993) and the ancient nature of the trait in question both augur well for successful translation of genetics findings from mice to humans. The mouse is specifically advantageous over the rat in that genetic models of specific traits not only can be identified and studied (e.g., spontaneous mutants, high and low responding strains) but also can be produced by transgenesis. Transgenic technology, to be discussed in detail later, allows the researcher an unsurpassed level of control, as mice are produced that differ only at desired genetic loci.

Differences between defined genetic populations of mice (and rats) in pain-related traits have been reported for many years (see Belknap and O'Toole 1991; Mogil et al. 1996b; Mogil 1999). Especially well known are the myriad differences between the inbred DBA/2 strain, which is pain resistant and sensitive to opioid analgesia, and the C57BL/6 strain, which is pain sensitive and resistant to opioid analgesia (see Frischknecht et al. 1988; Belknap and O'Toole 1991). However, the utility of well-defined inbred mouse strains becomes most apparent when one systematically compares such strains on different tests of nociceptive sensitivity. Our group has tested a common set of 12 inbred mouse strains on a large number of nociceptive and analgesic assays (Mogil et al. 1999a,b; Lariviere et al. 2002; Wilson et al. 2003). A pattern of differences between strains is readily observed for any single pain stimulus; however, a different pattern may emerge using other stimuli (Mogil 1999).

Observed strain differences are not only quantitative in nature; in some cases, distinct pain-modulating circuitry seems to underlie some differences. For example, stress produces analgesia in some mouse strains by activation of the opioid analgesic system, while in other strains similar levels of analgesia are produced through a non-opioid (naloxone-insensitive) pathway (Urca et al. 1985; Mogil and Belknap 1997). The analgesic effects of heroin are mediated variously by μ-, δ-, or κ-opioid receptors in different strains of mice (Rady et al. 1991, 1998). Even mice of the same strain but obtained from different suppliers (and hence, different breeding pools) can exhibit robust differences in pain-related traits. For example, the α_2-adrenergic antagonists reverse electrical stimulation-produced analgesia in Sprague Dawley rats from Harlan Sprague Dawley in Indianapolis, but not in rats of the same strain obtained from the now defunct Sasco Inc. (West et al. 1993). The suggestion that ceruleospinal noradrenergic neurons have different physiological functions in these substrains is supported by anatomical evidence. Clark and Proudfit (1992) observed, rather remarkably, that the ceruleospinal pathway projects bilaterally to the spinal cord in Harlan rats, terminating in dorsal horn laminae I–IV, but ipsilaterally in Sasco rats, terminating in laminae VII–VIII.

GENETIC CORRELATION AMONG PAIN TRAITS

This section describes the ongoing search for the identity of function of pain-related genes. It is important to note, however, that genetic approaches can be useful in furthering our understanding of pain physiology in advance of gene identification. Genetic correlation among pain traits is a perfect example of this utility.

Given a finite number of genes and a practically infinite number of genetically influenced traits, most genes influence several different traits. This property of genes, known as pleiotropy, is responsible for correlation among pain traits. Consequently, it is possible to determine whether traits share genetic mediation—and thus, presumably, physiological mediation—by measuring their correlation, because allelic variation in a gene will influence all traits in which that gene participates. Our laboratory has made extensive efforts to establish the nature and degree of these genetic correlations among and between nociceptive assays and analgesic modalities.

It has been well established that mice that have a high baseline sensitivity to nociception tend to show lower levels of morphine analgesia against that nociceptive stimulus, and vice versa (Panocka et al. 1986b; Mogil et al. 1996a; Elmer et al. 1997). By comparing several strains, the correlation between initial pain sensitivity and morphine analgesia was estimated to be between –0.63 and –0.85 in one study (Elmer et al. 1997), and –0.61 in a different study (Kest et al. 1999). We have recently replicated and extended these findings (Wilson et al. 2003). In a set of 12 inbred strains, we compared baseline sensitivity and morphine analgesia with analgesia from U50,488 (a κ-opioid agonist), clonidine (an α_2-adrenergic agonist), WIN55,212-2 (a cannabinoid CB1-receptor agonist), and epibatidine (a nicotinic receptor agonist). Although each drug activates a different receptor, the levels of analgesia produced were significantly correlated between drugs (r = 0.39 to 0.77). This surprising finding suggests that there are "master" genes responsible for a large proportion of the genetic variability in analgesic response, regardless of the specific mode of induction of that analgesic state. We also found that for each analgesic, initial sensitivity on the tail-withdrawal test correlated highly with analgesic sensitivity ($r = -0.33$ to -0.68), replicating and extending the phenomenon beyond morphine. This latter observation suggests that perhaps the "master" gene is really a pain sensitivity gene, having everything to do with the nociceptive assay and little to do with the specific analgesic involved. These findings generalize beyond the tail-withdrawal assay, because we replicated both phenomena on the more clinically relevant formalin test (Wilson et al. 2003). The unfortunate clinical implications of this study, should it be relevant to humans, is that patients who fail to respond sufficiently to one class of pain reliever are not likely to find adequate relief with any other class, although it should be stressed that only analgesics acting on classic descending modulatory circuits were tested.

Another line of research conducted in our laboratory concerns genetic correlations among strain sensitivities on separate nociceptive assays (Mogil et al. 1999a,b; Lariviere et al. 2002). Pain researchers employ a wide variety of painful experimental stimuli, which can be characterized along a number of dimensions, such as etiology (nociceptive, inflammatory, neuropathic),

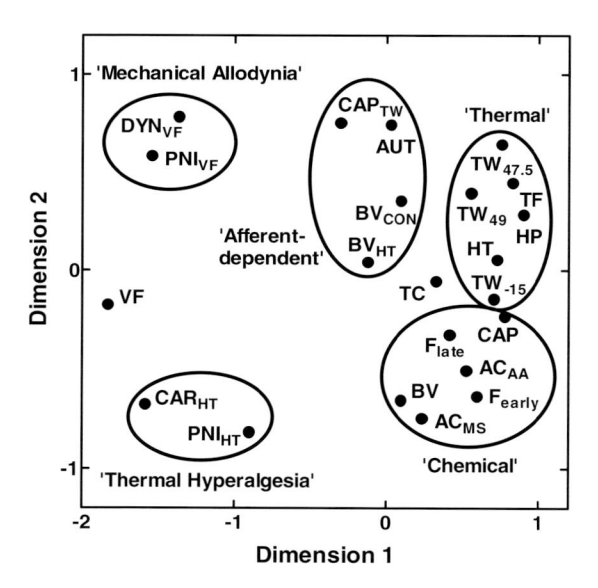

Fig. 1. Multidimensional scaling plot illustrating cross-correlations among inbred strain means for 22 assays of nociception and hypersensitivity. In this plot, Euclidean distances between objects are representative of their genetic correlation; objects with higher positive correlations are closer. The proportion of total variance accounted for is 0.83. See Table I for assay abbreviations. Reprinted from Lariviere et al. (2002), with permission.

Table I
Assay abbreviations used in Fig. 1

AC_{AA}	Abdominal constriction (writhing) test—acetic acid
AC_{MS}	Abdominal constriction (writhing) test—magnesium sulfate
AUT	Autotomy following sciatic and saphenous nerve transection
BV	Bee venom-induced spontaneous pain behavior (licking)
BV_{HT}	Bee venom-induced thermal hypersensitivity assessed with Hargreaves' test (ipsilateral)
BV_{CON}	Bee venom-induced thermal hypersensitivity assessed with Hargreaves' test (contralateral)
CAP	Capsaicin-induced spontaneous pain behavior (licking)
CAP_{TW}	Capsaicin-induced thermal hypersensitivity assessed with tail-withdrawal test
CAR_{HT}	Carrageenan-induced thermal hypersensitivity assessed with Hargreaves' test
DYN_{VF}	Dynorphin-induced mechanical hypersensitivity assessed with von Frey monofilament test
F_{early}	Early/acute phase of formalin test
F_{late}	Late/tonic phase of formalin test
HP	Hot-plate test
HT	Hargreaves et al.'s thermal paw-withdrawal test
PNI_{HT}	Peripheral nerve injury-induced thermal hypersensitivity assessed with Hargreaves' test
PNI_{VF}	Peripheral nerve injury-induced mechanical hypersensitivity assessed with von Frey monofilament test
TC	Tail-clip test
TF	Tail-flick from radiant heat source
TW_{-15}	Tail withdrawal from –15°C ethanol
$TW_{47.5}$	Tail withdrawal from 47.5°C water
TW_{49}	Tail withdrawal from 49°C water
VF	von Frey monofilament test

modality (thermal, chemical, mechanical), duration (acute, tonic, chronic), and location (cutaneous, subcutaneous, visceral). The literature contains multiple demonstrations of dissociations among pain assays (see Mogil et al. 1996a). Is the physiological basis of every different pain test dissociable? Can some assays be substituted for others? We addressed this issue by considering the following question: If a mouse strain is sensitive (or resistant) on one assay of nociception, on which others is it also sensitive (or resistant)? Using multivariate analysis, we showed that most of 23 nociceptive assays group into five distinct clusters based largely on stimulus modality (Lariviere et al. 2002) (see Fig. 1, Table I). Assays within each cluster share a high degree of genetic codetermination, implying common physiological mediation. For example, the "thermal" cluster includes the hot-plate, tail-flick/withdrawal, and Hargreaves' (paw-withdrawal) tests, whereas the "chemical" cluster includes the acetic acid and magnesium sulfate abdominal constriction tests, the formalin test, and bee venom tests. The other assays cluster into groups characterized as "mechanical hypersensitivity," "thermal hypersensitivity," and "afferent-dependent thermal hypersensitivity." This finding is important, because it suggests that a search for "neuropathic pain genes" may be misguided. In the mouse, it appears that the nature of the precipitating injury (i.e., inflammatory or neuropathic) does not confer genetic specificity. Rather, it is different pain *symptoms* that are mediated by separate sets of genes.

ARE GENETIC DIFFERENCES DEPENDENT ON AGE?

The genomic DNA polymorphisms (i.e., allelic variants) that give rise to strain differences in pain and analgesia traits are, of course, present at conception. Nonetheless, it is conceivable that their functional expression might be dependent on developmental status. Some strain differences may not emerge until adulthood, for instance. It is also entirely possible that genetic differences may be uncovered that are relevant only to the reproductively immature animal, only to disappear in adulthood.

Unfortunately, no such data have, to our knowledge, ever been collected. The animal genetics literature is unanimously based on the study of adult subjects. However, we have recently collected data that might represent an interaction between genetics and development. A survey of gabapentin analgesia on the late-phase formalin test in 14 inbred mouse strains revealed analgesic potencies (ED_{50}s) ranging from about 20 mg/kg (in C57BL/6 mice) to 100 mg/kg (in CBA mice). In a related study, we were evaluating the effect of a spontaneous mutation of a calcium channel subunit gene on gabapentin analgesia. Because the mutant mice did not survive to adulthood, we tested mutants and their wild-type counterparts as juveniles (3–4 weeks old). To our surprise, wild-type mice displayed a gabapentin analgesic ED_{50} of 5 mg/kg. It is possible that this increased sensitivity can be attributed to the hybrid genetic background of the wild-type animals, but we suspect that their young age may better explain the data. Experiments are currently under way to follow up on this finding.

IDENTIFICATION OF PAIN GENES

There are two complementary foci in pain and analgesia genetics. One task is to identify genes that produce proteins involved in the mediation of pain and analgesia. The second task is to determine which subset of those genes are responsible for individual differences observed in pain-related traits, and to identify allelic variants of genes predisposing the individual to or causing painful pathology. A few painful conditions are caused by single gene polymorphisms or mutations, such as congenital insensitivity to pain (Indo et al. 1996) and familial hemiplegic migraine (Ophoff et al. 1996). However, most pain traits are more complex, arising from interactions between multiple genes and environmental or developmental factors. Linkage and association studies in humans face serious statistical power challenges in such a context (Risch and Merikangas 1996). The task of identifying "pain genes" in humans is also complicated by definitional issues. For example, is the gene predisposing an individual to sickle cell anemia, which is frequently painful, a pain gene? How about the unidentified gene or genes predisposing individuals to the development of idiopathic migraine or fibromyalgia? It is very likely that certain genes are related to the probability of developing a painful clinical condition, whereas entirely different genes are related to how much pain is experienced by sufferers of that condition. For these reasons and others described above, most pain gene identification programs feature laboratory animals, especially the mouse.

Gene identification techniques can be characterized as either "top-down" or "bottom-up." In the former strategy, genes of relevance to pain are identified by first identifying subpopulations of a species (such as inbred strains, spontaneous mutants, and selected lines) that exhibit differential sensitivity, and then determining which genes are responsible for those differences. This process, known as quantitative trait locus (QTL) mapping and discussed in detail below, is of note because it is the only gene identification method that can account for normal individual variability in pain phenotypes. Top-down gene identification can also be accomplished by comparing the activity of genes, using mRNA quantification or other expression-profiling technologies, in nociceptive versus non-nociceptive states. DNA microarray technology, in which the expression of thousands of genes may be quantified simultaneously, is a promising new method for the rapid survey of the entire genome (see Watson and Akil 1999); researchers are now beginning to apply this method to pain models (Xiao et al. 2002). Bottom-up approaches attempt to confirm known genes as being related to pain. By adding, deleting, or otherwise altering the expression of such genes, researchers hope to characterize the normal function of their protein products. Techniques such as transgenic knockouts and mutagenesis attempt to simplify immensely the complex interactions among multiple genes by examining the effects of manipulating a single genetic target. A few of the most popular and effective techniques in current use are discussed below (also see Mogil and McCarson 2000).

SELECTIVE BREEDING

In this oldest of genetic approaches, mice are bred (or not bred) based on their sensitivity to a trait of interest. Also known as artificial selection, the technique involves the pairing of extremely high and low responders to produce lines of divergently responding offspring. This process does not alter the genes themselves, of course, but it does change the allelic frequencies of the genes that affect the traits under study in each line. It is thus possible to distinguish the particular effects of genes associated with the trait, because they are the only loci that will be systematically affected by the selection. Artificial selection is useful for identifying pleiotropic effects of these genes, because any other trait that segregates alongside the primary phenotype is most likely under their influence as well. If the trait cannot be modified by selection, variability in that trait cannot be genetically mediated.

High-analgesia/low-analgesia mouse strains. Mice submitted to a stressor, such as a 3-minute forced swim, exhibit an analgesic effect that can be attributed at least partially to activation of endogenous opioid systems. This stress-induced analgesia (SIA) paradigm was used to divide outbred Swiss-Webster mice into high-analgesia and low-analgesia groups based on post-swim hot-plate test latencies. Selected mice from each group that exhibited the extreme responsiveness of the line were intermated for several generations. Significant phenotypic division was achieved in the first filial generation, which suggests that few genes are involved in SIA variation (Panocka et al. 1986b). Other traits that correlate with SIA magnitude in these lines, and therefore possibly share genetic mediation, include baseline nociceptive sensitivity to thermal stimuli (Panocka et al. 1986b; Mogil et al. 1996a), morphine analgesia (Panocka and Marek 1986; Panocka et al. 1986a; Mogil et al. 1996a), U50,488H analgesia (Kest et al. 1993), opioid-mediated footshock SIA (Marek et al. 1987; Panocka and Sadowski 1990), and ethanol-induced analgesia (Mogil et al. 1993).

High-analgesic-response/low-analgesic-response mouse strains. These lines were conceived from a heterogeneous stock, this time with reference to hot-plate latencies following treatment with levorphanol, an opioid receptor agonist (Belknap et al. 1983). This model has been used to evaluate the similarity of other drug effects to those of levorphanol; if high-analgesic-response (HAR) mice respond well to a drug while low-analgesic-response (LAR) mice respond poorly, it is reasonable to assume similar genetic mediation between the novel drug and levorphanol. One study devised a hierarchy of drugs on the basis of divergence in HAR versus LAR dose-response curves: morphine > levorphanol > pentazocine > ethylketocyclazocine >

U50,488H > clonidine (Belknap et al. 1987). These data suggest that selection has predominantly affected μ-opioid over κ-opioid and non-opioid receptor mechanisms. Another study similarly ranked μ-opioid mechanisms over δ-opioid mechanisms: DAMGO > DADLE > DSLET > DPDPE (Belknap and Laursen 1987).

High-autotomy/low-autotomy rat strains. Starting with outbred Sabra rats, Devor and Raber (1990) selected for high and low autotomy (i.e., self-mutilation) behavior after sciatic and saphenous nerve transection, a model of anesthesia dolorosa (Wall et al. 1979). Virtually asymptotic selection was achieved within one or two generations, suggesting that variability in autotomy may be inherited as a single gene trait. The selected lines have been tremendously useful in testing hypotheses about the physiological mediation of autotomy (Cohn and Seltzer 1991; Shir et al. 1991, 2001; Liu et al. 2001) and about environmental factors that affect this behavior (Belfer et al. 1998; Raber and Devor 2002).

One disadvantage of selected lines is that they represent poor starting genotypes for QTL mapping, because they are not yet inbred. Because of this limitation, little progress has been made in identifying the genes whose frequencies were altered by these selection projects.

INBRED STRAIN COMPARISON

Through successive brother-sister matings, it is possible to create inbred strains in which every member is genetically identical to every other. Each pairing "fixes" roughly half of the genes in the next generation, ensuring that after 20 mating rounds each offspring will possess identical homozygous alleles at virtually all (99.9%) genetic loci. However, the particular allele that becomes fixed and is passed down in homozygous form to each successive generation is randomly selected from the various alleles segregating in the founding population. A usual first step when investigating genetic variation involves comparing a panel of inbred strains (a "strain survey") on the desired trait. All variation among members of a strain must by definition be caused by environmental effects, because the animals are genetically identical. Variation between strains can be attributed to genetic effects, if care is taken to minimize differences in animal care and experimental protocols between strains.

For purposes of gene identification, surveys of inbred strains can reveal the most useful, extreme-responding progenitor strains from which to begin QTL mapping efforts. In a mapping study, a backcross or F_2 (filial second generation) intercross between high- and low-responding strains is produced, in which alleles at trait-relevant genes are segregating (i.e., existing in homozygous *or* heterozygous form). This generation is tested for phenotypic variation on the relevant nociceptive assay. The animals are then genotyped for their inheritance of a number of polymorphic markers spaced across the genome, such as microsatellites or single nucleotide polymorphisms (SNPs). These markers are co-inherited with nearby genes and can establish linkage relationships; markers that correlate highly with an observed trait must be located near genes responsible for this trait. This technique is powerful enough, at least in theory, to identify loci that contribute only a small fraction to the variability of a trait, a more complex procedure than identifying single-gene-mediated traits (Soller et al. 1976; Lander and Schork 1994). Unfortunately, QTL mapping is not able to pinpoint the precise genes in question. A number of subsequent techniques, collectively known as "positional cloning," can be employed to narrow the confidence interval containing the QTL. Alternatively, or at any point during the positional cloning process, "candidate" genes within the current confidence interval can be assessed functionally or with respect to differential gene expression or sequence alterations (Collins 1997).

RECOMBINANT INBRED STRAINS

A more sophisticated version of the inbred strain model, a recombinant inbred (RI) set, consists of the inbred descendants of a single F_2 intercross between two inbred progenitor strains. These sets are standardized and commercially available, eliminating (for QTLs of large enough effect) the need for new test crosses.

CXB mice. This set of 11 RI strains was created from BALB/c and C57BL/6 progenitors, and contains seven RI strains and two reciprocal F_1 hybrids in addition to the original parent strains. One of the RI strains, CXBK, was found to display an abnormally low responsiveness to morphine compared to its sibling strains (Baran et al. 1975); this characteristic was later described as specific to μ_1-opioid-receptor binding relative to other opioid-binding sites (Moskowitz and Goodman 1985). CXBK mice have been used as a model of μ_1-opioid-receptor deficiency in a large number of studies of opioid-mediated effects, such as morphine hyperlocomotion (Moskowitz et al. 1985a), opioid footshock SIA (Moskowitz et al. 1985b), opioid swim SIA (Marek et al. 1988), and acupuncture analgesia (Peets and Pomeranz 1978).

BXD mice. The BXD set comprises 30 strains resulting from a cross of C57BL/6 and DBA/2 mice. This cross is particularly advantageous because the parent strains are divergent on a number of pain-relevant traits, as noted above. BXD mice have been extensively used to map QTLs for various drug effects (see Crabbe et al. 1994). Using this resource as a starting point, we found a QTL on proximal chromosome 10 that accounts for 28–33% of the variance in systemic morphine analgesic sensitivity (Belknap and Crabbe 1992; Belknap et al. 1995). The μ-opioid receptor gene, *Oprm*, is located within this region (Kozak et al. 1994) and is a strong candidate for the QTL. Another QTL for morphine analgesia using BXD mice was found on chromosome 9 (Belknap and Crabbe 1992); we have provided compelling pharmacological evidence that the gene in question may be *Htr1b*, which codes for the serotonin-1B receptor subtype (Hain et al. 1999). Finally, we used BXD mice to identify an apparently male-specific QTL mediating hot-plate nociception; concurrently obtained pharmacological evidence suggests that the gene in question may be *Oprd1*, coding for the δ_2-opioid receptor (Mogil et al. 1997). In what may be the first successful translation of a pain genetics finding from mouse to human, Kim and colleagues from the National Institute of Dental and Craniofacial Research reported preliminary data in humans (at the 2002 Society for Neuroscience annual meeting in San Diego, California) showing an association, in males only, between a DNA variant of the human *OPRD1* gene and thermal pain sensitivity.

SPONTANEOUS MUTANTS

In large, homogenous populations of inbred mice, such as those maintained by commercial suppliers, mutations are occasionally identified by observing pigmentation or behavioral anomalies in an animal that should appear identical to its cagemates. Many of these mutations have been maintained, bred true, and are commercially available. Some of these mutants have been observed to display altered phenotypes on pain-relevant traits compared to their background strain. The *sepia* and *gunmetal* mutants were reported to be more sensitive to morphine analgesia (Shuster 1989), for example. *Beige*-J mice (C57BL/6J-bg^J) exhibit less opioid analgesia (Mathiasen et al. 1987; Muraki et al. 1991), possibly due to an abnormal circulating splenic factor (Raffa et al. 1988). Our laboratory is currently investigating the properties of recessive yellow (C57BL/6-$Mc1r^{e/e}$) mice, which display a null mutation of the gene encoding the melanocortin-1 receptor, based on the hypothesis that this receptor may play a sex-specific role in the modulation of κ-opioid analgesia.

TARGETED MUTATIONS

Detecting spontaneous mutations is little more than a matter of luck, and so researchers have developed several methods to produce mutant models on a more reliable timetable. Mutagenesis is one procedure useful for creating mutations de novo; radiation or chemical agents are used to induce random base pair changes in the DNA sequence, and the resultant offspring are carefully screened for signs of novel phenotypic features. While this method has proved quite valuable in *Drosophila*, it is extraordinarily time-consuming and expensive in mammals used in pain research. Nonetheless, at least two large mutagenesis screens are underway that will be screening for alterations in nociceptive sensitivity (Hrabe de Angelis et al. 2000; Nolan et al. 2000), although no published reports have claimed success in producing mutants with pain-related phenotypes.

Advances in molecular biology have facilitated the manipulation of individual genes. It is now possible to introduce new genes into the genome of a living embryo, as well as to delete endogenous genes. Such "transgenic" studies have already identified a large number of genes as "pain genes" (for review see Mogil and Grisel 1998; Mogil et al. 2000).

Transgenesis. The term "transgenesis" commonly refers to the addition of an exogenous gene into the DNA sequence, although it more properly designates any alteration of the genome. The addition of a gene involves injecting a vector containing the desired DNA sequence into a fertilized embryo. In about 20% of cells so treated (Capecchi 1980), the exogenous gene will randomly insert itself into the host DNA, along with the regulatory sites included on the vector. Mice homozygous for the transgene can then be produced by screening for the added allele and mating affected individuals. However, the number of insertion sites can vary from one to hundreds, and a vector may disrupt other genes by inserting itself inside a coding region.

Knockout mice. Rather than inserting functional genetic material, the vector used in creating "knockout" mice is designed to interfere with an endogenous gene, thereby eliminating its expression. The insertion may replace essential coding regions, cause a frameshift error, or interject a premature stop codon. Complete inactivation of the gene is usually the goal, although other mutational effects can be created as well (Rubinstein et al. 1993; Bronson and Smithies 1994). Genes that are critical for proper development of the animal are not suitable for deletion studies, but most genes involved in pain are not quite so vital to survival. The advantage of the knockout mouse over more conventional pharmacological techniques is that eliminating a protein (such as a receptor or enzyme) is far more selective than merely inhibiting its action with drugs. It is not always simple to interpret the results of knockout studies, however (see Crusio 1996; Gerlai 1996; Lariviere et al. 2001). The genome of complex mammals contains a great amount of redundancy, and other genes may compensate for the deficiency. This redundancy may dilute or mask the effect of knockouts, such as in the β-endorphin knockout mouse, where the non-opioid SIA system upregulates to counter the lack of opioid SIA (Rubinstein et al. 1996). Pleiotropic properties of the inactivated gene can also complicate interpretation; a gene deficiency can interfere unexpectedly with other traits that can influence nociceptive behavior, such as locomotor activity or emotionality.

GENETICS AND PEDIATRIC PAIN

Allelic variants are known or suspected to underlie a number of human pathological states, but the contribution of heritable factors to susceptibility is as yet undetermined for most diseases. Although we currently know very little about the role that genetics plays in many disease etiologies, powerful associative techniques combined with increasingly dense genomic maps and high-throughput genotyping have opened a new era in medical genetics. We will limit the discussion below to genetic diseases featuring pain and a pediatric onset. All relevant cases are caused by single-gene mutations; perhaps in the near future this topic will also include more subtle developmental or multi-gene effects that increase susceptibility or exacerbate symptoms.

The investigation of a suspected genetic disease follows an orderly course. Genetic diseases are most readily identified by family or population studies. Family studies are used to establish patterns of heritability, while population studies are useful to determine the prevalence of pathogenic alleles within an interrelated or heterogeneous group. Once the heritability of a trait or disorder is verified using twin studies, linkage analysis and positional cloning can localize the responsible gene to increasingly specific chromosome regions until its identity is confirmed. The location of the base pair substitutions that constitute the "mutation" may be within exons, resulting in amino acid changes in the final protein product or the insertion of a premature stop codon, but they may also be found in introns or regulatory regions thousands of base pairs distant from the coding regions. Such changes in transcriptional regulation are potentially as devastating as protein structural changes; they may cause gene overexpression, or may result in the loss of expression of the gene altogether. Because a mutant gene may include several different allelic polymorphisms representing numerous mutation sites in different subjects, haplotype analysis is performed to correlate disease states with defined DNA sequences.

FAMILIAL MEDITERRANEAN FEVER

Familial Mediterranean fever (FMF) is a heritable disease with onset during childhood. As the name denotes, FMF occurs most frequently in populations of eastern Mediterranean descent, specifically Arabs, non-Ashkenazi Jews, Armenians, and Turks (Sohar et al. 1967; Khachadurian and Armenian 1974). It is the most common and best understood of the hereditary fever syndromes (Samuels et al. 1998), and allelic frequencies for the disease can be very high in these groups. A population study in Jordan found 192 cases of pediatric FMF in a total population of 494,000 children, which indicates a homozygote frequency of about 1:2600, and an allele frequency of about 1:50 (Rawashdeh and Majeed 1996). Similar studies have estimated the carrier frequency to be between 1:5 and 1:16 among Sephardic Jews (Daniels et al. 1995; Yuval et al. 1995), and 1:7 among Armenian-Americans (Rogers et al. 1989).

Heller (1958) described the symptoms of FMF in 1958; these include acute attacks of chest and abdominal pain, fever, and inflammation, as well as arthritis, splenomegaly, hepatomegaly, pleurisy, and amyloidosis. An attack can last from 12 to 72 hours and recur at variable intervals. The age of onset is usually before 16 years, and can be as early as 4 months. Early investigations recognized the familial pattern of the disease and established an autosomal recessive mode of inheritance. The fact that the disease displays full concordance in monozygotic twins implies that a single gene is responsible for the phenotype (Shohat et al. 1992).

The search for this gene (see Kastner 1998) required positional cloning, a difficult and tedious process, especially before the completion of the Human Genome Project. The nature of the disease led early researchers to believe that the relevant gene must encode a protein involved in regulating inflammation. This approach is limited, however, by the fact that inflammatory effects are often secondary products of a genetic malfunction, not directly linked to the gene itself. Positional cloning conveys the advantage of being hypothesis-neutral, able to find the gene regardless of the nature of the protein it produces. Researchers at the U.S. National Institutes of Health (NIH), using a panel of affected non-Ashkenazi Jewish families, found a linkage to a region on the short arm of chromosome 16 (Pras et al. 1992). In 1997 this group (International FMF Consortium 1997) and a French team (French FMF Consortium 1997) simultaneously discovered the *MEFV* gene, a 115-kb sequence containing 10 exons. These groups found several mutations in this gene, all of which were simple missense mutations resulting in an amino acid substitution. The *MEFV* gene product was termed pyrin by the NIH group, for its pro-inflammatory actions, and marenostrin by the

French group. Although its exact pathogenic mechanism is unknown, it may mediate the actions of neutrophils, which are commonly recruited during inflammation. Other researchers have postulated that pyrin/marenostrin is a transcription factor involved in regulating other inflammatory molecules (Babior and Matzner 1997).

JUVENILE PRIMARY FIBROMYALGIA AND CHRONIC FATIGUE SYNDROME

Fibromyalgia and chronic fatigue syndrome (CFS) are both disorders involving generalized pain and weariness. Both occur in children, and it has been hypothesized that they are alternative diagnoses of the same underlying pathology because a significant portion of CFS patients meet the criteria for fibromyalgia as well (Bell et al. 1994; Buchwald 1994). Researchers have found familial links among patients with the two diseases. In one small study, about half of the children with both fibromyalgia and CFS had a family member with CFS, while 42% of the children with only CFS had a family member with the same disease (Bell et al. 1994). In another study of 34 children with fibromyalgia, 71% had a mother with fibromyalgia (Roizenblatt et al. 1997).

The etiology of both diseases is unknown, and we lack conclusive proof that they are genetic in nature. However, evidence is mounting that implicates immunological or serotonergic mechanisms. Two genetic predictors have been linked to CFS: the presence of chronic fatigue in another family member, and a history of allergies or asthma, which could indicate a genetic immune dysfunction (Bell et al. 1991). Pellagrino and colleagues (1989) analyzed the frequency of fibromyalgia in close relatives of 17 current fibromyalgia patients; over half (52%) of the relatives also exhibited symptoms of the disease, indicating an autosomal dominant mode of inheritance. These researchers found an especially high incidence of fibromyalgia in females, suggesting an unknown sex-specific factor. Familial aggregation was also observed in two subsequent studies, one confirming an autosomal dominant pattern (Stormorken and Brosstad 1992), and the other suggesting the influence of polygenic factors (Yunus et al. 1995). Buskila et al. (1996) found a 1:1 male female ratio among the youngest fibromyalgia cohort, this ratio shifting heavily toward the females in later age groups. They conjectured that a major gene with a possible autosomal dominant pattern underlies the disease, but that in males it exhibits a lower penetrance or milder expressivity due to unknown age-related factors (Buskila et al. 1996).

Several groups have attempted to identify fibromyalgia-related genes using associative techniques. Fibromyalgia has been linked with the human lymphocyte antigen (HLA) locus (Burda et al. 1986), and Yunus and colleagues (1999) hypothesized that a gene located in or near the HLA region contributes to the disease. Serotonergic mechanisms may be at work in fibromyalgia, because abnormal serotonin (5-HT) activity has been noted in patients (Russell et al. 1992; Wolfe et al. 1997), and 5-HT reuptake inhibitors can be effective in the treatment of chronic pain (Jung et al. 1997). The 5-HT transporter is encoded by a gene (SLC6A4) located on chromosome 17q12; a 44-base pair deletion in the promotor region of this gene reduces transcriptional efficiency. This mutation has been linked to fibromyalgia; compared to normal controls, a higher proportion of fibromyalgia patients are homozygous for the short allele (Offenbaecher et al. 1999). Another possible factor may be linked to the 5–HT_A receptor gene; a silent polymorphism of this gene, while not itself responsible for changes in protein structure, may be in linkage disequilibrium with the actual functional variant (Bondy et al. 1999).

THE FUTURE OF PAIN GENETICS

We stand at the verge of major breakthroughs in the field of pain genetics. It will not be long before all the genetic "players" in pain are known, although it will of course take far longer to gain a deep understanding of their function and interactions. Single-gene diseases have already yielded to genetic dissection, and may be amenable to gene therapy in the near future. More complex pain traits will take longer, but animal studies provide theoretically unlimited statistical power toward gene identification. Once the genes predisposing to pain sensitivity and chronic pain susceptibility are known, the important work of determining their interaction with environmental factors can begin. Eventually, we will understand the causes of variability in pain-related traits, and use this knowledge to improve therapy for children and adults alike.

ACKNOWLEDGMENTS

This work is supported by NIH grants DA15191 and DE12735 to J.S. Mogil.

REFERENCES

Babior BM, Matzner Y. The familial Mediterranean fever gene—cloned at last. *N Engl J Med* 1997; 337:1548–1549.

Baran A, Shuster L, Eleftheriou BE, Bailey DW. Opiate receptors in mice: genetic differences. *Life Sci* 1975; 17:633–640.

Belfer I, Davidson E, Ratner A, et al. Dietary supplementation with the inhibitory amino acid taurine suppresses autotomy in HA rats. *Neuroreport* 1998; 9:3103–3107.

Belknap JK, Crabbe JC. Chromosome mapping of gene loci affecting morphine and amphetamine responses in BXD recombinant inbred mice. *Ann NY Acad Sci* 1992; 654:311–323.

Belknap JK, Laursen SE. DSLET (D-Ser^2-Leu^5-Enkephalin-Thr^6) produces analgesia on the hot plate by mechanisms largely different from DAGO and morphine-like opioids. *Life Sci* 1987; 41:391–395.

Belknap JK, O'Toole LA. Studies of genetic differences in response to opioid drugs. In: Harris RA, Crabbe JC (Eds). *The Genetic Basis of Alcohol and Drug Actions*. New York: Plenum Press, 1991, pp 225–252.

Belknap JK, Haltli NR, Goebel DM, Lamé M. Selective breeding for high and low levels of opiate-induced analgesia in mice. *Behav Genet* 1983; 13:383–396.

Belknap JK, Danielson PW, Laursen SE, Noordewier B. Selective breeding for levorphanol-induced antinociception on the hot-plate assay: commonalities in mechanism of action with morphine, pentazocine, ethylketocyclazocine, U-50488H and clonidine in mice. *J Pharmacol Exp Ther* 1987; 241:477–481.

Belknap JK, Mogil JS, Helms ML, et al. Localization to proximal Chromosome 10 of a locus influencing morphine-induced analgesia in crosses derived from C57BL/6 and DBA/2 mouse strains. *Life Sci* 1995; 57:PL117–124.

Bell DS, Bell KM, Cheney PR. Primary juvenile fibromyalgia syndrome and chronic fatigue syndrome in adolescents. *Clin Infect Dis* 1994; 18:S21–S23.

Bell KM, Cookfair D, Bell DS, et al. Risk factors associated with chronic fatigue syndrome in a cluster of pediatric cases. *Rev Infect Dis* 1991; 13:213–223.

Bellamy N. Variance in NSAID studies: contribution of patient variance. *Agents Actions Suppl* 1985; 17:21–28.

Bengtsson B, Thorson J. Back pain: a study of twins. *Acta Genet Med Gemellol (Roma)* 1991; 40:83–90.

Bondy B, Spaeth M, Offenbaecher M, et al. The T102C polymorphism of the 5-HT2A-receptor gene in fibromyalgia. *Neurobiol Dis* 1999; 6:433–439.

Bonica JJ. Causalgia and other reflex sympathetic dystrophies. In: Bonica JJ (Ed). *The Management of Pain,* 2nd ed. Philadelphia: Lea and Febiger, 1990.

Brennum J, Kjeldsen M, Jensen K, Jensen TS. Measurements of human pressure-pain thresholds on fingers and toes. *Pain* 1989; 38:211–217.

Bronson SK, Smithies O. Altering mice by homologous recombination using embryonic stem cells. *J Biol Chem* 1994; 269:27155–27158.

Buchsbaum MS, Davis GC, Coppola R, Naber D. Opiate pharmacology and individual differences. I. Psychophysical pain measurements. *Pain* 1981; 10:357–366.

Buchwald D. Comparison of patients with chronic fatigue syndrome, fibromyalgia, and multiple chemical sensitivities. *Arch Intern Med* 1994; 154:2049–2053.

Burda CD, Cox FR, Osborne P. Histocompatability antigens in the fibrositis (fibromyalgia) syndrome. *Clin Exp Rheumatol* 1986; 4:355–357.

Buskila D, Neumann L, Hazanov I, Carmi R. Familial aggregation in the fibromyalgia syndrome. *Semin Arthritis Rheum* 1996; 26:605–611.

Capecchi MR. High efficiency transformation of DNA into cultured mammalian cells. *Cell* 1980; 244:1288–1292.

Chapman CR, Hill HF, Saeger L, Gavrin J. Profiles of opioid analgesia in humans after intravenous bolus administration: alfentanil, fentanyl and morphine compared on experimental pain. *Pain* 1990; 43:47–55.

Chapman WP, Jones CM. Variations in cutaneous and visceral pain sensitivity in normal subjects. *J Clin Invest* 1944; 23:81–91.

Chen ACN, Dworkin SF, Haug J. Human pain responsivity in a tonic pain model: psychological determinants. *Pain* 1989; 37:143–160.

Clark FM, Proudfit HK. Anatomical evidence for genetic differences in the innervation of the rat spinal cord by noradrenergic locus coeruleus neurons. *Brain Res* 1992; 591:44–53.

Clark JW, Bindra D. Individual differences in pain thresholds. *Can J Psychol* 1956; 10:69–76.

Cohn S, Seltzer Z. Inherited propensity for neuropathic pain is mediated by sensitivity to injury discharge. *Neuroreport* 1991; 2:647–650.

Collins FS. Positional cloning moves from perditional to traditional. *Nat Genet* 1997; 9:347–350.

Copeland NG, Jenkins NA, Gilbert DJ, et al. A genetic linkage map of the mouse: current applications and future prospects. *Science* 1993; 262:57–66.

Crabbe JC, Belknap JK, Buck KJ. Genetic animal models of alcohol and drug abuse. *Science* 1994; 264:1715–1723.

Crusio WE. Gene-targeting studies: new methods, old problems. *Trends Neurol Sci* 1996; 19:186–187.

Daniels M, Shohat T, Brenner-Ullman A, Shohat M. Familial Mediterranean fever: high gene frequency among the non-Ashkenazic and Ashkenazic Jewish populations in Israel. *Am J Med Genet* 1995; 55:311–314.

Day RO. Variability in response to NSAIDs: what progress? *Agents Actions Suppl* 1993; 44:3–6.

Dearborn GVN. A case of congenital pure analgesia. *J Nerv Ment Dis* 1932; 75:612–615.

Devor M, Raber P. Heritability of symptoms in an experimental model of neuropathic pain. *Pain* 1990; 42:51–67.

Elmer GI, Pieper JO, Negus SS, Woods JH. Genetic variance in nociception and its relationship to the potency of morphine-induced analgesia in thermal and chemical tests. *Pain* 1997; 75:129–140.

French FMF Consortium. A candidate gene for familial Mediterranean fever. *Nat Genet* 1997; 17:25–31.

Frischknecht H-R, Siegfried B, Waser PG. Opioids and behavior: genetic aspects. *Experientia* 1988; 44:473–481.

Galer BS, Coyle N, Pasternak GW, Portenoy RK. Individual variability in the response to different opioids: report of five cases. *Pain* 1992; 49:87–91.

Gerlai R. Gene-targeting studies of mammalian behavior: is it the mutation or the background genotype? *Trends Neurol Sci* 1996; 19:177–181.

Gonzales FJ, Skoda RC, Kimura S, et al. Characterization of the common genetic defect in humans deficient in debrisoquine metabolism. *Nature* 1988; 331:442–446.

Hain HS, Belknap JK, Mogil JS. Pharmacogenetic evidence for the involvement of 5-hydroxytryptamine (serotonin)-1B receptors in the mediation of morphine antinociceptive sensitivity. *J Pharmacol Exp Ther* 1999; 291:444–449.

Hakim AJ, Cherkas L, El Zayat S, et al. The genetic contribution to carpal tunnel syndrome in women: a twin study. *Arthritis Rheum* 2002; 47:275–279.

Heikkila JK, Koskenvuo M, Heliovaara M, et al. Genetic and environmental factors in sciatica: evidence from a nationwide panel of 9365 adult twin pairs. *Ann Med* 1989; 21:393–398.

Heller H, Sohar E, Sherf L. Familial Mediterranean fever. *Arch Intern Med* 1958; 102:50–56.

Honkasalo M-L, Kaprio J, Winter T, et al. Migraine and concomitant symptoms among 8167 adult twin pairs. *Headache* 1995; 35:70–78.

Hrabe de Angelis M, Flaswinkel H, Fuchs H, et al. Genome-wide, large-scale production of mutant mice by ENU mutagenesis. *Nature* 2000; 25:444–447.

IASP Subcommittee on Taxonomy. Pain terms: a list with definitions and notes on usage. *Pain* 1979; 6:249.

Indo Y, Tsurata Y, Karim MA, et al. Mutations in the TRKA/NGF receptor gene in patients with congenital insensitivity to pain with anhidrosis. *Nat Genet* 1996; 13:485–488.

International FMF Consortium. Ancient missense mutations in a new member of the *RoRet* gene family are likely to cause familial Mediterranean fever. *Cell* 1997; 90:797–807.

Isselee H, De Laat A, Lesaffre E, Lysens R. Short-term reproducibility of pressure pain thresholds in masseter and temporalis muscles of symptom-free subjects. *Eur J Oral Sci* 1997; 105:583–587.

Jacobs JWG, Geenan R, van der Heide A, et al. Are tender point scores assessed by manual palpation in fibromyalgia reliable? *Scand J Rheumatol* 1995; 24:243–247.

Jensen TS, Krebs B, Nielsen J, Rasmussen P. Immediate and long-term phantom limb pain in amputees: incidence, clinical characteristics and relationship to pre-amputation limb pain. *Pain* 1985; 21:267–278.

Joutel A, Bousser M-G, Biousse V, et al. A gene for familial hemiplegic migraine maps to chromosome 19. *Nat Genet* 1993; 5:40–45.

Jung AC, Staiger T, Sullivan M. The efficacy of selective serotonin reuptake inhibitors for the management of chronic pain. *J Gen Intern Med* 1997; 12:384–389.

Kastner DL. Familial Mediterranean fever: the genetics of inflammation. *Hosp Pract* 1998; April 15:131–158.

Kest B, Mogil JS, Sternberg WF, et al. Evidence for the up-regulation of kappa opiate mechanisms in mice selectively bred for high analgesia. *Proc West Pharmacol Soc* 1993; 36:249–253.

Kest B, Wilson SG, Mogil JS. Sex differences in supraspinal morphine analgesia are dependent on genotype. *J Pharmacol Exp Ther* 1999; 289:1370–1375.

Khachadurian AK, Armenian HK. Familial paroxysmal polyserositis (familial Mediterranean fever). Incidence of amyloidosis and mode of inheritance. *Birth Defects* 1974; 10:62–64.

Kozak CA, Filie J, Adamson MC, et al. Murine chromosomal location of the μ and κ opioid receptor genes. *Genomics* 1994; 21:659–661.

Kraus RL, Sinneger MJ, Glossmann H, et al. Familial hemiplegic migraine mutations change α_{1A} Ca^{2+} channel kinetics. *J Biol Chem* 1998; 273:5586–5590.

Lander ES, Schork NJ. Genetic dissection of complex traits. *Science* 1994; 265:2037–2048.

Lanier LH. Variability in the pain threshold. *Science* 1943; 97:49–50.

Lariviere WR, Chesler EJ, Mogil JS. Transgenic studies of pain and analgesia: mutation or background phenotype? *J Pharmacol Exp Ther* 2001; 297:467–473.

Lariviere WR, Wilson SG, Laughlin TM, et al. Heritability of nociception. III. Genetic relationships among commonly used assays of nociception and hypersensitivity. *Pain* 2002; 97:75–86.

Larsson B, Bille B, Pedersen NL. Genetic influence in headaches: a Swedish twin study. *Headache* 1995; 35:513–519.

Lasagna L, Beecher HK. The optimal dose of morphine. *JAMA* 1954; 156:230–234.

Levine JD, Gordon NC, Smith R, Fields HL. Analgesic responses to morphine and placebo in individuals with postoperative pain. *Pain* 1981; 10:379–389.

Libman E. Observations on individual sensitiveness to pain. *JAMA* 1934; 102:335–341.

Liu C-N, Raber P, Ziv-Sefer S, Devor M. Hyperexcitability in sensory neurons of rats selected for high versus low neuropathic pain phenotype. *Neuroscience* 2001; 105:265–275.

Maier C, Hildebrandt J, Klinger R, et al. Morphine responsiveness, efficacy and tolerability in patients with chronic non-tumor associated pain—results of a double-blind placebo-controlled trial (MONTAS). *Pain* 2002; 97:223–233.

Marek P, Panocka I, Sadowski B. Selective breeding of mice for high and low swim analgesia: differential effect on discrete forms of footshock analgesia. *Pain* 1987; 29:393–396.

Marek P, Yirmiya R, Liebeskind JC. Strain differences in the magnitude of stress-induced analgesia correlate with brain opiate receptor concentration. *Brain Res* 1988; 447:188–190.

Martin N, Boomsma D, Machin G. A twin-pronged attack on complex traits. *Nat Genet* 1997; 17:387–392.

Mathiasen JR, Raffa RB, Vaught JL. C57BL/6J-bgJ (Beige) mice: differential sensitivity in the tail flick test to centrally administered mu- and delta-opioid receptor agonists. *Life Sci* 1987; 40:1989–1994.

Michalowicz BS, Pihlstrom BL, Hodges JS, Bouchard TJ Jr. No heritability of temporomandibular joint signs and symptoms. *J Dent Res* 2000; 79:1573–1578.

Mogil JS. The genetic mediation of individual differences in sensitivity to pain and its inhibition. *Proc Natl Acad Sci USA* 1999; 96:7744–7751.

Mogil JS, Belknap JK. Sex and genotype determine the selective activation of neurochemically-distinct mechanisms of swim stress-induced analgesia. *Pharmacol Biochem Behav* 1997; 56:61–66.

Mogil JS, McCarson KE. Finding pain genes: bottom-up and top-down approaches. *J Pain* 2000; 1(Suppl 1):66–80.

Mogil JS, Marek P, Yirmiya R, et al. Antagonism of the non-opioid component of ethanol-induced analgesia by the NMDA receptor antagonist MK-801. *Brain Res* 1993; 602:126–130.

Mogil JS, Kest B, Sadowski B, Belknap JK. Differential genetic mediation of sensitivity to morphine in genetic models of opiate antinociception: influence of nociceptive assay. *J Pharmacol Exp Ther* 1996a; 276:532–544.

Mogil JS, Sternberg WF, Marek P, et al. The genetics of pain and pain inhibition. *Proc Natl Acad Sci USA* 1996b; 93:3048–3055.

Mogil JS, Richards SP, O'Toole LA, et al. Genetic sensitivity to hot-plate nociception in DBA/2J and C57BL/6J inbred mouse strains: possible sex-specific mediation by δ_2-opioid receptors. *Pain* 1997; 70:267–277.

Mogil JS, Grisel JE. Transgenic studies of pain. *Pain* 1998; 77:107–128.

Mogil JS, Wilson SG, Bon K, et al. Heritability of nociception. I. Responses of eleven inbred mouse strains on twelve measures of nociception. *Pain* 1999a; 80:67–82.

Mogil JS, Wilson SG, Bon K, et al. Heritability of nociception. II. "Types" of nociception revealed by genetic correlation analysis. *Pain* 1999b; 80:83–93.

Mogil JS, Yu L, Basbaum AI. Pain genes?: natural variation and transgenic mutants. *Annu Rev Neurosci* 2000; 23:777–811.

Moskowitz AS, Goodman RR. Autoradiographic analysis of mu_1, mu_2, and delta opioid binding in the central nervous system of C57BL/6BY and CXBK (opioid receptor-deficient) mice. *Brain Res* 1985; 360:108–116.

Moskowitz AS, Terman GW, Carter KR, et al. Analgesic, locomotor and lethal effects of morphine in the mouse: strain comparisons. *Brain Res* 1985a; 361:46–51.

Moskowitz AS, Terman GW, Liebeskind JC. Stress-induced analgesia in the mouse: strain comparisons. *Pain* 1985b; 23:67–72.

Muraki T, Oike N, Shibata Y, Nomoto T. Analgesic effect of μ- and κ-opioid agonists in beige and CXBK mice. *J Pharm Pharmacol* 1991; 43:210–212.

Nolan PM, Peters J, Strivens M, et al. A systematic, genome-wide, phenotype-driven mutagenesis programme for gene function studies in the mouse. *Nature* 2000; 25:440–443.

Offenbaecher M, Bondy B, de Jonge S, et al. Possible association of fibromyalgia with a polymorphism in the serotonin transporter gene regulatory region. *Arthritis Rheum* 1999; 42:2482–2488.

Ophoff RA, Terwindt GM, Vergouwe MN, et al. Familial hemiplegic migraine and episodic ataxia type-2 are caused by mutations in the Ca^{2+} channel gene CACNL1A4. *Cell* 1996; 87:543–552.

Panocka I, Marek P. Inheritance of stress-induced analgesia in mice. *Ann NY Acad Sci* 1986; 467:441–443.

Panocka I, Sadowski B. Correlation between magnitude and opioid mediation of stress-induced analgesia: individual differences and the effect of selective breeding. *Acta Neurobiol Exp* 1990; 50:535–548.

Panocka I, Marek P, Sadowski B. Differentiation of neurochemical basis of stress-induced analgesia in mice by selective breeding. *Brain Res* 1986a; 397:156–160.

Panocka I, Marek P, Sadowski B. Inheritance of stress-induced analgesia in mice: selective breeding study. *Brain Res* 1986b; 397:152–155.

Peets JM, Pomeranz B. CXBK mice deficient in opiate receptors show poor electroacupuncture analgesia. *Nature* 1978; 273:675–676.

Pellagrino MJ, Waylonis GW, Sommer A. Familial occurrence of primary fibromyalgia. *Arch Phys Med Rehabil* 1989; 70:61–63.

Pras E, Aksentijevich I, Gruberg L, et al. Mapping of a gene causing familial Mediterranean fever to the short arm of chromosome 16. *N Engl J Med* 1992; 326:1509–1513.

Raber P, Devor M. Social variables affect phenotype in the neuroma model of neuropathic pain. *Pain* 2002; 97:139–150.

Rady JJ, Roerig SC, Fujimoto JM. Heroin acts on different opioid receptors than morphine in Swiss Webster and ICR mice to produce antinociception. *J Pharmacol Exp Ther* 1991; 256:448–457.

Rady JJ, Elmer GI, Fujimoto JM. Opioid receptor selectivity of heroin given intracerebroventricularly differs in six strains of inbred mice. *J Pharmacol Exp Ther* 1998; 288:438–445.

Raffa RB, Kimball ES, Mathiasen JR. The analgesic defect of C57BL/6J-bgJ/bgJ (beige-J; Chediak-Higashi syndrome) mice transmitted by adoptive transfer of spleen cells to normal littermates. *Life Sci* 1988; 42:1231–1236.

Raphael KG, Marbach JJ, Gallagher RM, Dohrenwend BP. Myofascial TMD does not run in families. *Pain* 1999; 80:15–22.

Rawashdeh MO, Majeed HA. Familial Mediterranean fever in Arab children: the high prevalence and gene frequency. *Eur J Pediatr* 1996; 155:540–544.

Richards RL. Causalgia: a centennial review. *Arch Neurol* 1967; 16:339–350.

Risch N, Merikangas K. The future of genetic studies of complex human diseases. *Science* 1996; 273:1516–1517.

Rogers DB, Shohat M, Petersen GM, et al. Familial Mediterranean fever in Armenians: autosomal recessive inheritance with high gene frequency. *Am J Med Genet* 1989; 34:168–172.

Roizenblatt S, Tufik S, Goldenberg J, et al. Juvenile fibromyalgia: clinical and polysomnographic aspects. *J Rheumatol* 1997; 24:579–585.

Rubinstein M, Japon M, Low MJ. Introduction of a point mutation into the mouse genome by homologous recombination in embryonic stem cells using a replacement type vector with a selectable marker. *Nucleic Acids Res* 1993; 21:2613–2617.

Rubinstein M, Mogil JS, Japon M, et al. Absence of opioid stress-induced analgesia in mice lacking β-endorphin by site-directed mutagenesis. *Proc Natl Acad Sci USA* 1996; 93:3995–4000.

Russell IJ, Vaeroy H, Javors M, Nyberg F. Cerebrospinal fluid biogenic amine metabolites in fibromyalgia/fibrositis syndrome and rheumatoid arthritis. *Arthritis Rheum* 1992; 35:550–556.

Samuels J, Aksentijevich I, Torosyan Y, et al. Familial Mediterranean fever at the millenium: clinical spectrum, ancient mutations, and a survey of 100 American referrals to the National Institutes of Health. *Medicine* 1998; 77:268–297.

Sherman ED. Sensitivity to pain. *CMAJ* 1943; 45:437–441.

Shir Y, Raber P, Devor M, Seltzer Z. Mechano- and thermo-sensitivity in rats genetically prone to developing neuropathic pain. *Neuroreport* 1991; 2:313–316.

Shir Y, Zeltser R, Vatine J-J, et al. Correlation of intact sensibility and neuropathic pain-related behaviors in eight inbred and outbred rat strains and selection lines. *Pain* 2001; 90:75–82.

Shohat M, Livneh A, Zemer D, et al. Twin studies in familial Mediterranean fever. *Am J Med Genet* 1992; 44:179–182.

Shuster L. Pharmacogenetics of drugs of abuse. *Ann NY Acad Sci* 1989; 562:56–73.

Sindrup SH, Brosen K. The pharmacogenetics of codeine hypoalgesia. *Pharmacogenetics* 1995; 5:335–346.

Sindrup SH, Poulsen L, Brosen K, et al. Are poor metabolisers of sparteine/debrisoquine less pain tolerant than extensive metabolisers? *Pain* 1993; 53:335–349.

Sohar E, Gafni J, Pras M, Heller H. Familial Mediterranean fever. A survey of 470 cases and review of literature. *Am J Med Gen* 1967; 44:179–182.

Soller M, Brody T, Genizi A. On the power of experimental designs for the detection of linkage between marker loci and quantitative loci in crosses between inbred lines. *Theor Appl Genet* 1976; 47:35–39.

Stormorken H, Brosstad F. Fibromyalgia: family clustering and sensory urgency with early onset indicate genetic predisposition and thus a "true" disease. *Scand J Rheumatol* 1992; 21:207.

Thrush DC. Congenital insensitivity to pain: a clinical, genetic and neurophysiological study of four children from the same family. *Brain* 1973; 96:369–386.

Treloar SA, Martin NG, Heath AC. Longitudinal genetic analysis of menstrual flow, pain, and limitation in a sample of Australian twins. *Behav Genet* 1998; 28:107–116.

Urca G, Segev S, Sarne Y. Footshock-induced analgesia: its opioid nature depends on the strain of rat. *Brain Res* 1985; 329:109–116.

Walker JS, Nguyen TV, Day RO. Clinical response to non-steroidal anti-inflammatory drugs in urate-crystal induced inflammation: a simultaneous study of intersubject and intrasubject variability. *Br J Clin Pharm* 1994; 38:341–347.

Walker JS, Sheather-Reid RB, Carmody JJ, et al. Nonsteroidal antiinflammatory drugs in rheumatoid arthritis and osteoarthritis. *Arthritis Rheum* 1997; 40:1944–1954.

Wall PD, Devor M, Inbal R, et al. Autotomy following peripheral nerve lesions: experimental anaesthesia dolorosa. *Pain* 1979; 7:103–113.

Watson SJ, Akil H. Gene chips and arrays revealed: a primer on their power and their uses. *Biol Psychiatry* 1999; 45:533–543.

West WL, Yeomans DC, Proudfit HK. The function of noradrenergic neurons in mediating antinociception induced by electrical stimulation of the locus coeruleus in two different sources of Sprague-Dawley rats. *Brain Res* 1993; 626:127–135.

Wilson SG, Smith SB, Chesler EJ, et al. The heritability of antinociception: common pharmacogenetic mediation of five neurochemically distinct analgesics. *J Pharmacol Exp Ther* 2003; 304:547–549.

Wolfe F, Russell IJ, Vipraio G, et al. Serotonin levels, pain threshold, and fibromyalgia symptoms in the general population. *J Rheumatol* 1997; 24.

Wolff BB, Jarvik ME. Variations in cutaneous and deep somatic pain sensitivity. *Can J Psychol* 1963; 17:37–44.

Wolff BB, Jarvik ME. Relationship between superficial and deep somatic thresholds of pain with a note on handedness. *Am J Psychol* 1964; 77:589–599.

Wolff BB, Kantor TG, Jarvik ME, Laska E. Response of experimental pain to analgesic drugs. I. Morphine, aspirin, and placebo. *Clin Pharmacol Ther* 1965; 7:224–238.

Xiao H-S, Huang Q-H, Zhang F-X, et al. Identification of gene expression profile of dorsal root ganglion in the rat peripheral axotomy model of neuropathic pain. *Proc Natl Acad Sci USA* 2002; 99:8360–8365.

Yunus MB, Rawlings KK, Khan MA, et al. Genetic studies of multicase families with fibromyalgia syndrome (FMS) with HLA typing. *Arthritis Rheum* 1995; 38:S247.

Yunus MB, Khan MA, Rawlings KK, et al. Genetic linkage analysis of multicase families with fibromyalgia syndrome. *J Rheumatol* 1999; 26:408–412.

Yuval Y, Hemo-Zisser M, Zemer D, et al. Dominant inheritance in two families with familial Mediterranean fever (FMF). *Am J Med Genet* 1995; 57:973–977.

Ziegler DK, Hur Y-M, Bouchard Jr TJ, et al. Migraine in twins raised together and apart. *Headache* 1998; 38:417–422.

Correspondence to: Jeffrey S. Mogil, PhD, Department of Psychology, McGill University, 1205 Dr Penfield Avenue, Montreal, PQ, Canada H3A 1B1. Email: jeff@hebb.psych.mcgill.ca.

4

Social Development and Pain in Children

Carl L. von Baeyer and Lara J. Spagrud

Department of Psychology, University of Saskatchewan, Saskatoon, Saskatchewan, Canada

Pain, from birth onward, is a product of the interplay among biological maturation, experience with minor and major physical insults, and socially mediated learning of pain behavior. The interaction of maturation and experience produces dramatic changes from infancy through adolescence in the developing child's understanding, experience, and expression of pain. This chapter discusses healthy or normative child development as well as disordered development in children who are exposed to frequent or severe pain as a result of early illness, injury, or medical procedures.

In considering socio-emotional development from infancy through adolescence, we will relate pain to the following variables: attachment, temperament, socialization and social learning, emotion regulation, and the development of pain expression. We also will address the social consequences of early, prolonged, or frequent pain. Pain management for children is improved when it is based on a sound understanding of development. In a final section, we will give examples of clinical applications of this understanding. (One of the most significant aspects of social development, pain in the context of the family, is reviewed by Chambers in this volume.)

ATTACHMENT

Social living is fundamental to the human condition, and its complexity has played an important role in the development of higher brain functions, making possible abilities such as language. Thus, one would expect the social context to be important from the earliest moments of life. Babies are born with the capacity to learn, within hours or days of birth, to recognize and respond differentially to their primary caregiver, a phenomenon known as attachment.

Attachment behaviors are those that help to elicit the attention of and maintain proximity to the primary caregiver. Bowlby (1988) theorized that these innately organized behaviors intensify when a baby or child is under stress due to separation from the primary attachment figure, exposure to an unfamiliar person or situation, or physical distress such as hunger or pain. The common expressions of anticipatory distress and pain in young children (crying, clinging to the parent, and distressed facial expression) can be seen as having survival value in that they elicit protection by the parent. When the primary attachment relationship is disrupted, for example by prolonged separation or inconsistent parenting, then disordered attachment behaviors such as despair, withdrawal, anger, or disorganized responses to unfamiliar situations are seen in the child. The experience of hospitalization is often fraught with the stressors identified by Bowlby: separation, strangers, and physical distress.

Based on observation or ratings of children's behavior during separation from parents and encounters with strangers, children can be classified as having secure or insecure attachments (Ainsworth et al. 1978). A securely attached child is thought to have an internal representation or working model in which the caregiver is trusted to be available to provide help whenever needed—in other words, to be a secure base for the child's exploration of the world. The securely attached child expresses distress openly when faced with a stressor, and seeks proximity with the caregiver, but as the child grows older, he or she deals with mild threats independently and confidently. Insecure attachment is thought to have a number of forms, including anxious-ambivalent, anxious-avoidant, and disorganized types of attachment, which are associated with less adaptive reactions to stress and greater likelihood of maladjustment in later childhood and adulthood.

Attachment theory provokes important questions about pain in childhood, which we will discuss in the remainder of this section. First, what is the effect of painful experiences on attachment? It might be expected that long-term and/or severe pain would disrupt the formation of attachment in infants, with possible consequences in other domains of their social development. Second, what is the influence of a pre-existing secure versus insecure attachment on a child's reaction to pain? It might be expected that securely attached infants would express their distress more intensely or efficiently, resulting in quicker efforts to comfort the child by the caregiver, while insecurely attached infants would respond to pain in a less organized, less persistent way, resulting in suboptimal caregiving.

To date, little research has focused on attachment in relation to pain, although many studies have examined attachment in relation to prematurity, developmental delay, hospitalization, parental deprivation (as in studies of children raised in orphanages; Chisholm 1998), and problems in parental adjustment (e.g., Van Ijzendoorn et al. 1992). In general, an early secure attachment between child and parent leads to good outcomes for the child's social development. With a secure base, the child is able to explore the world and to cope with stress with gradually increasing independence. However, when a stressor such as chronic pain leads in the long term to repeated activation of the attachment-caregiving system in older children, it may be counter-productive, as parents' caregiving efforts discourage the child from coping independently with pain and instead reward dependency and disability. In other words, attachment behaviors such as crying, clinging, and protesting at separation, which are adaptive in infancy and in short-term illness, may be maladaptive in older children with chronic illness, who in many cases would fare better if they were encouraged to be as active and independent as possible. Marvin (1992) reported that in 17 out of 19 clinical cases, changing attachment patterns in families with a child with chronic pain was an important factor in the symptom-free status of the children 6 months after their treatment. Specifically, children in the treatment program were given privileges and responsibilities to encourage independence from their parents. Some researchers have suggested that the genesis of later somatization disorders derives from early attachment problems (Stuart and Noyes 1999). Grunau et al. (1994) described a follow-up study of children born extremely prematurely, who were therefore exposed to prolonged hospitalization and repeated medical procedures. These children at the age of 4 years had higher somatization scores, which was attributed in part to disruption of the parent-child relationship (see Grunau, this volume).

   In a recent study, Walsh and colleagues (in press) reviewed literature linking attachment and pain, and predicted significant concordance between reactions to separation from parents and reactions to anticipated painful events. They studied 60 children aged 4 and 5 years, obtaining verbal responses to pictures of separation incidents (the Separation Anxiety Test) and pain incidents (the Charleston Pediatric Pain Pictures, with parent figures added). As predicted, children classified as securely attached were better able to express vulnerability or need for support with respect to more severe pain incidents, as well as greater self-confidence about handling milder pain situations independently, than were children classified as having ambivalent or avoidant attachment. The results supported Bowlby's description of internal working models of attachment relationships, and were not accounted for by individual differences in receptive language ability, emotional awareness, or emotion regulation.

Beyond those mentioned above, few studies have directly tested predictions concerning pain based on attachment theory. One potential direction for future research would be to follow children whose attachment has been directly assessed as secure or nonsecure during their toddler years, in order to identify later differences in their reactions to everyday pain and to medical procedures.

Attachment, as shown above, refers to the relationship of the child and caregiver. Also of importance are individual difference variables thought to be largely innate. Of these, the most prominent influence on early social development is termed "temperament."

TEMPERAMENT

Temperament refers to stable individual differences in the quality and intensity of activity level, attention, and emotional reactivity. Many children have a temperament that is described as "easy," meaning that they are generally cheerful, adapt easily to new experiences, and establish regular routines. A minority of children who are described as having a "difficult" temperament, by contrast, tend to react warily and intensely to new experiences and to have irregular daily routines. Temperamental differences can be identified in early infancy and tend to persist, although they can be magnified or attenuated by parenting practices (Thomas and Chess 1977). Temperament plays an important role in determining a child's reaction to emotional and physical stressors, so one would expect temperament to affect both the experience and expression of pain (Schechter et al. 1991). A temperamental dimension of particular relevance to pain is termed "threshold," that is, the minimum intensity of a stimulus to which a child will typically react. Children who are described by their parents as typically reacting to low-threshold stimuli in general appear to be more sensitive to pain stimuli in particular (Lee and White-Traut 1996; Bournaki 1997).

Some researchers have used a standardized measure of temperament called the Behavioral Style Questionnaire (McDevitt and Carey 1978) to investigate the role of various dimensions of temperament in young children's responses to pain. This questionnaire consists of 100 items rated by parents that measure nine dimensions of temperament: activity, rhythmicity, approach, adaptability, intensity, mood, persistence, distractibility, and threshold. Schechter et al. (1991) correlated ratings on the Behavioral Style Questionnaire with observed distress during immunization injections in 65 children aged 4–5 years. These authors reported that children categorized as "difficult" based on the mother's temperament rating had distress scores two to three times the means of the children in the other temperament clusters. They suggested that preparation of children for painful procedures may need to be individualized based on temperamental characteristics.

There are consistent sex differences in temperament, with boys tending on average to be more active and daring and girls tending to be more anxious and timid from toddler age on. These differences in temperament, which cannot be explained by purely environmental factors, are reflected in boys' higher rates of accidental injury (e.g., Hedlund and Lindgren 1986) and in girls' higher rates of recurrent pain problems, which are presumed to be influenced by anxiety (e.g., Perquin et al. 2000). Boys who were stable in their temperamental aggressiveness across the 6- to 12-year age span have been reported to show lower pain sensitivity (Séguin et al. 1996). Also linking temperamental characteristics with pain, Chung and Evans (2000) compared self-reports and parents' diary records of health complaints for 32 children (mean age 7 years), classified as shy or non-shy. Because shy children had more emotional upset and more gastrointestinal symptoms, the authors suggested that they might be more sensitive to internal states.

Sensitivity to pain may be one of the components that make up a child's temperament. Reports that some children are constitutionally or temperamentally sensitive to pain date back at least to 1913, when Moro reviewed a series of children with recurrent abdominal pain. He described the majority of these children as fussy, anxious, and demanding; many were perturbed by events that would seem minor to most children. Levels of pain sensitivity differed between children with fibromyalgia and controls (Conte 1999); those with fibromyalgia had a more difficult temperament and greater levels of depression and anxiety as well as pain sensitivity. In another study of the "pain-sensitive temperament" in children with cancer, higher levels of pain sensitivity were associated with greater anxiety and pain, both during and after the painful procedure of lumbar puncture (Chen et al. 2000). The authors suggested targeting pain-sensitive children for special psychological preventative intervention prior to painful procedures.

While temperament is thought to reflect largely innate differences in children's ways of reacting to the world, learning also plays an important role.

SOCIALIZATION AND SOCIAL LEARNING

Children's social environment is filled with people from whom they learn how to react to painful events. Considerable evidence indicates that the social behavior of parents and peers can influence the development of children's experience and expression of pain. These influences can be generally classified as antecedents (e.g., modeling) and consequences (e.g., reinforcement of illness behavior).

Both experimental and clinical evidence shows that children's pain behavior is influenced by models and particularly by mothers (Craig 1986; Osborne et al. 1989; Bonner and Finney 1996; Mikail and von Baeyer 1990; Garralda 2000). Parents who have persistent pain complaints of their own, or who are highly expressive of pain, are likely to have children who follow suit. For example, our clinic treated a 10-year-old boy whose disabling pains, which had no known medical explanation, occurred at various times in his head, neck, shoulders, legs, feet, chest, belly, or back, and were manifested in dramatic ways. Both of his parents were highly expressive of pain, one with ulcers and angina and the other with back pain and headaches; pain was a common topic of conversation in the household.

In an intriguing recent experimental study allowing for causal inferences (Goodman and McGrath, in press), children first observed their mothers immerse one arm in iced water (the cold pressor task). The mothers were randomly assigned to one of three conditions: they were asked to exaggerate or minimize their pain, or they were given no instruction. The children then performed the cold pressor task on their own. Results are shown in Fig. 1.

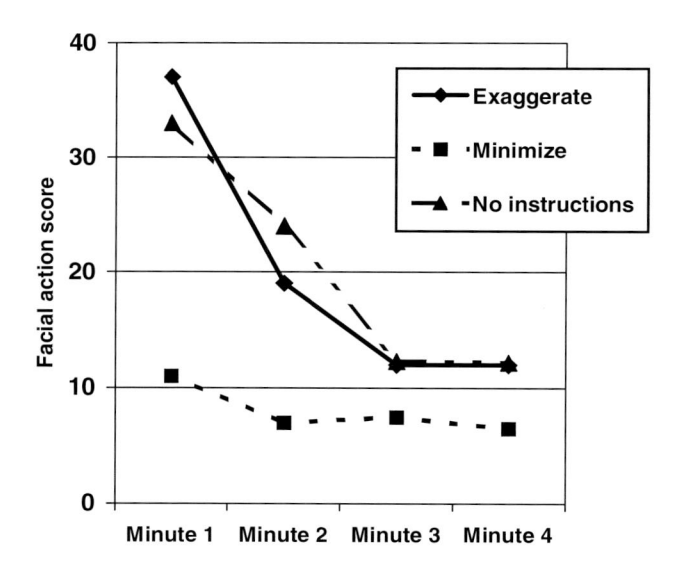

Fig. 1. Child's facial action pain scores during the cold pressor test, after watching the mother perform the same test under one of three conditions of expressiveness.

The children in the minimize condition showed fewer facial actions reflecting pain compared to the exaggerate and control conditions, indicating that mothers' suppression of their own pain behavior led their children to express less pain when exposed to the same stimulus.

Modeling is one among a number of social *antecedents* of pain (e.g., social referencing, reinforcement). Pain behavior also has *consequences* that may alter children's future behavior. An important example of such a mechanism is encouragement of illness behavior (Walker et al. 1993). If parents provide permission to stay home from school, to stay in bed, or to avoid chores contingent on pain behavior, then some children will respond to this inadvertent reinforcement of disability by functioning poorly at school and by avoiding social contact, withdrawing instead into a sick role. Walker and Zeman (1992) used the Illness Behavior Encouragement Scale to evaluate influences on parents' encouragement of their child's illness behavior. They found that parents encourage gastrointestinal symptoms more than colds, and that girls were encouraged for illness behavior more than boys. Unruh and Campbell (1999) reviewed these and other gender differences associated with pain, drawing attention to sex role stereotypes such as those imputing more psychological rather than physical causal attributions to pain experienced by girls compared with boys. These authors also suggested that "[s]ocialization practices may influence boys to inhibit expressions of pain, while giving girls more freedom to express or inhibit pain responsivity."

The studies mentioned above concerning modeling and social reinforcement suggest a familial route for transmission of norms and values regarding the appraisal of the meaning of painful events. Appropriate ways to express pain are negotiated in recurring interactions between children and family members: children learn ways of expressing or suppressing their pain through modeling and reinforcement, and parents' behavior is in turn reinforced by the child's reactions.

REGULATION OF EMOTION

The previous section emphasized external environmental factors (modeling and reinforcement) in children's reaction to pain. Another way to conceptualize pain is as a stressor that elicits the child's skills in emotion regulation, that is, in maintaining emotional homeostasis or balance rather than becoming disorganized under the influence of emotions. Babies have innate or learned strategies for self-comforting such as thumb sucking, rocking, and clutching a teddy bear. These emotion regulation strategies are highly relevant to children's handling both of pain and of anticipatory anxiety or fear of pain. By age 3 to 4 years, children learn a number of strategies to modulate their expression of emotion. For example, they know that they can blunt the impact of a scary movie by covering their eyes or ears, and they can survive a brief separation using self-talk (e.g., "Daddy said he'd be back soon").

The development of emotion regulation is influenced both by parenting practices and by temperament. For example, maternal sensitivity to child cues observed at 3 years of age has been shown to predict somatization in children at school entry, suggesting that expression of distress through bodily complaints versus other means may be socialized in the preschool years (Grunau et al. 1994).

Parents may interact with their child during a painful event in ways that magnify the child's distress or attenuate it. Table I lists parental behaviors that have been associated with increases or decreases in children's pain during brief painful medical procedures (Blount et al. 1989; Frank et al. 1995; Manimala et al. 2000; Piira and von Baeyer 2001).

Numerous studies have examined the development of emotion regulation in the context of immunization injections (e.g., Izard et al. 1983; Craig et al. 1984). While facial actions characteristic of pain predominate in younger infants' response to inoculation, by the second year of life their pain expression becomes briefer, being largely converted to expression of other emotions such as anger or sadness. Axia and Bonichini (1998) reported that the duration of facial expressions of pain (during a 90-second postinoculation interval) decreased almost linearly from 3 to 18 months of age, lasting for

Table I
Parental behaviors associated with decreases and increases in children's distress during painful procedures

Decrease Child's Distress	Increase Child's Distress
Using nonprocedural talk and distraction methods (e.g., facilitating play with toys, bubble-blowing, party blowers; encouraging the child to watch cartoons)	Making reassuring or empathetic statements
	Apologizing
	Criticizing
	Bargaining with the child
Giving commands to engage in coping	Providing explanations during the procedure
Using breathing techniques	Giving the child control over when to start the procedure
Using humor	Catastrophizing
Giving sensory and procedural information before the procedure	Becoming agitated

Source: Blount et al. (1989), Frank et al. (1995), Manimala et al. (2000), Piira and von Baeyer (2001).

52, 34, 14, and 6 seconds at ages 3, 5, 11, and 18 months, respectively. During the same period, expressions of anger, sadness, and interest increased, although not in a linear fashion. Also noteworthy in this study was that more than half of the 3-month-olds, but only 7% of the 18-month-olds, showed recurrence of crying after initial soothing, again suggesting that the effectiveness of internalized emotion regulation increases as children mature.

The development of internalized emotion regulation may also be revealed by the attenuation of overt expression of pain when pain is prolonged: children's self-reports of postoperative pain follow expected patterns of response to movement and analgesics, but these self-reports show low correlation with observational measures of pain, and even children reporting severe pain may show few observable signs (e.g., Beyer et al. 1990).

Clues to children's understanding and regulation of emotion also come from studies of language. Wellman et al. (1995) examined preschoolers' use of emotion terms such as happy, sad, mad, and cry, as well as pain terms such as burn, sting, and hurt. They found that terms for most basic emotions were present by age 2 years, and that from age 2 to 5 years the children's emotion vocabulary expanded. The authors concluded that preschool-age children refer to emotions and physical pains differently, and that they distinguish such feelings from the external situations that elicit them.

Studies of older children's and adolescents' coping with pain have differentiated between emotion-focused and problem-focused coping strategies, techniques involving approach such as information-seeking, and involuntary responses (Reid et al. 1998; Compas and Boyer 2001). In general, emotion-focused reactions to stress such as catastrophizing (dwelling on the negative aspects of a situation and its possible dangers) have less positive outcomes than problem-focused and approach strategies such as working to change the situation, using humor, or attending to some outside distraction. In work with children who had headaches or arthritis, Reid et al. (1998) reported that those who employed mainly emotion-focused and avoidance strategies such as catastrophizing had greater distress and pain, while higher levels of approach coping were related to less disability.

DEVELOPMENT OF PAIN EXPRESSION

Throughout the course of early child development, systematic transformations can be observed in the ways in which pain is expressed or communicated. Anand and Craig (1996) suggest that a child's specific reactions to pain at any stage in life are the optimal adaptations given the child's experience and competence. Reactions to aversive stimuli (e.g., physiological changes, withdrawal of a limb, crying, and facial expressions) are essentially automatic in early life; there is presumed to be little discontinuity in infancy between private experience and outward expression (Hadjistavropoulos and Craig 2002). However, during the toddler and preschool years the expression of pain is increasingly shaped by the child's growing understanding of emotions and ability to anticipate outcomes and feelings. For example, babies under 1 year of age rarely cry *before* an inoculation injection, but almost always cry *afterward*. By contrast, about 50% of 3-year-olds cry *before* an injection, suggesting that, because of their previous experience, they anticipate and fear the pain of the imminent needle puncture (Negayama 1999). By the age of 4 weeks, eye contact plays a role in calming a distressed infant (Zeifman et al. 1996). By preschool age, children are developing an ability to feign, exaggerate, or suppress outward signs of pain, if doing so carries some gain for the child (e.g., resuming play after a fall, or making it look as if another child is to blame for an injury). This development makes sense in light of research on "theory of mind," which addresses children's development of awareness that other people have thoughts and perspectives that may differ from their own (Wellman 1990).

Everyday pain—that is, the ordinary bumps, bruises, and scrapes that are a normal part of children's lives—provides a powerful training experience insofar as the child learns how others will react. Every incident provides a lesson in the display of pain and in coping with pain. In two studies (Fearon et al. 1996; von Baeyer et al. 1998), preschool-aged children were observed during active play at their day care centers. Minor painful incidents occurred on average around 0.3 times per child per hour. The severity of incidents was measured, as well as the intensity and duration of the child's response (e.g., crying) and the nature of the adult response that followed (e.g., ignoring or cuddling the child). Interestingly, the adult response was predicted by the child's expression of distress but not by the severity of the incident itself, so that a child who cried about a very minor incident was more likely to receive care than a child who responded stoically to a more severe incident (von Baeyer et al. 1998). This finding suggests that individual differences in children's response to pain may be maintained and magnified by differential adult responses.

Other data on the socialization of pain expression were provided by Craig et al. (1984), who analyzed the reactions of mothers to immunization injections in children under 24 months of age. The authors found that physical soothing was more frequently provided for younger children and distraction more frequently for older children. This finding suggests that as children get older, mothers move away from providing physical soothing when their children cry in response to pain, and instead they begin encouraging their toddlers to shift their attention away from pain as a way of having them cope on their own. Similarly, Negayama (1999) found that Japanese mothers smiled more (and reproved the children more for their weakness) when older preschool children cried after a needle than when younger children cried. The smiling was taken as a non-empathetic response to the older children's pain, which would be consistent with the mothers' making an effort to teach their children to suppress their pain expression.

Children's expression of pain is influenced both by age and by social context. Zeman and Garber (1996) showed the interactive effects of these factors in a study of "display rules" governing the expression of negative emotions and pain. Children at Grades 1, 3, and 5 were asked how they would express pain in the presence of their peers, their mothers, their fathers, and when alone. The results are shown in Fig. 2. In comparison with the situation of being alone, the presence of peers reduces pain expression and that of mothers increases it; the effect of fathers depends on the child's age, with older children being less likely to display their pain with fathers present. This study was limited by being based on self-report of the child's typical reactions to pain rather than on direct observation. The study by

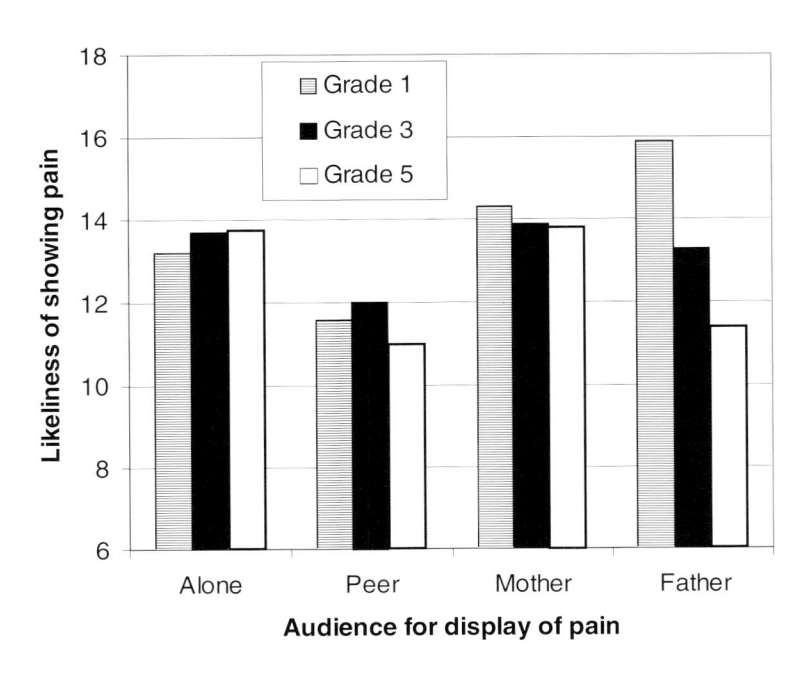

Fig. 2. Display rules: the effect of audience on children's self-reported display of pain. Adapted from Zeman and Garber (1996), with permission. Note that the origin of the graph is not set at zero.

Zeman and Garber (1996) suggests that children implement emotion self-regulation in part by eliciting external social support that is dependent upon who witnesses their pain.

Social influences on pain expression also occur in the hospital, in interaction with health care providers. For example, Byrne et al. (2001) showed that nurses in an orthopedic ward actively discouraged children from displaying their pain: they frequently "construed pain as unreal, unwarranted or not deserving help." Children who did not complain of pain or ask for analgesics were described by nurses as "very good" or "great." Children who showed a lot of pain were appraised as malign, unmotivated, not coping, or even as engaging in dramatic acting: one child, according to the nurse, "deserved an Oscar for her performance." Byrne's team understood these attributions as ways for nurses themselves to cope with the emotional threat presented by patients' pain. However, the impact of these reactions on patients was to increase rather than decrease their distress. Faced with a nurse's denial of his pain, a child intensifies his expression of pain in order to be believed, to obtain analgesics, or to try to avoid a feared procedure.

CONSEQUENCES OF PROLONGED PAIN

To this point we have emphasized studies of normally developing children exposed to painful events. We now turn to some comments on the social development of children and adolescents who have long-term pain. What are the effects of prolonged pain on the child's emotions, relationships, and school life?

The quality of data available to answer these questions is not as good as for procedural and other brief painful experiences. Because experimental designs are not possible, we can only compare children who have suffered prolonged pain with controls who have not. Differences between the groups could be due to the pain or to associated factors such as greater physical impairment or general ill-health in the group with prolonged pain. However, it would be expected that persistent pain would interfere with mid-childhood and adolescent social development, in particular by keeping young people away from activities with their peers and by encouraging dependence on the parents.

Hunfield and colleagues (2002) provide a recent example of research on these issues. These investigators interviewed adolescents from a population study whose chronic or recurrent pain continued throughout a 3-year study period. Pain had marked consequences for many of these young people. They frequently "structured their activities and sleeping hours to prevent aggravation of pain." Those with headaches reported problems with cognitive activities, while those with limb and back pain had problems with physical exertion. In studies of this type, it is difficult to determine whether these other problems are consequences of the pain, or whether both the pain and the other difficulties have common origins in a primary psychological problem such as somatization, anxiety, or depression.

Exposure to painful and stressful medical procedures carries long-term socio-emotional consequences. For example, children aged 6–17 years who had spent at least 24 hours in a pediatric intensive care unit were the subjects of a recent prospective cohort study with a 6-month follow-up (Rennick et al. 2002). The authors summarized their findings as follows: "[C]hildren who were younger, more severely ill, and who endured more invasive procedures had significantly more medical fears, a lower sense of control over their health, and ongoing posttraumatic stress responses for 6 months postdischarge."

Rhee (2001) reviewed earlier research on the presumed consequences of chronic pediatric headache. Headache pain has been associated with difficulties in school attendance, completion of homework, participation in free-time activities, perceived stressfulness of peer relationships and schoolwork, and self-confidence. Although the causal direction of these associations remains unclear in most studies (e.g., difficulty in school might cause stress, thus triggering headache), it is likely that prolonged pain has a long-term harmful effect on social development.

CLINICAL IMPLICATIONS

This chapter has touched on a variety of evidence bearing on the reciprocal relationships among children's temperament, experience with pain, modes of expressing and coping with pain, and various social influences. The studies cited, while far from definitive, do suggest some speculative implications for parenting and clinical practice. Promotion of secure attachment in infants and toddlers requires stable, consistent, and sensitive caregiving. Caregivers can promote secure attachment in the early years of a child's life by being continuously available and by being quick to respond with aid to the child's expressions of distress. A child who thus develops a secure base, that is, a representation of the world in which caregivers are seen as trustworthy and supportive, will later be able to cope with mild and moderate stressors (including painful events) more independently than a child who has experienced insensitive, inconsistent, or inadequate care. One might expect, then, that in adolescence and adulthood, necessary painful medical procedures such as blood tests would be avoided to a lesser extent by people who developed secure attachments in their early years. Interestingly, the predictions and evidence from attachment theory contradict predictions from traditional operant (behaviorist) theory. The latter would hold that a baby's expressions of distress should not be reinforced but rather ignored whenever possible so that they will extinguish. The evidence favors the predictions made from attachment theory rather than the behaviorist predictions.

Parents who overtly and dramatically express their own pain may unwittingly promote pain behavior in their children through the process of modeling. For parents who require repeated painful procedures or who have chronic pain, clinicians might develop strategies to help the parents minimize or at least refrain from exaggerating their distress in front of their children. Painful events may be less threatening for children if they have been exposed to calm, confident coping by their parents and significant others.

Given the strong evidence for modeling of reactions to pain, the infrequent use of peer models in helping children to cope with painful procedures is surprising. Some institutions employ videotapes showing confident child models for preparation for hospitalization or for common surgical procedures. Extending those methods, it would be possible to show young patients a videotape of other children undergoing venipuncture and other feared procedures in a nonthreatening, child-friendly social environment, while employing effective distraction and imagery techniques. Based on social learning theory, such approaches would be expected to be more effective than distraction or imagery by itself. There are many opportunities for research comparing such interventions.

Parents of children with recurrent pain should be made aware of the role of reinforcement in maintaining pain behavior, as well as its social consequences. While breakfast in bed, staying home from school to watch television, and special snacks may be appropriate caregiving for occasional, brief, acute illnesses, such indulgence is usually counterproductive when pain is recurrent. Clinical practice with children's recurrent pain must include a component of parent education that stresses a matter-of-fact, unexcited parental reaction that attenuates rather than amplifies the child's agitated or frightened response to a painful event.

Finally, knowledge of social development may inform tertiary prevention efforts, that is, efforts to prevent the negative long-term consequences of recurrent or chronic pain. Social isolation, often resulting from school avoidance, is an important contributing factor in depression and discouragement about pain. Health care providers may achieve better results by broadening their focus: instead of considering treatment of the patient's symptoms in isolation, it may be important to emphasize ways to normalize interactions with peers by helping children with painful medical conditions return to school (part-time if necessary) or by offering innovative interventions involving groups, friends, or peer counselors. Such approaches would call for health care providers to contact and establish collaboration with educators and leaders of community recreational and religious programs.

The way children experience and express a painful event is shaped by the interactions between their biological makeup, their immediate environment, their thoughts and appraisals of the event, and especially by their history of social learning. This chapter has reviewed the evidence for the social developmental aspects of that complex interconnected web of influences, and has drawn some implications for clinical practice with children and their parents and peers.

ACKNOWLEDGMENTS

The authors appreciate assistance offered by Kenneth D. Craig, G. Allen Finley, Carrie L. Hicks, Patrick J. McGrath, Tammy Marche, Tiina Piira, John Taplin, Trudi Walsh, and Liesle Young.

REFERENCES

Ainsworth MDS, Blehar MC, Waters E, Wall S. *Patterns of Attachment: A Psychological Study of the Strange Situation*. Hillsdale, NJ: Erlbaum, 1978.

Anand KJS, Craig KD. Editorial: new perspectives on the definition of pain. *Pain* 1996; 67:3–6.

Axia G, Bonichini S. Regulation of emotion after acute pain from 3 to 18 months: a longitudinal study. *Early Dev Parenting* 1998; 7:203–210.

Beyer J, McGrath P, Berde C. Discordance between self-report and behavioral pain measures in children aged 3–7 years after surgery. *J Pain Symptom Manage* 1990; 5:350–356.

Blount RL, Corbin SM, Sturger JW, et al. The relationship between adults' behavior and child coping and distress during BMA/LP procedures: a sequential analysis. *Behav Ther* 1989; 20:585–601.

Bonner MJ, Finney JW. A psychosocial model of children's health status. In: Ollendick TH, Prinz RJ (Eds). *Advances in Clinical Child Psychology*, Vol. 18. New York: Plenum Press, 1996, pp 231–282.

Bournaki M. Correlates of pain-related responses to venipunctures in school-age children. *Nurs Res* 1997; 46:147–154.

Bowlby J. *A Secure Base: Parent-Child Attachment and Healthy Human Development*. New York: Basic Books, 1988.

Byrne A, Morton J, Salmon P. Defending against patients' pain: a quantitative analysis of nurses' responses to children's postoperative pain. *J Psychosom Res* 2001; 20:69–76.

Chen E, Craske MG, Katz ER, Schwartz E, Zeltzer LK. Pain-sensitive temperament: does it predict procedural distress and response to psychological treatment among children with cancer? *J Pediatr Psychol* 2000; 25:269–278.

Chisholm K. A three year follow-up of attachment and indiscriminate friendliness in children adopted from Romanian orphanages. *Child Dev* 1998; 69:1092–1106.

Chung JYY, Evans MA. Shyness and symptoms of illness in young children. *Can J Behav Sci* 2000; 32:49–57.

Compas BE, Boyer MC. Coping and attention: implications for child health and pediatric conditions. *J Dev Behav Pediatr* 2001; 22:323–333.

Conte PM. Temperament and stress response in children with fibromyalgia. Dissertation. Yeshiva University, 1999.

Craig KD. Social modeling influences: pain in context. In: Sternbach R (Ed). *The Psychology of Pain*, 2nd ed. New York: Raven Press, 1986, pp 67–96.

Craig KD, McMahon RJ, Morison JD, Zaskow C. Developmental changes in infant pain expression during immunization injections. *Soc Sci Med* 1984; 19:1331–1337.

Fearon I, McGrath PJ, Achat H. "Booboos": the study of everyday pain among young children. *Pain* 1996; 68:55–62.

Frank NC, Blount RL, Smith AJ, Manimala MR, Martin JK. Parent and staff behavior, previous child medical experience, and maternal anxiety as they relate to child procedural distress and coping. *J Pediatr Psychol* 1995; 20:277–289.

Garralda ME. The links between somatisation in children and in adults. In: Reder PM, Jolley A, McClure M (Eds). *Family Matters: Interfaces between Child and Adult Mental Health*. London: Routledge, 2000, pp 122–134.

Goodman JE, McGrath PJ. Mother's modeling influences children's pain during a cold pressor task. *Pain*; in press.

Grunau RVE, Whitfield MF, Petrie JH, Fryer EL. Early pain experience, child and family factors, as precursors of somatization: a prospective study of extremely premature and fullterm children. *Pain* 1994; 56:353–359.

Hadjistavropoulos T, Craig KD. A theoretical model for understanding self-report and observational measures of pain: a communications model. *Behav Res Ther* 2002; 40:551–570.

Hedlund R, Lindgren U. The incidence of femoral shaft fractures in children and adolescents. *J Pediatr Orthop* 1986; 6:47–50.

Hunfield JA, Perquin CW, Bertina W, et al. Stability of pain parameters and pain-related quality of life in adolescents with persistent pain: a three-year follow-up. *Clin J Pain* 2002; 18:99–106.

Izard C, Hembree E, Dougherty L, Spizirri C. Changes in facial expressions of 2- to 19-month-old infants following acute pain. *Dev Psychol* 1983; 19:418–426.

Lee L, White-Traut R. The role of temperament in pediatric pain response. *Issues Comprehensive Pediatr Nurs* 1996; 19:49–63.

Manimala MR, Blount RL, Cohen LL. The effects of parental reassurance versus distraction on child distress and coping during immunizations. *Children's Health Care* 2000; 29:161–177.

Marvin RS. Attachment- and family systems-based intervention in developmental psychopathology. *Dev Psychopathol* 1992; 4:697–711.

McDevitt SC, Carey WB. The measurement of temperament in 3-7 year old children. *J Child Psychol Psychiatry* 1978; 19:245–253.

Mikail SF, von Baeyer CL. Pain, somatic focus, and emotional adjustment in children of chronic headache sufferers and controls. *Soc Sci Med* 1990; 31:51–59.

Moro E. Über rezidivierende Nabelkoliken bei älteren Kindern [Recurrent umbilical colics in older children]. *Münchener Med Wochenschr* 1913; 23:2827–2829.

Negayama K. Development of reactions to pain of inoculation in children and their mothers. *Int J Behav Dev* 1999; 23:731–746.

Osborne R, Hatcher JW, Richtsmeier A. The role of social modeling in unexplained pediatric pain. *J Pediatr Psychol* 1989; 14:43–61.

Perquin CW, Hazebroek-Kampschreur AA, Hunfeld JA, et al. Pain in children and adolescents: a common experience. *Pain* 2000; 87:51–58.

Piira T, von Baeyer CL. Parent's behaviour in helping children to cope with painful procedures. *Pediatr Pain Lett* 2001; 5:13–17.

Reid GJ, Gilbert CA, McGrath PJ. The Pain Coping Questionnaire: preliminary validation. *Pain* 1998; 76:83–96.

Rennick J, Johnston C, Dougherty G, Platt R, Ritchie J. Children's psychological responses after critical illness and exposure to invasive technology. *J Dev Behav Pediatrics* 2002; 23:133–144.

Rhee H. Risk factors for and sequelae of headaches in schoolchildren with clinical implications from a psychosocial perspective. *J Pediatr Nurs* 2001; 16:392–401.

Schechter N, Bernstein B, Beck A, Hart L, Scherzer L. Individual differences in children's response to pain: role of temperament and parental characteristics. *Pediatrics* 1991; 87:171–177.

Séguin JR, Pihl RO, Boulerice B, Tremblay RE, Harden PW. Pain sensitivity and stability of physical aggression in boys. *J Child Psychol Psychiatry* 1996; 37:823–834.

Stuart S, Noyes R. Attachment and interpersonal communication in somatization. *Psychosomatics* 1999; 40:34–43.

Thomas A, Chess S. *Temperament and Development.* New York: Brunner/Mazel, 1977.

Unruh AM, Campbell MA. Gender variation in children's pain experiences. In: McGrath PJ, Finley GA (Eds). *Chronic and Recurrent Pain in Children and Adolescents,* Progress in Pain Research and Management, Vol. 13. Seattle: IASP Press, 1999, pp 199–241.

Van Ijzendoorn M, Goldberg S, Kroonenberg P, Frenkel O. The relative effects of maternal and child problems on the quality of attachment: a meta-analysis of attachment in clinical samples. *Child Develop* 1992; 63:840–858.

von Baeyer CL, Baskerville S, McGrath PJ. Everyday pain in three- to five-year-old children in day care. *Pain Res Manage* 1998; 3:111–116.

Walker LS, Zeman JL. Parental response to child illness behavior. *J Pediatr Psychol* 1992; 17:49–71.

Walker LS, Garber J, Greene JW. Psychosocial correlates of recurrent abdominal pain: a comparison of pediatric patients with recurrent abdominal pain, organic illness, and psychiatric disorders. *J Abnorm Psychol* 1993; 102:248–258.

Walsh TM, Symons DK, McGrath PJ. Continuity of internal working models of relationships during separation from parents and pain experience. *Attachment Hum Dev*; in press.

Wellman HM. *The Child's Theory of Mind.* Cambridge, MA: MIT Press, 1990.

Wellman HM, Harris PL, Banerjee M, Sinclair A. Early understanding of emotion: evidence from natural language. *Cognition Emotion* 1995; 9:117–149.

Zeifman D, Delaney S, Blass E. Sweet taste, looking, and calm in 2- and 4-week-old infants: the eyes have it. *Dev Psychol* 1996; 32:1090–1099.

Zeman J, Garber J. Display rules for anger, sadness, and pain: it depends on who is watching. *Child Dev* 1996; 67:957–973.

Correspondence to: Carl L. von Baeyer, PhD, Department of Psychology, University of Saskatchewan, 9 Campus Drive, Saskatoon, SK, Canada S7N 5A5. Fax: 306-966-6630; email: carl.vonbaeyer@usask.ca.

5

The Role of Family Factors in Pediatric Pain

Christine T. Chambers

Department of Pediatrics, University of British Columbia; Centre for Community Child Health Research, British Columbia Research Institute for Children's and Women's Health; and Department of Psychology, British Columbia's Children's Hospital, Vancouver, British Columbia, Canada

The family provides a rich and important source of information about pain for children. Parents are often present when their children experience pain. As a result, parents hold the primary responsibility for responding to pain symptoms and deciding on further courses of action as necessary. In addition, children are often witnesses to episodes of pain and illness in their parents. Not surprisingly, clinical lore, in the form of speculation by physicians and other health professionals, and psychological theory have pointed to the important role that the family may play in influencing children's pain experiences (Craig 1983, 1986). In considering the important psychological and social factors that contribute to pain beyond physical pathology (Merskey and Bogduk 1994), it is clear that consideration of family factors must play a central role in our understanding of children's pain.

This chapter will review research describing the role of family factors in pediatric pain, including both acute and chronic pain. For the purposes of this chapter, acute pain will be defined as pain of variable duration typically characterized by sudden onset; a demonstrable etiology, such as noxious or tissue damaging stimulation produced by trauma, disease, or treatment; and a limited and predictable course (American Academy of Pediatrics and American Pain Society 2001). Chronic pain will be defined as repeated or continuous episodes of pain that are experienced either as a component of a well-characterized medical disorder or by otherwise healthy children in the absence of a well-defined organic etiology (American Pain Society 2001). I will examine several research themes addressing family factors in acute and chronic pain. Within acute pain, the review will include research on parental presence during painful medical procedures, parental behaviors during painful medical procedures, interventions with parents for painful medical procedures, and parental assessment and management of postoperative pain. For chronic pain, I will review research examining aggregation of pain complaints within families, parent behavior among children with chronic pain, and interventions for parents of children with chronic pain.

Operant conditioning, classical conditioning, social learning theory, attachment theory, psychodynamic theory, and family systems theory have been used to explain the role of family factors in pain. A comprehensive review of each of these theories is beyond the scope of this chapter; however, they will be acknowledged throughout the chapter. Although no one theory can explain all aspects of familial issues in pediatric pain, a broad social learning perspective encompassing vicarious learning, modeling, and reinforcement is most widely used. Several general reviews of family factors on adults' pain supplement this review of the family and children's pain (e.g., Payne and Norfleet 1986; Flor et al. 1987; Turk et al. 1987; Hertzman et al. 1989; Roy 1989, 1990; Snelling 1990; Kerns and Weiss 1994; Kerns 1999). Finally, although this chapter focuses on psychological and social factors that might explain the role of the family in pediatric pain, I also acknowledge the potentially predisposing and interactive effects of genetic and shared environmental/lifestyle factors (see the chapter by Smith and Mogil in this volume for a discussion of genetic factors).

PARENTAL PRESENCE DURING PAINFUL MEDICAL PROCEDURES

The question of whether parents should be present during painful medical procedures has been a hotly debated and extensively researched topic since the late 1960s, when the first studies began to emerge (Schulman et al. 1967; Vernon et al. 1967). Additional research examining the role of parental presence was prompted by a letter from a physician published in the *British Medical Journal* in the mid 1980s expressing his dissatisfaction with the denial of his request to be present during the anesthesia induction of his 3-year-old daughter (While 1985). The exclusion of parents from their children's procedures stems from the belief that parents interfere with the completion of procedures and that children react more adversely when their parents are present. Many hospitals do not have a policy regarding parental presence and leave this decision up to the discretion of the individual health professional (Baines and Overton 1995; McCormick and Spargo 1996).

Most research examining parental presence has been conducted for anesthesia induction in children prior to surgery (for editorials, see Hannallah 1994; Kain 1995). However, studies have also examined the role of parental presence for a variety of other medical procedures (e.g., venipuncture or immunization) and in diverse settings (e.g., the emergency department or the intensive care unit). Parental presence during anesthesia induction typically involves having the parent don hospital scrubs and accompany the child into the operating room until the induction is complete. Although anesthesia induction tends to be more stressful than painful for children, the substantial amount of work conducted in this area is helpful in understanding the role of parental presence for other procedures for which pain is a common feature. Numerous studies have surveyed parents' and professionals' attitudes regarding parental presence at anesthesia induction (Braude et al. 1990; Ryder and Spargo 1991; Henderson et al. 1993; Roman et al. 1993; Baines and Overton 1995; Bosenberg et al. 1996; Kain et al. 1996b; McCormick and Spargo 1996). Across these studies, most parents report that they prefer to be present during their child's induction and that they feel that their presence is of benefit to their child (Braude et al. 1990; Ryder and Spargo 1991; Henderson et al. 1993). Despite their preference for being present during induction, parents do report a number of upsetting factors associated with being present, including seeing the child upset prior to the induction, watching their child go limp during the induction, and being separated from the child after induction of anesthesia (Vessey et al. 1994). When surveyed, most anesthetists report that they are in favor of parental presence during induction (Roman et al. 1993; Bosenberg et al. 1996); however, anesthetists usually see parents as less helpful to the child than do parents (McEwen et al. 1994). Interesting international differences in attitudes toward parental presence during anesthesia induction have been reported. For example, Kain et al. (1996a) found that, while 82% of the anesthetists surveyed from Great Britain believed that parental presence during induction decreased child anxiety and improved cooperation, only 64% of respondents from the United States agreed with these statements. International variations in concerns regarding legal ramifications and use of induction techniques have been offered as explanations for these disparities in findings (Kain et al. 1996a).

A number of studies have examined the impact of parental presence versus absence during anesthesia induction for children (for a review, see Palermo et al. 1999). Outcome measures typically include perioperative measures of child anxiety, distress, and cooperation. Studies in which parents were not randomly assigned to be present or absent, but were permitted to choose for themselves, tend to report positive effects for parental presence, including lower levels of child anxiety and distress (Hannallah and Rosales

1983; Cameron et al. 1996). However, studies that systematically or randomly assigned parents to be present or absent typically report less favorable results. For example, Hickmott and colleagues (1989) found no differences in 1- to 9-year-old children's moods or cooperation during induction as a function of parental presence versus absence. Similarly, in the only study to date to examine parental presence at anesthesia induction among infants, Palermo and colleagues (2000) demonstrated no impact of parental presence on the infants' behavioral distress.

Kain and colleagues (1996b, 1998, 2000) have conducted an excellent series of controlled investigations. In their first study, they randomly assigned children between the ages of 1 and 6 years to either a parental presence or parental absence condition. Several behavioral and physiological measures were used to assess the children's anxiety and distress. Reliable self-reports of distress were unavailable due to the young age of the participants. Overall, there were no significant differences between the groups on any of the outcome measures. However, Kain and colleagues (1996b) identified three groups of children who showed a diminished stress response with parental presence: children older than 4 years of age, children whose parents had low levels of general anxiety, and children who were temperamentally less active. Other research has indicated that child distress during induction may indeed vary as a function of the parents' level of anxiety (Johnston et al. 1988; Bevan et al. 1990; Glazebrook et al. 1994; Cameron et al. 1996) as well as the child's age and temperament (Lumley et al. 1990; Glazebrook et al. 1994). These findings highlight the important role that individual child and parent factors may play in predicting positive response to parental presence during anesthesia induction.

Another study by Kain and colleagues (1998) contrasted parental presence during induction with the use of oral midazolam, a sedative premedication, and found that the medication was more effective than parental presence for managing both child and parent distress during the preoperative period. A subsequent study contrasted the effects of oral midazolam alone versus oral midazolam plus parental presence during induction (Kain et al. 2000). While there were no differences in child distress between the two groups, parents who were present reported that they were less anxious and more satisfied with the separation process and overall care provided (Kain et al. 2000). A more recent study found no significant differences in parental self-reported anxiety or electrocardiogram abnormalities, but the authors noted increased parental heart rate and skin conductance levels for parents who were present during anesthesia induction (Kain et al. 2003). This research indicates that, while parental presence may not produce lower levels of child distress and anxiety during anesthesia induction, parents who would like to be present may benefit from the opportunity to attend their child's induction. Far less research has examined parental presence in the post-anesthesia care unit. It appears that parental presence in this setting is associated with lower levels of parent anxiety, but does not necessarily provide any significant direct benefit to the child (Diniaco and Ingoldsby 1983; Bru et al. 1993; Hall et al. 1995).

Research examining parental presence during other painful medical procedures shows even less benefit than do studies on anesthesia induction. While a trend is apparent among children, parents, and medical staff that parental presence is preferred during painful medical procedures (Shaw and Routh 1982; Haimi-Cohen et al. 1996; Sacchetti et al. 1996), the research examining this issue is quite mixed. A randomized controlled trial of parental presence for children 3 years of age and younger undergoing either venipuncture, intravenous cannulation, or urethral catheterization in a pediatric emergency department found that parents who were present reported significantly less anxiety than did parents who were not present, but there was no significant difference in pain responses, as measured by cry analysis and observer reports of pain (Bauchner et al. 1996). Parental presence did not negatively affect the ability of the clinician to complete the procedure. Other studies have similarly reported no differences in child pain or distress as a function of parental presence or absence during dental treatment (Fenlon et al. 1993), lumbar punctures (Haimi-Cohen et al. 1996), and burn care procedures (Doctor 1994).

Several studies report positive effects of parental presence during painful procedures. For example, in two studies, Wolfram and colleagues (Wolfram and Turner 1996; Wolfram et al. 1997) found lower levels of distress and pain on the part of children and lower levels of parent distress when children aged 1–18 years were randomly assigned to either a parent present or parent absent condition for venipuncture in a pediatric emergency department. The distress of the health professional performing the venipuncture did not differ across the two groups. A pilot study examining parental presence during invasive medical procedures in the pediatric intensive care unit similarly found that presence significantly reduced parental anxiety and that most parents and health professionals reported that parental presence was helpful to the child (Powers and Rubenstein 1999).

A few studies have supported the belief that parental presence may negatively affect child behavior during procedures. For example, Shaw and Routh (1982) found that, while 18-month-olds in a parent-absent condition protested upon their mother's departure, it was the 18-month-olds in the parent-present condition whose behavior was rated as significantly more negative during routine immunization. In the same study, the behavior of

5-year-old children was more negative during injection if the parent was present (Shaw and Routh 1982). Gonzalez and colleagues (1993) similarly reported significantly more behavioral distress during routine injections when parents were present for children aged 4–7 years, but found no differences in distress levels for the children under 4 years of age. For some young children, parental presence may serve to facilitate the release of negative emotions and anxiety during painful procedures. Expression of distress in the presence of the parent could be positive (e.g., reflecting appropriate attachment behavior) or negative (e.g., indicating amplification of distress).

In summary, while parental presence may be of benefit for some during anesthesia induction, its impact on child behavior during other painful procedures is not as clear. There is no evidence that parental presence interferes with either procedure completion or staff anxiety. The effectiveness of parental presence is likely to vary as a function of individual child and parent characteristics, what the parents do during the procedure, and the type of procedure and medical setting. Research has yet to systematically address these issues, some of which are described in more detail below. Meanwhile, if appropriate, it seems reasonable that parents who would prefer to be present during their children's procedures should be encouraged to be there. However, a subgroup of parents prefer not to be present during procedures (Braude et al. 1990), and health professionals should respect this preference. The decision for a parent to be present or absent should be reached in discussions between the parent and the health professionals (Bauchner et al. 1991). Research needs to move beyond simple examinations of the effects of parental presence or absence to delineating the types of families for which parental presence works best and to better understanding what parents do and how they can be instructed to help their children during painful medical procedures (von Baeyer 1997).

PARENTAL BEHAVIOR DURING PAINFUL MEDICAL PROCEDURES

There has been a surprising lack of coordination between research examining parental presence during medical procedures and studies that describe and quantify what parents actually do during these procedures. It may not be the mere physical presence or absence of the parent that is critically important, but rather what the parent says or does when present (von Baeyer 1997). While some valuable information regarding the behaviors parents engage in during children's medical procedures has emerged from interviews and questionnaires (e.g., Caty et al. 1989; Kazak et al. 1996b), recent research has found significant discrepancies between what parents report doing during procedures and what they actually do (Cohen et al. 2000). Therefore, it would appear that descriptive studies that include direct observation and quantification of parent behavior during procedures would provide the most rich and valid source of information in this area.

Bush and colleagues (1986) conducted one of the first studies to examine parent-child interactions during painful medical procedures. They observed 50 children ranging from 4 to 10 years of age and their mothers during painful medical procedures. Four classes of child behavior (prosocial behavior, distress, attachment, and exploration) and six classes of parental behavior (distraction, reassurance, ignoring, informing, agitation, and restraining) were coded. Results showed that maternal agitation was linked to increased child distress, and that maternal distraction was linked to decreased child distress. Surprisingly, although one might expect maternal reassurance to be linked to decreased child distress, the reverse was true. A study by Manne and colleagues (1992) confirmed that adult distraction resulted in increased child coping and a reduction in distress and crying for children with cancer undergoing venipuncture. Jacobsen and colleagues (1990) found that parental explanations regarding the procedures were associated with increases in child distress.

Most of the recent research examining parent-child interactions during painful procedures has been conducted by Ronald Blount and his colleagues. In their first study, Blount et al. (1989) made audiotapes and transcripts of verbal interactions among 23 sets of 5- to 13-year-old children, their parents, and medical staff during bone marrow aspirations and lumbar punctures. Child and adult behaviors were coded using a measure developed for use in the study called the Child-Adult Medical Procedure Interaction Scale (CAMPIS), which includes codes for 19 adult behaviors and 16 child behaviors (described below). A group of trained raters coded behaviors from the audiotapes and transcripts. Particular adult behaviors were closely associated with either coping or distress behaviors in the children undergoing painful procedures. Specifically, adults' reassuring comments, apologies to the child, indications of empathy, giving control to the child, and criticism of the child typically preceded child distress. In contrast, adult commands to engage in coping procedures, nonprocedural talk to the child, and humor directed to the child preceded successful efforts by the child to cope with the pain.

A revised version of the CAMPIS, the CAMPIS-R (Child-Adult Medical Procedure Interaction Scale—Revised), was subsequently developed (Blount et al. 1997). The revised measure grouped the adult CAMPIS codes into three general categories: coping promoting (i.e., nonprocedural talk to the child, commands to use coping strategy, use of humor), distress promoting (i.e., reassuring comments, criticism, apologies, giving control, empathy), and adult neutral (e.g., checking the child's status). Similarly, the child CAMPIS codes were classified into three categories: child coping (e.g., making coping statements, nonprocedural talk by the child), child distress (e.g., crying, verbalizing pain), and child neutral (e.g., requests for relief from nonprocedural discomfort). Follow-up studies examining patterns of adult-child interaction coded behaviors using the CAMPIS-R during different phases of medical procedures (Blount et al. 1990). Comparisons of adult behaviors as a function of whether the child could be classified as a "high coper" or "low coper" (Blount et al. 1991) have provided further support for the pattern of parent-child interactions found in this team's initial study. Numerous independent studies have found support for the role of parental distress-promoting and coping-promoting behaviors in influencing child distress and coping (e.g., Kleiber and McCarthy 1999; Miller et al. 2001; Salmon and Pereira 2002). A short form of the CAMPIS-R is now available (Blount et al. 2001).

While much less research has examined parent-child interactions during procedures for infants, evidence indicates that behaviors such as reassurance are linked with increases in pain behaviors in even very young infants during immunization (Sweet and McGrath 1998). Behaviors found to be related to increases or decreases in child distress are exhibited not only by parents, but by health professionals such as physical therapists (Miller et al. 2001), nurses (Blount et al. 1989), and physicians (Dahlquist et al. 1995), although differences have been reported in the specific nature and relative importance of parental versus medical staff behaviors (Dahlquist et al. 1995; Sweet and McGrath 1998). Regardless, the powerful influence of adult behavior was evident in a study of children undergoing immunizations, where 38% of the variance in children's coping behaviors and 55% of the variance in children's distress behaviors could be predicted from adults' coping-promoting and distress-promoting behaviors (Frank et al. 1995). Parent and child behaviors during acute painful medical procedures are strongly associated. Although the research has not been conducted from a deliberate theoretical perspective, it can be readily interpreted as supporting the importance of reinforcement in children's pain.

A limitation of this excellent descriptive work is that it is correlational (Peterson et al. 1997). While parental behaviors are related to increases and decreases in child distress and coping, it is impossible to ascertain from this research whether certain parent behaviors are causally related to child outcomes. To address this limitation, we conducted an experimental investigation of the impact of maternal behaviors on children's pain experiences

(Chambers et al. 2002). Mothers of 8- to 12-year-old children were randomly assigned to a pain-promoting, pain-reducing, or control (no training) interaction condition while their children completed an experimental pain paradigm, the cold pressor task. Mothers were trained to interact with their children in the assigned manner through use of verbal instruction, videotaped demonstration, and role-playing practice. Training was based on behaviors that were linked with either increases or decreases in child pain in previous research by Blount and colleagues (1989). As a result, mothers in the pain-promoting condition were trained to interact with their children using reassurance, empathy, apologies, giving control, and mild criticism. Mothers in the pain-reducing condition were trained to interact with their child using nonprocedural talk (distraction), suggestions on how to cope, and humor. Children's pain experiences during the cold pressor task were assessed using self-reports of intensity and affect, coding of facial activity, tolerance, and heart rate responsiveness. Results indicated that girls whose mothers interacted with them in the pain-promoting manner reported more pain than did daughters of mothers in the control group, who in turn reported more pain than girls whose mothers interacted with them in the pain-reducing manner (Chambers et al. 2002). This effect was not significant for boys. Maternal interaction had no effect on children's pain affect, facial activity, tolerance, or heart rate. The results of this study were interpreted as indicating that maternal behavior can have a direct impact on daughters' subjective reports of pain. Other studies that involved direct manipulations of parental behavior designed to produce systematic increases or decreases in child distress have yielded similar findings (Gonzalez et al. 1993; Manimala and Blount 2000).

In summary, parental behavior plays an important role in influencing children's pain during medical procedures. The consistent finding that parental behaviors such as reassurance are linked to increases in child distress (Blount et al. 1989) is intriguing and not in keeping with common-sense assumptions about the therapeutic benefits of reassurance. However, it is congruent with a reinforcement model. The finding is of concern because research has indicated that reassurance is the mostly common strategy employed by parents during procedures (Broome and Endsley 1989; Blount et al. 1997). Consistent with a social learning perspective (Craig 1986), parental verbalizations and nonverbal behavior may function primarily as signals for parental anxiety or concern and thus precipitate children's behavioral distress. In addition, these particular parental behaviors may serve to reinforce children's pain and distress behaviors as the interaction progresses. A quotation from a recent award-winning children's novel illustrates this phenomenon: "If an adult tells you not to worry, and you weren't worried before, you better hurry up and start because you're already running late" (Curtis 1999). Research is needed to examine the exact qualities of reassuring comments (e.g., timing, content, vocal tone, etc.) that could account for the increase in pain and distress associated with these types of comments. In addition, research is needed to examine factors that may influence the relationship between parent behaviors and child outcomes during procedures, such as child temperament, coping, and self-efficacy. Regardless, the solid descriptive research in this area provides an excellent foundation upon which to cultivate interventions to help parents learn to better support their children during procedures.

INTERVENTIONS WITH PARENTS FOR PAINFUL MEDICAL PROCEDURES

The policy statement on the assessment and management of acute pain in children written by the American Academy of Pediatrics and the American Pain Society (2001) advises that families be involved in the care of children's acute pain; however, there is no discussion of exactly how parents should assist their child during painful procedures. Indeed, parents often report that they want to be involved in their child's medical care, but frequently experience frustration, communication problems with professionals, and a desire for more information regarding how they might best help their child (Neill 1996a,b; Simons et al. 2001). While staff are generally supportive of parental involvement in the care of children in medical settings (Johnson and Lindschau 1996), an understanding of parents' needs, expectations, and experiences is critical (Kristensson-Hallstrom 2000). Our ability to appropriately involve parents in their children's medical procedures would be facilitated through the development and testing of specific interventions for parents that are clinically feasible and related to significant improvements in child outcomes.

Recent years have seen excellent progress in the pharmacological and psychological management of pain from medical procedures (Finley and McGrath 2001). For example, a recent systematic review of treatments for procedure-related pain in children (Powers 1999) concluded that cognitive-behavioral therapy (e.g., relaxation exercises, distraction, imagery, filmed modeling, reinforcement/incentive, and behavioral rehearsal) was a well-established treatment for procedure-related pain in children. Parents were involved as coaches to provide adjunct support in many of the studies included in the review (e.g., Jay and Elliott 1990; Manne et al. 1990, 1994; Blount et al. 1992; Powers et al. 1993). Recent studies have continued to include parents in intervention programs for procedural pain in children (Zelikovsky et al. 2000; Kleiber et al. 2001; Pringle et al. 2001; Dahlquist et al. 2002).

Intervention programs that include parents as coaches typically involve a brief information session during which a therapist provides a rationale for the training, introduction of specific techniques (e.g., using a party blower, blowing bubbles, or telling favorite stories), an opportunity for modeling the techniques, and feedback and praise for the parent. Results of research using this approach have generally been positive, often with reductions in child and parent distress, but not necessarily with changes in children's pain. For example, Blount and colleagues (1992) found that children of trained parents used distraction more during immunization and showed less observable distress than did children of untrained parents. While trained parents and children reported that they felt less distressed than they normally would, there were no differences in children's self-reports of pain. A more recent study by Kleiber and colleagues (2001) examined the role of parents as distraction coaches during intravenous insertion for preschoolers. Parents and children were alternately assigned to a distraction education or a standard care condition. While there was a trend for the parent intervention group to show decreased distress over time, there were no group differences for child behavioral distress or pain. Studies that involve simultaneous training of both the parent and child by a therapist tend to report more positive findings. For example, Manne and colleagues (1990) found that an intervention with both children and parents significantly reduced observed child distress, parent-rated child distress, and parents' ratings of their own distress, and that these changes were maintained across the course of several procedures. Evidence also indicates that parents can play an important role in combined psychological and pharmacological interventions for procedural distress (Kazak et al. 1996a, 1998).

Only one study to date has examined the effectiveness of instructing parents to help their infants during immunization (Felt et al. 2000). The intervention consisted of providing parents with information about techniques that included visual, auditory, oral, and kinesthetic modalities (e.g., toys, the parent's voice, and a pacifier). Results of this study found that parents who received the information were more likely to use such a technique with their infant and that their infants showed shorter durations of distress, were rated as more comfortable by their parents immediately after the immunization, and had lower salivary cortisol levels in the hour following immunization.

Despite the evidence that parents can play an important role in assisting their children during painful medical procedures, it is very rare to find standard use of training programs for parents in clinical settings. Involvement of coaches during children's medical procedures may be necessary for children to benefit optimally from cognitive-behavioral interventions (Cohen et al. 2002). Furthermore, descriptive research examining parental behavior during procedures (Blount et al. 1989; Cohen et al. 2002) shows that parents need guidance from professionals to be able to take a more active and constructive role in assisting their child during procedures, rather than simply being an ineffectual provider of comfort and reassurance. Dissemination of effective treatments for involving parents and reducing child pain during procedures should be a priority.

PARENTAL ASSESSMENT AND MANAGEMENT OF POSTOPERATIVE PAIN

Pediatric surgeries are increasingly being performed on an outpatient or "day surgery" basis. As a result, parents have become more involved in the postoperative care of their children, including pain assessment and management. Recent research examining parental management of children's postoperative pain following outpatient surgery has revealed less than adequate medication practices (Knight 1994; Finley et al. 1996; Romsing and Walther-Larsen 1996; Sutters and Miaskowski 1997). For example, Finley and colleagues (1996) found that 60–75% of children judged to be experiencing clinically significant pain following outpatient surgery were administered inadequate pain medication (i.e., three or fewer doses) at home by parents on each of three days following surgery. This finding is of concern because children with poor pain relief are more likely to experience postoperative nausea and vomiting and are more challenging to care for at home (Munro et al. 1999). The tendency for parents to undermedicate their children's postoperative pain may be related to negative attitudes about the use of analgesic medications, including concerns about drug addiction or side effects (Gedaly-Duff and Ziebarth 1994; Knight 1994; Forward et al. 1996). For example, in the study by Finley et al. (1996), over 40% of parents believed that pain medications should be used only as a last resort.

While interventions designed to prepare children and their families for day surgeries have been quite successful in reducing child and parent anxiety (Visintainer and Wolfer 1975; Wolfer and Visintainer 1979; Ellerton and Merriam 1994), few studies have explored specific interventions for improving parental management of their children's pain following surgery. We conducted a randomized trial to evaluate the effectiveness of a pain education booklet titled *Pain, Pain, Go Away: Helping Children with Pain* on parents' attitudes and management of their children's postoperative pain (Chambers et al. 1997). While parents who received this booklet had fewer concerns about the use of acetaminophen for children compared to parents who did not receive this information, the intervention did not have a significant impact on the amount of medication parents administered to their children following surgery (Chambers et al. 1997). A surgical preparation program for parents, including information about children's postoperative behavior, resulted in parents who felt well-prepared to care for their children postoperatively (Kristensson-Hallstrom et al. 1997). The children of these parents experienced less pain and fewer side effects in the postoperative period than did a group of control children.

Parents may also undermedicate their children's pain because of difficulty in accurately identifying and assessing it. Several studies have examined the relationship between parents' and children's ratings of postoperative pain. While most studies report significant correlations between parent and child ratings (O'Hara et al. 1987; Bennett-Branson and Craig 1993; Miller 1996; Romsing 1996; Chambers et al. 1998; Goodenough et al. 1999; Demyttenaere et al. 2001), when parent and child mean scores are compared or level of agreement is computed it is clear that parents significantly underestimate their children's pain and that parental global ratings of pain show generally poor levels of agreement with their children's self-reports (for a review, see Chambers et al. 1998). No research has attempted to discover reasons for this. Perhaps parental minimization of children's pain represents a coping strategy or denial mechanism that shields parents from fully acknowledging and experiencing their children's suffering. Studies examining factors associated with the accuracy of family caregiver estimates of patient pain among adults reveal that caregiver experience of patient pain is significantly related to disparities in pain ratings (Redinbaugh et al. 2002). Given that discrepancies in the perception of pain experience between patients and their caregivers are associated with deleterious outcomes and poorer quality of life among adult patients (Miaskowski et al. 1997; Redinbaugh et al. 2002), studies that are able to predict what types of parents are likely to underestimate their children's pain, and what the specific consequences of underestimation are, should be areas of future research in pediatric pain assessment.

In response to the documented parental difficulties assessing pain in children, we developed the Parents' Postoperative Pain Measure (PPPM; Chambers et al. 1996), a 15-item behavioral checklist based on nonverbal pain cues that children show following surgery (e.g., whining or complaining more than usual, holding the sore part of the body, and groaning or moaning more than usual; Reid et al. 1995). In the preliminary study describing the development of the measure among a sample of 7–12-year-olds, the measure showed excellent psychometric properties (Chambers et al. 1996). Correlations between PPPM scores and child-rated pain were high, while PPPM scores were only moderately related to scores on a measure of more general emotional distress. Scores on the PPPM showed significant decreases from the first to second postoperative day, and the measure was successful in discriminating between children who had undergone surgeries that resulted in no or low pain and children whose surgeries caused moderate to high pain. Using a cut-off score of 6 out of 15, the PPPM showed excellent levels of sensitivity and specificity in detecting children who independently reported clinically significant levels of pain (Chambers et al. 1996).

More recently, a series of additional validation studies for the measure have shown that the PPPM is specific to pain, and not anxiety, and that scores on the PPPM are sensitive to analgesic intervention (Finley et al., in press). The measure has been shown to be valid for use by parents of children from the ages of 2 to 12 years of age (Chambers et al., in press). The measure has been used successfully by a team of independent investigators with children experiencing chronic pain (Hunfeld et al. 1997, 2001) and has been incorporated into clinical practice guidelines (Royal College of Nursing 1999). It has also been translated into several languages including Thai (Khusongkiet et al. 1999), Korean (Shin and Jung 2000), and Finnish (Kokki et al. 2003). Additional research is needed to examine whether use of the PPPM can improve parental pain management practices following surgery. However, a home-based, parent-directed pain management protocol consisting of a pain assessment instrument and an algorithm relating pain scores to appropriate pain medication was successful in improving pain-related outcomes (e.g., earlier to return to school) following day surgery (Seid and Varni 1999).

In summary, parental management and assessment of children's pain is an area that deserves futures attention. Although the studies reviewed in this section refer to "parental" assessment and management of children's postoperative pain, in reality these studies have included almost exclusively samples of mothers. The generalizability of the findings to fathers has yet to be determined. Regardless, the tendency for some parents to underestimate and undermedicate their children's pain is an intriguing mystery that deserves unraveling.

AGGREGATION OF PAIN COMPLAINTS WITHIN FAMILIES

Given the common and salient nature of pain in our everyday lives, it should not be surprising that research has found a striking similarly in the pain experiences of children and their parents. For example, children with recurrent abdominal pain are more likely to have parents who report similar pain problems (Apley and Naish 1958; Apley 1975; Zuckerman et al. 1987). Furthermore, persons with recurrent pain often come from families with a positive family history for pain (Turkat et al. 1984; Ehde et al. 1991).

While most research examining aggregation of pain in families has relied on retrospective reports, a recent prospective community-based study of over 500 families found that children whose parents reported a large number of painful incidents during the 1-week study period were more likely to also report a large number of painful incidents themselves (Goodman et al. 1997). The simple aggregation of pain complaints and problems among family members is not sufficient to show that family factors play a causal role in their etiology (Goodman et al. 1994). Aggregation of pain complaints in families may occur due to biological factors such as genetics or other shared lifestyle factors such as nutrition (Goodman et al. 1997). However, this research does highlight the family as a worthwhile context to consider in children's pain experiences.

Children may learn how to interpret symptoms of pain and determine what type of response is appropriate by observing how parents respond to their own episodes of pain. Some support for this mechanism comes from studies that have demonstrated that children with recurrent pain of unknown medical origin are more likely to have been exposed to salient "pain models" than are children with pain that has an identified organic basis (Routh and Ernst 1984; Osborne et al. 1989; Robinson et al. 1990). For example, Osborne et al. (1989) interviewed 20 children with recurrent unexplained pain and 20 children with recurrent explained pain secondary to sickle cell anemia, as well as their parents, to determine the presence of models of pain or illness behavior in the child's environment. The children with unexplained pain identified more pain models than did children with explained pain. Individuals most commonly identified as "pain models" were parents, followed by siblings, classmates, and other extended family members. In addition, children perceived the frequency and intensity of their own pain to be similar to their models' pain experiences. A study comparing the responses of healthy children and juvenile arthritis patients and their parents to the cold pressor task found remarkable similarity in terms of pain threshold, intensity, and tolerance between parents and children (Thastum et al. 1997). The results of these studies, and others (Routh and Ernst 1984; Robinson et al. 1990; Merlijn et al. 2003), appear to support a social learning perspective by indicating that "pain models" are present in the daily environment of children who develop functional pains, and that the children's experience of these pains closely follows that of their identified model. In addition to the pain-specific research, similar studies examining children's adjustment to more general medical conditions like diabetes have supported the importance of familial modeling influences (e.g., Turkat 1982).

Chronic pain conditions are highly prevalent among adults (Blyth et al. 2001). As a result, it is reasonable to assume that a large number of children are raised by parents for whom chronic pain and pain-related disability play a significant role. Because of the power of social learning influences in shaping children's pain responses, children of adults with chronic pain might represent an at-risk population for developing pain and possibly other difficulties. A number of studies have attempted to describe the health and wellbeing of children of parents with chronic pain (Chaturvedi and Kanakalatha 1988; Dura and Beck 1988; Rickard 1988; Mikail and von Baeyer 1990; Chun et al. 1993; Roy et al. 1994). While the results of these studies are restricted due to various methodological limitations, such as small sample size and reliance on parent report (Chambers and Smith 2002), the findings generally indicate that children of parents with chronic pain appear at risk for a variety of somatic, behavioral, and emotional issues. However, studies differ in the specific variables identified to be problematic for these children. For the most part, studies have ignored the role of parental disability, which may be a more powerful predictor of child adjustment than the parents' type, intensity, and frequency of pain. Study of the children of adults with chronic pain provides an important context for advancing knowledge regarding the role of the family in pediatric pain. Additional research addressing previous methodological limitations could inform the creation of programs to prevent the development of pain and disability among children of adults with chronic pain.

HOW PARENTAL BEHAVIOR AFFECTS CHILDREN WITH CHRONIC PAIN

This chapter has described the powerful role parents play in influencing children's acute pain. Given that chronic pain conditions often consist of a series of recurring acutely painful incidents such as repeated headaches or stomachaches, parental behavior should also play an important role in pediatric chronic pain. Parent-child interactions are transactional in their nature, and child-to-parent and reciprocating effects often occur over time with many pathways of influence. When considering the families of children with chronic pain, researchers have studied many potentially important variables, including family functioning, parenting practices, parent characteristics, and parent behaviors.

Research examining the family functioning of children with chronic pain has generally found poorer family environments than for children without chronic pain. For example, one study found that the family atmosphere of children with tension-type headache was more often unhappy and that the relationship between parents was more often distant (Aromaa et al. 2000). Other studies have found that adolescents who perceived their families as disorganized and less cohesive were more likely to report somatic complaints (Terre and Ghiselli 1997). Among children with painful gastrointestinal disorders, family factors such as marital dysfunction, triangulation, enmeshment, overprotection, rigidity, conflict avoidance, and poor conflict resolution were highly predictive of disease activity (Wood et al. 1989). Family environment is also correlated with the health status of adolescents with juvenile fibromyalgia (Schanberg et al. 1998) and with pain among children with juvenile rheumatoid arthritis (Ross et al. 1993). However, not all studies find differences in family functioning when comparing children with chronic pain to those who are pain-free, and these studies are often correlational in nature, limiting conclusions in regard to causality. For example, Brace and colleagues (2000) found no significant difference among their samples of children with chronic fatigue syndrome, juvenile rheumatoid arthritis, and healthy controls on measures of family cohesion, adaptability, or family type. In terms of parenting styles, some evidence shows that parents may excuse children's misbehavior when children exhibit symptoms of physical illness, particularly when the physical symptoms are associated with a medical diagnosis (Walker and Van Slyke 1995). Certain parent characteristics, such as the parents' physical state and their own method of coping with pain, are related to disability among children with fibromyalgia (Reid et al. 1997).

Most research examining the role of the family in pediatric chronic pain has focused on assessment and exploration of parent behaviors that occur specifically in response to children's chronic pains, particularly recurrent abdominal pain. As a result, the remainder of this section will be devoted to a review of this literature. Given that epidemiological studies indicate that recurrent pains are commonplace for children (Goodman and McGrath 1991), one might expect that parent-child interactions during these pain episodes would provide a primary arena for the socialization of pain responses in children. Children's pain responses may become subject to principles of reinforcement, whereby the pain behavior is either positively reinforced by favorable outcomes or negatively reinforced if the pain expression leads to the removal of aversive events (Craig 1983). As the responsibility usually rests with parents to administer consequences for child behavior, both positive and negative, it follows that parents would hold considerable power in influencing their children's pain experiences. In some cases, children's pain complaints may serve to distract the family from other problems or provide parents with the opportunity to spend "special time" with their children (Minuchin et al. 1978). To reflect its potentially powerful impact on children's pain experiences, parental reinforcement of pain behavior has been hypothesized as a critical factor that might discriminate between children with pain conditions who become disabled by their pain, as opposed to those children who either recover from the pain or learn to cope effectively (Walker 1999). An early study to examine such issues was conducted by Dunn-Geier et al. (1986), who investigated differences in mother-child interactions between a group of 10 adolescents who were coping well with chronic benign intractable pain and a group of 10 adolescents (matched as to age, sex, and pain location) who were not coping well. "Copers" and "non-copers" were classified based on school attendance. Mother-child interaction was videotaped during a 15-minute interaction task in which the adolescent was asked to engage in physical exercise (e.g., sit-ups, step-ups, and arm curls) under the mother's supervision. Mother-child interaction was scored using a variation of Mash and Terdal's (1981) response class matrix, which provides information about the antecedents and consequences of a given behavior. Results showed that "non-copers" had mothers who were significantly more likely to exhibit behavior that discouraged the adolescents' efforts at coping with the exercise task and were generally over-involved with their children's behavior. The authors concluded in their discussion that, "although these results do not demonstrate a causal relationship between parent-child interactions and coping, the data are consistent with the clinical impression that parental behavior may influence child coping" (Dunn-Geier et al. 1986). A social learning perspective emphasizing reinforcement of sick role behavior and a family systems approach that included unhealthy enmeshment are both supportable with these data.

Another investigation examined environmental consequences of pain among a sample of 20 children with recurrent unexplained pain and 20 children with recurrent medically explained pain (Osborne et al. 1989). The school-aged children were asked two questions about the positive and negative consequences of their pain: (1) "What do other people do for you when you have your pain?" and (2) "What things that you like to do does the pain keep you from doing?" The responses of each child to both questions were categorized by trained raters as either being positive consequences, negative consequences, or neutral consequences. Positive consequences were defined as those that would increase the probability of the behavior being repeated, while negative consequences were defined as those that would decrease the probability of the behavior being repeated. Neutral consequences were defined as those that would not clearly lead to a change in the probability that the behavior would be repeated. Children with explained pain were more likely to report negative consequences of their pain, while children with unexplained pain were more likely to report positive or neutral consequences. Using the same questions, parents were also interviewed regarding what they felt were the consequences of their children's pain; their responses yielded a similar pattern of results. While the interview did not ask children to specify who was responsible for administering consequences, it seems reasonable to assume, given the nature of the consequences provided (e.g., being allowed to stay home from school), that parents were generally responsible for making these decisions.

In an attempt to better quantify parental responses to child illness and pain behavior, Walker and Zeman (1992) developed the Illness Behaviour Encouragement Scale (IBES), a 12-item measure of parental responses to children's episodes of pain and other illness behaviors. Examples of items on this scale include: "How often do you let your child stay home from school when he/she has (symptom)?" and "How often do you spend more time than usual with your child when he/she has (symptom)?" The items all reflect reinforcement or encouragement of sick role behavior. A child form was also created to obtain child perceptions of the degree to which their parents engaged in the various actions that encouraged pain and illness behavior. In their initial validation study (Walker and Zeman 1992), the measure was administered to a sample of 58 pediatric patients ranging in age from 9 to 12 years and their mothers, along with a series of other questionnaires. Parents and children completed the IBES twice, once in response to times when the children experienced symptoms of the common cold and once when they experienced gastrointestinal pains. Results showed significant positive correlations between children's and mothers' reports on the IBES, suggesting that mothers and children had similar perceptions of parental encouragement of sick role behaviors during episodes of child pain and illness. Further, correlations between IBES scores and scores on other measures of illness behavior for colds and gastrointestinal symptoms tended to be positive and significant, providing further evidence for the construct validity of the IBES.

In a second study, described in the same paper, Walker and Zeman (1992) used the IBES in a community sample of 7–17-year-old children to evaluate the extent to which child age and gender, parent gender, and type of child illness influenced parental encouragement of child illness behavior. Girls reported more parental encouragement of their pain and illness behavior than did boys. Further, children perceived mothers and fathers to be similar in their encouragement of illness behavior for colds, but mothers were perceived to encourage illness behavior for gastrointestinal symptoms and pain significantly more than fathers. Analyses using parent IBES scores revealed similar patterns of results, with the exception that parents' reports of illness behavior encouragement did not vary as a function of the gender of the child. The lack of parent-rated corroboration of differential illness behavior encouragement among girls in comparison to boys could be interpreted as indicating that, although the frequency with which parents encourage illness behavior in girls and boys may not differ, girls may be more aware of and sensitive to their parents' behavior. The authors concluded that the IBES, and other applications of social learning theory to the study of parent-child interaction during child illness and pain episodes, should be used to identify parental behaviors that could be effectively targeted in promoting child health. Interesting recent research has found that child characteristics such as low self-worth and poor academic competence may influence the effect of social factors, such as family encouragement of illness, on symptom maintenance (Walker et al. 2002).

In an additional study, Walker and colleagues (1993) examined parental encouragement of illness behavior, using the IBES, among a sample of pediatric patients with recurrent abdominal pain (RAP), patients with peptic disease (a painful condition), patients with psychiatric disorders, and a group of healthy children. Results showed that children with RAP and children with peptic disease reported receiving more encouragement for pain-related behavior (e.g., responding with increased attention and special privileges to symptom complaints) in comparison to children in the psychiatric or healthy group. The investigators concluded that operant learning may have played a role in the onset or maintenance of illness behavior in the RAP and peptic disease patients. However, they also acknowledged that "additional work is needed to examine the extent to which these parental behaviours are causes versus consequences of child behaviours" (Walker et al. 1993).

In summary, positive consequences of pain (Osborne et al. 1989) and parental discouragement of adaptive coping (Dunn-Geier et al. 1986) have been associated with the presence of unexplained pains and difficulties coping effectively with chronic pains. The research by Walker and Zeman (1992) adds to our knowledge of parental responses to child pain behavior by showing that the degree to which parents engage in reinforcement of pediatric symptoms varies as a function of the child's gender, the parent's gender, and the type of symptom being examined. Although most research has been conducted for recurrent abdominal pain, some evidence indicates that parental behavior may play a similar role in pediatric headache (Wall et al. 1997, 1998). However, a recent study examining psychosocial factors associated with chronic pain in adolescents (e.g., headache, back, limb, and abdominal pain) found that the chronic pain group reported less reinforcement for their pain behavior than did a pain-free control group (Merlijn et al. 2003). The study of parent-child interactions in pediatric chronic pain has relied almost exclusively on children's and parent's self-reports of parental behaviors. Because parent reports of children's pain behavior may not be valid (Cohen et al. 2000), descriptive research using observational methods of family assessment is greatly needed. However, the studies using the IBES strongly suggest that reinforcement of sick role behaviors by parents in an important factor in child pain.

THE IMPACT OF PAIN ON THE FAMILY

While it has been long recognized that serious pediatric conditions, such as childhood cancer, can have a significant impact on the family and increase caregiver burden associated with pain (Ferrell et al. 1993, 1994; Hoekstra-Weebers et al. 1998), only recently have researchers turned their attention to the impact of pediatric chronic pain on the family. Parents of children with chronic conditions must face a number of common adaptive tasks, including accepting the condition, managing it on a day-to-day basis, meeting the child's normal developmental needs, and coping with ongoing stress and periodic crises (Canam 1993). The families of children with chronic pain experience similar stressors. Although most chronic pain conditions are not life-threatening, for those children whose chronic pain is associated with no identified organic cause, the uncertainty regarding the etiology of their pain can be distressing for families. While parents commonly report that their children's pain interferes the most with school, sports, and leisure activities, a significant number of parents also report that pediatric chronic pain interferes with family outings (Bennett et al. 2000). Many parents also indicate that they have had to take time off from their own work and incur costs such as parking and other travel costs to accommodate multiple medical appointments to investigate and treat their children's pain (Bennett et al. 2000). A series of studies by Hunfeld and colleagues (2001, 2002b) reveals that mothers of adolescents with severe chronic pain report significant restrictions in their family's social life, family problems coping with the adolescent's pain, and personal strain as a result of the pain. Moreover, there is evidence that the impact of pain on the family remain stable even after several years (Hunfeld et al. 2002a). Clinicians working with children with chronic pain should be attentive to the potential family burden associated with caring for a child with chronic pain.

INTERVENTIONS WITH PARENTS FOR CHILDREN WITH CHRONIC PAIN

Many treatment programs have been developed to assist children with chronic pain (Holden et al. 1999; Janicke and Finney 1999; Walco et al. 1999). However, only a handful of studies examining the treatment of pediatric chronic pain have incorporated a parent training component. The inclusion of parent training seems to have arisen from clinical observations and an appreciation for the evidence, reviewed above, highlighting the importance of family functioning in influencing children's chronic pain. Indeed, several treatment researchers have emphasized that pain often serves to remove children from undesirable situations (e.g., school) or bring about desirable outcomes (e.g., parental attention), and that parents often are responsible for making decisions about, and administering, these consequences (Masek et al. 1984). Therefore, decreasing the frequency of child pain behaviors by changing the interaction patterns that are reinforcing the pain behaviors would be a logical step in a comprehensive pediatric pain treatment program. Parents generally acknowledge the contribution of psychosocial factors to their children's pain and as a result are often receptive to behavioral interventions (Claar and Walker 1999). General guidelines for modifying parental behavior in response to their children's pain often include such suggestions as: "provide frequent approval for maintaining normal activity" and "ignore excessive complaining, pain gestures, and requests for special treatment and assistance" (Masek et al. 1984).

Given the multitude of factors that contribute to children's pain, it is not surprising that the data suggest that pharmacological treatment alone is effective with only a minority of pediatric patients (Ramsden et al. 1983). While treatment outcome studies have typically included modifications in parent behavior as part of a larger package (e.g., relaxation, biofeedback), research has generally indicated that operant pain behavior management on the part of the parents is an effective adjunct method of treating pediatric pain conditions like migraine and recurrent abdominal pain (Mehegan et al. 1987; Sanders et al. 1989; Allen and McKeen 1991; Beames et al. 1992). For example, Sanders et al. (1994) compared a cognitive-behavioral family intervention to standard care among a sample of 7–14-year-old children with recurrent abdominal pain. The family intervention consisted of six sessions that included an explanation of RAP and a rationale for pain management procedures, contingency management training for parents, and self-management training for children. The authors found that children who received the family intervention had a higher rate of complete elimination of pain, lower levels of relapse at 6- and 12-month follow-up, and lower levels of interference with their activities as a result of pain (Sanders et al. 1994, 1996).

Similarly, Allen and Shriver (1998) explored the use of parent-mediated pain behavior management strategies as an adjunct to the biofeedback treatment of children with headaches. They randomly assigned 27 children between the ages of 7 and 18 years who met diagnostic criteria for migraine headache either to a biofeedback-only treatment group or to a biofeedback group that also included pain behavior management guidelines for parents. These guidelines included encouraging independent management of children's pain, encouraging normal activity during pain episodes, eliminating status checks, reducing parental response to pain behavior, reducing pharmacological dependence, treating pain requiring a reduction in activity as illness (e.g., requiring bed rest), and recruiting other family members to follow the same guidelines. These guidelines primarily involve positive reinforcement of healthy coping, elimination of reinforcement, and mild punishment of sick role behavior. Although no direct measures of parental compliance with treatment were obtained, results showed that children in both treatment groups improved, but that the children whose parents were assigned to follow the pain behavior management strategies were more likely to experience clinically significant improvements in headache activity, were more likely to be headache free, and showed better levels of adaptive functioning at a 3-month follow-up in comparison to children who received only the biofeedback treatment (Allen and Shriver 1998).

In summary, involving parents in the treatment of pediatric chronic pain is important in influencing positive outcome and in the maintenance of treatment gains. In addition to their involvement in the treatment of chronic pains such as headache and recurrent abdominal pain, parents also can play a key role in interventions targeting disease-related pain in children, such as juvenile rheumatoid arthritis (Barlow et al. 1999; Andre et al. 2002).

FAMILY AS AN IMPORTANT CONTEXT FOR PEDIATRIC PAIN

The family is an important context to bear in mind when considering pediatric pain. The family is involved in caring and responding to their children's pain across their development and in many different settings. Parents can exert both positive and negative influences on children's pain, and it is the responsibility of researchers and clinicians who work with children in pain to develop an appreciation and awareness of the complexities of parent-child interactions and how family relationships may influence, or be influenced by, children's pain. A broad social learning perspective, with an emphasis on modeling, reinforcement, and family systems can be helpful in understanding family influences on children's pain. Future research is clearly needed to advance our knowledge regarding the role of the family in pediatric pain in several important areas that have been highlighted throughout this chapter. The family is only one of many factors that play an important role in determining children's pain experiences. The potentially interactive effects of family aspects with other factors such as genetics, individual child characteristics, and broader societal influences remain to be explored.

ACKNOWLEDGMENTS

Dr. Chambers was supported by career awards from the Canadian Institutes of Health Research and the Michael Smith Foundation for Health Research during the preparation of this manuscript. Thanks are extended to Kelly Smith, Tara Mulldoon, and Kelly Hayton for their assistance with the preparation of this chapter and to Dr. Leora Kuttner, Dr. Carl von Baeyer, and Dr. Ken Craig for their comments on drafts of this manuscript.

REFERENCES

Allen KD, McKeen LR. Home-based multicomponent treatment of pediatric migraine. *Headache* 1991; 31:467–472.

Allen KD, Shriver MD. Role of parent-mediated pain behavior management strategies in biofeedback treatment of childhood migraines. *Behav Ther* 1998; 29:477–490.

American Academy of Pediatrics and American Pain Society. The assessment and management of acute pain in infants, children, and adolescents. American Academy of Pediatrics Committee on Psychosocial Aspects of Child and Family Health and American Pain Society Task Force on Pain in Infants, Children, and Adolescents. *Pediatrics* 2001; 108:793–797.

American Pain Society. *Pediatric Chronic Pain*. Glenview: American Pain Society, 2001.

Andre M, Hagelberg S, Stenstrom CH. Education in the management of juvenile chronic arthritis. *Scand J Rheumatol* 2002; 30:323–327.

Apley J. *The Child with Abdominal Pains*. Oxford: Blackwell Scientific, 1975.
Apley J, Naish N. Recurrent abdominal pains: a field survey of 1,000 school children. *Arch Dis Child* 1958; 33:165–170.
Aromaa M, Sillanpaa M, Rautava P, Helenius H. Pain experience of children with headache and their families: a controlled study. *Pediatrics* 2000; 106:270–275.
Baines D, Overton JH. Parental presence at induction of anaesthesia: a survey of N.S.W. hospitals and tertiary paediatric hospitals in Australia. *Anaesth Intensive Care* 1995; 23:191–195.
Barlow JH, Shaw KL, Harrison K. Consulting the 'experts': children's and parents' perceptions of psycho-educational interventions in the context of juvenile chronic arthritis. *Health Educ Res* 1999; 14:597–610.
Bauchner H, Waring C, Vinci R. Parental presence during procedures in an emergency room: results from 50 observations. *Pediatrics* 1991; 87:544–548.
Bauchner H, Vinci R, Bak S, Pearson C, Corwin MJ. Parents and procedures: a randomized controlled trial. *Pediatrics* 1996; 98:861–867.
Beames L, Sanders MR, Bor W. The role of parent training in the cognitive behavioral treatment of children's headaches. *Behav Psychother* 1992; 20:167–180.
Bennett SM, Hunstman E, Lilley CM. Parent perceptions of the impact of chronic pain in children and adolescents. *Child Health Care* 2000; 29:147–159.
Bennett-Branson SM, Craig KD. Postoperative pain in children: developmental and family influences on spontaneous coping strategies. *Can J Behav Sci* 1993; 25:355–383.
Bevan JC, Johnston C, Haig MJ, et al. Preoperative parental anxiety predicts behavioural and emotional responses to induction of anaesthesia in children. *Can J Anesth* 1990; 37:177–182.
Blount RL, Corbin SM, Sturges JW, et al. The relationship between adult's behavior and child coping and distress during BMA LP procedures: a sequential analysis. *Behav Ther* 1989; 20:585–601.
Blount RL, Sturges JW, Powers SW. Analysis of child and adult behavioral variations by phase of medical procedure. *Behav Ther* 1990; 21:33–48.
Blount RL, Landolffritsche B, Powers SW, Sturges JW. Differences between high and low coping children and between parent and staff behaviors during painful medical procedures. *J Pediatr Psychol* 1991; 16:795–809.
Blount RL, Bachanas PJ, Powers SW, et al. Training children to cope and parents to coach them during routine immunizations: effects of child, parent and staff behaviours. *Behav Ther* 1992; 23:689–705.
Blount RL, Cohen LL, Frank NC, et al. The Child-Adult Medical Procedure Interaction Scale-Revised: an assessment of validity. *J Pediatr Psychol* 1997; 22:73–88.
Blount RL, Bunke V, Cohen LL, Forbes CJ. The Child-Adult Medical Procedure Interaction Scale-Short Form (CAMPIS-SF): validation of a rating scale for children's and adults' behaviors during painful medical procedures. *J Pain Symptom Manage* 2001; 22:591–599.
Blyth FM, March LM, Brnabic AJM, et al. Chronic pain in Australia: a prevalence study. *Pain* 2001; 89:127–134.
Bosenberg AT, Williams GD, Reddy D. Attitudes towards parental presence at induction of anaesthesia. *S Afr Med J* 1996; 86:664–667.
Brace MJ, Smith MS, McCauley E, Sherry DD. Family reinforcement of illness behavior: a comparison of adolescents with chronic fatigue syndrome, juvenile arthritis, and healthy controls. *Dev Behav Pediatr* 2000; 21:332–339.
Braude N, Ridley SA, Sumner E. Parents and paediatric anaesthesia: a prospective survey of parental attitudes to their presence at induction. *Ann R Coll Surg Engl* 1990; 72:41–44.
Broome ME, Endsley R. Parent and child behavior during immunization. *Pain* 1989; 37:85–92.
Bru G, Carmody S, Donohue-Sword B, Bookbinder M. Parental visitation in the post-anesthesia care unit: a means to lessen anxiety. *Child Health Care* 1993; 22:217–226.

Bush JP, Melamed BG, Sheras PL, Greenbaum PE. Mother-child patterns of coping with anticipatory medical stress. *Health Psychol* 1986; 5:137–157.

Cameron JA, Bond MJ, Pointer SC. Reducing the anxiety of children undergoing surgery: parental presence during anaesthetic induction. *J Paediatr Child Health* 1996; 32:51–56.

Canam C. Common adaptive tasks facing parents of children with chronic conditions. *J Adv Nurs* 1993; 18:46–53.

Caty S, Ritchie JA, Ellerton M. Helping hospitalized preschoolers manage stressful situations: the mother's role. *Child Health Care* 1989; 18:202–209.

Chambers CT, Smith KB. Children of parents with chronic pain: an at-risk population? *Pediatr Pain Lett* 2002; 6:1–5.

Chambers CT, Reid GJ, McGrath PJ, Finley GA. Development and preliminary validation of a postoperative pain measure for parents. *Pain* 1996; 68:307–313.

Chambers CT, Reid GJ, McGrath PJ, Finley GA, Ellerton ML. A randomized trial of a pain education booklet: effects on parents attitudes and postoperative pain management. *Child Health Care* 1997; 26:1–13.

Chambers CT, Reid GJ, Craig KD, McGrath PJ, Finley GA. Agreement between child and parent reports of pain. *Clin J Pain* 1998; 14:336–342.

Chambers CT, Craig KD, Bennett SM. The impact of maternal behavior on children's pain experiences: an experimental analysis. *J Pediatr Psychol* 2002; 27:293–301.

Chambers CT, Finley GA, McGrath PJ, Walsh TM. The Parents' Postoperative Pain Measure: replication and extension to 2- to 6-year-old children. *Pain;* in press.

Chaturvedi SK, Kanakalatha P. Pain in children of chronic pain patients. *Pain Clinic* 1988; 2:195–199.

Chun DY, Turner JA, Romano JM. Children of chronic pain patients: risk factors for maladjustment. *Pain* 1993; 52:311–317.

Claar RL, Walker LS. Maternal attributions for the causes and remedies of their children's abdominal pain. *J Pediatr Psychol* 1999; 24:345–354.

Cohen LL, Manimala R, Blount RL. Easier said than done: what parents say they do and what they do during children's immunizations. *Child Health Care* 2000; 29:79–86.

Cohen LL, Bernard RS, Greco LA, McClellan CB. A child-focused intervention for coping with procedural pain: are parent and nurse coaches necessary? *J Pediatr Psychol* 2002; 27:749–757.

Craig KD. Modeling and social learning factors in chronic pain. In: Bonica JJ, Lindblom U, Iggo A (Eds). *Proceedings of the Third World Congress on Pain,* Advances in Pain Research and Therapy, Vol. 5. New York: Raven Press, 1983, pp 813–827.

Craig KD. Social modeling influences: pain in context. In: Sternbach RA (Ed). *The Psychology of Pain.* New York: Raven Press, 1986, pp 67–95.

Curtis CP. *Bud, not Buddy.* New York: Delacorte Press, 1999.

Dahlquist LM, Power TG, Carlson L. Physician and parent behavior during invasive pediatric cancer procedures: relationships to child behavioral distress. *J Pediatr Psychol* 1995; 20:477–490.

Dahlquist LM, Busby SM, Slifer KJ, et al. Distraction for children of different ages who undergo repeated needle sticks. *J Pediatr Oncol Nurs* 2002; 19:22–34.

Demyttenaere S, Finley GA, Johnston CC, McGrath PJ. Pain treatment thresholds in children following minor surgery. *Clin J Pain* 2001; 17:173–177.

Diniaco MJ, Ingoldsby BB. Parental presence in the recovery room. *AORN J* 1983; 38:685–693.

Doctor ME. Parent participation during painful wound care procedures. *J Burn Care Rehabil* 1994; 15:288–292.

Dunn-Geier BJ, McGrath PJ, Rourke BP, Latter J, D'Astous J. Adolescent chronic pain: the ability to cope. *Pain* 1986; 26:23–32.

Dura JR, Beck SJ. A comparison of family functioning when mothers have chronic pain. *Pain* 1988; 35:79–89.

Ehde DM, Holm JE, Metzger DL. The role of family structure, functioning, and pain modeling in headache. *Headache* 1991; 31:35–40.
Ellerton M, Merriam C. Preparing children and families psychologically for day surgery: an evaluation. *J Adv Nurs* 1994; 19:1057–1062.
Felt BT, Mollen E, Diaz S, et al. Behavioral interventions reduce infant distress at immunization. *Arch Pediatr Adolesc Med* 2000; 154:719–724.
Fenlon WL, Dobbs AR, Curzon MEJ. Parental presence during treatment of the child patient: a study with British patients. *Br Dent J* 1993; 174:23–28.
Ferrell B, Rhiner M, Rivera LM. Development and evaluation of the family pain questionnaire. *J Psychosoc Oncol* 1993; 10:21–35.
Ferrell BR, Rhiner M, Shapiro B, Strause L. The family experience of cancer pain management in children. *Cancer Practice* 1994; 2:441–446.
Finley GA, McGrath PJ (Eds). *Acute and Procedure Pain in Infants and Children,* Progress in Pain Research and Management, Vol. 20. Seattle: IASP Press, 2001.
Finley GA, McGrath PJ, Forward SP, McNeill G, Fitzgerald P. Parents' management of children's pain following 'minor' surgery. *Pain* 1996; 64:83–87.
Finley GA, Chambers CT, McGrath PJ, Walsh T. Construct validity of the Parents' Postoperative Pain Measure. *Clin J Pain;* in press.
Flor H, Turk DC, Rudy TE. Pain and families. II. Assessment and treatment. *Pain* 1987; 30:29–45.
Forward SP, Brown TL, McGrath PJ. Mothers' attitudes and behavior toward medicating children's pain. *Pain* 1996; 67:469–474.
Frank NC, Blount RL, Smith AJ, Manimala MR, Martin JK. Parent and staff behavior, previous child medical experience, and maternal anxiety as they relate to child procedural distress and coping. *J Pediatr Psychol* 1995; 20:277–289.
Gedaly-Duff V, Ziebarth D. Mothers' management of adenoid-tonsillectomy pain in 4- to 8-year-olds: a preliminary study. *Pain* 1994; 57:299.
Glazebrook CP, Lim E, Sheard CE, Standen PJ. Child temperament and reaction to induction of anaesthesia: implications for maternal presence in the anaesthetic room. *Psychol Health* 1994; 10:55–67.
Gonzalez JC, Routh DK, Armstrong FD. Effects of maternal distraction versus reassurance on children's reactions to injections. *J Pediatr Psychol* 1993; 18:593–604.
Goodenough B, Thomas W, Champion GD, et al. Unravelling age effects and sex differences in needle pain: ratings of sensory intensity and unpleasantness of venipuncture pain by children and their parents. *Pain* 1999; 80:179–190.
Goodman JE, McGrath PJ. The epidemiology of pain in children and adolescents: a review. *Pain* 1991; 46:247–264.
Goodman JE, Gidron Y, McGrath PJ. Pain proneness in children: toward a new conceptual framework. In: Grzesiak RC, Ciccone DS (Eds). *Psychological Vulnerability to Chronic Pain.* New York: Springer, 1994, pp 90–115.
Goodman JE, McGrath PJ, Forward SP. Aggregation of pain complaints and pain-related disability and handicap in a community sample of families. In: Jensen TS, Turner JA, Wiesenfeld-Hallin Z (Eds). *Proceedings of the 8th World Congress on Pain,* Progress in Pain Research and Management, Vol. 8. Seattle: IASP Press,1997, pp 673–682.
Haimi-Cohen Y, Amir J, Harel L, Straussberg R, Varsano Y. Parental presence during lumbar puncture: anxiety and attitude toward the procedure. *Clin Pediatr* 1996; 35:2–4.
Hall PA, Payne JF, Stack CG, Stokes MA. Parents in the recovery room: survey of parental and staff attitudes. *BMJ* 1995; 310:163–164.
Hannallah RS. Who benefits when parents are present during anaesthesia induction in their children? *Can J Anesth* 1994; 41:271–275.
Hannallah RS, Rosales JK. Experience with parents' presence during anaesthesia induction in children. *Can Anaesth Soc J* 1983; 30:286–289.
Henderson MA, Baines DB, Overton JH. Parental attitudes to presence at induction of paediatric anaesthesia. *Anaesth Intensive Care* 1993; 21:324–327.

Hertzman M, Williams J, Sigafoos A, et al. The family in chronic pain. *Psychiatr Forum* 1989:24–36.

Hickmott KC, Shaw EA, Goodyer I, Baker RD. Anaesthetic induction in children: the effects of maternal presence on mood and subsequent behaviour. *Eur J Anaesthesiol* 1989; 6:145–155.

Hoekstra-Weebers J, Heuvel F, Jaspers JPC, Kamps WA, Klip EC. Brief report: an intervention program for parents of pediatric cancer patients: a randomized controlled trial. *J Pediatr Psychol* 1998; 23:207–214.

Holden EW, Deichmann MM, Levy JD. Empirically supported treatments in pediatric psychology: recurrent pediatric headache. *J Pediatr Psychol* 1999; 24:91–109.

Hunfeld JAM, van der Wouden JC, den Deurwaarder ESG, van Suijlekom-Smit LWA, Hazebroek-Kampschreur AAJM. Measuring chronic pain in children: an exploration. *Percept Mot Skills* 1997; 84:1176–1178.

Hunfeld JAM, Perquin CW, Duivenvoorden HJ, et al. Chronic pain and its impact on quality of life in adolescents and their families. *J Pediatr Psychol* 2001; 26:145–153.

Hunfeld JAM, Perquin CW, Bertina W, et al. Stability of pain parameters and pain-related quality of life in adolescents with persistent pain: a three-year follow-up. *Clin J Pain* 2002a; 18:99–106.

Hunfeld JAM, Perquin CW, Hazebroek-Kampschreur AAJM, et al. Physically unexplained chronic pain and its impact on children and their families: the mother's perception. *Psychol Psychother* 2002b; 75:251–260.

Jacobsen PB, Manne SL, Gorfinkle K, et al. Analysis of child and parent behavior during painful medical procedures. *Health Psychol* 1990; 9:559–576.

Janicke DM, Finney JW. Empirically supported treatments in pediatric psychology: recurrent abdominal pain. *J Pediatr Psychol* 1999; 24:115–127.

Jay SM, Elliott CH. A stress inoculation program for parents whose children are undergoing painful medical procedures. *J Consult Clin Psychol* 1990; 58:799–804.

Johnson A, Lindschau A. Staff attitudes toward parent participation in the care of children who are hospitalized. *Pediatr Nurs* 1996; 22:99–102.

Johnston CC, Bevan JC, Haig MJ, Kirnon V, Tousignant G. Parental presence during anesthesia induction: a research study. *AORN J* 1988; 47:187–194.

Kain ZN. Parental presence during induction of anaesthesia. *Paediatr Anaesth* 1995; 5:209–212.

Kain ZN, Ferris CA, Mayes LC, Rimar S. Parental presence during induction of anaesthesia: practice differences between the United States and Great Britain. *Paediatr Anaesth* 1996a; 6:187–193.

Kain ZN, Mayes L, Caramico LA, et al. Parental presence during induction of anesthesia: a randomized controlled trial. *Anesthesiology* 1996b; 84:1060–1067.

Kain ZN, Mayes L, Wang S-M, Caramico LA, Hofstadter MB. Parental presence during induction of anesthesia versus sedative premedication: which intervention is more effective? *Anesthesiology* 1998; 89:1147–1156.

Kain ZN, Mayes LC, Wang S-M, et al. Parental presence and a sedative premedicant for children undergoing surgery: a hierarchical study. *Anesthesiology* 2000; 92:939–946.

Kain ZN, Caldwell-Andrews AA, Mayes LC, et al. Parental presence during induction of anesthesia: physiological effects on parents. *Anesthesiology* 2003; 98:58–64.

Kazak AE, Penati B, Boyer BA, et al. A randomized controlled prospective outcome study of a psychological and pharmacological intervention protocol for procedural distress in pediatric leukemia. *J Pediatr Psychol* 1996a; 21:615–631.

Kazak AE, Penati B, Waibel MK, Blackall GF. The Perception of Procedures Questionnaire: psychometric properties of a brief parent report measure of procedural distress. *J Pediatr Psychol* 1996b; 21:195–207.

Kazak AE, Penati B, Brophy P, Himelstein B. Pharmacologic and psychologic interventions for procedural pain. *Pediatrics* 1998; 102:59–66.

Kerns RD. Family therapy for adults with chronic pain. In: Gatchel RJ, Turk DC (Eds). *Psychosocial Factors in Pain.* New York: Guilford Press, 1999, pp. 445–456.

Kerns RD, Weiss LH. Family influences on the course of chronic illness: a cognitive-behavioral transactional model. *Soc Behav Med* 1994; 16:116–121.

Khunsongkiet P, Finley GA, Chambers CT, McGrath PJ. Attempted cross-cultural validation of the Parents' Postoperative Pain Measure. *Abstracts: 9th World Congress on Pain.* Seattle: IASP Press, 1999, p 199.

Kleiber C, McCarthy AM. Parent behavior and child distress during urethral catheterization. *J Soc Pediatr Nurs* 1999; 4:95–104.

Kleiber C, Craft-Rosenberg M, Harper DC. Parents as distraction coaches during IV insertion: a randomized study. *J Pain Symptom Manage* 2001; 22:851–861.

Knight JC. Post-operative pain in children after day case surgery. *Paediatr Anaesth* 1994; 4:45–51.

Kokki A, Kankkunen P, Pietila A, Vehvilainen-Julkunen K. Validation of the Parents' Postoperative Pain Measure in Finnish children. *Scand J Caring Sci* 2003; 17:12–18.

Kristensson-Hallstrom I. Parental participation in pediatric surgical care. *AORN J* 2000; 71:1021–1029.

Kristensson-Hallstrom I, Elander G, Malmfors G. Increased parental participation in a paediatric surgical day-care unit. *J Clin Nurs* 1997; 6:297–302.

Lumley MA, Abeles LA, Melamed BG, Pistone LM, Johnson JH. Coping outcomes in children undergoing stressful medical procedures: the role of child-environmental variables. *Behav Assessment* 1990; 12:223–238.

Manimala MR, Blount RL. The effects of parental reassurance versus distraction on child distress and coping during immunizations. *Child Health Care* 2000; 29:161–177.

Manne SL, Redd WH, Jacobsen PB, Gorfinkle K, Schorr O. Behavioral intervention to reduce child and parent distress during venipuncture. *J Consult Clin Psychol* 1990; 58:565–572.

Manne SL, Bakeman R, Jacobsen PB, et al. Adult child interaction during invasive medical procedures. *Health Psychol* 1992; 11:241–249.

Manne SL, Bakeman R, Jacobsen PB, Gorfinkle K, Redd WH. An analysis of a behavioral intervention for children undergoing venipuncture. *Health Psychol* 1994; 13:556–566.

Masek BJ, Russo DC, Varni JW. Behavioral approaches to the management of chronic pain in children. *Pediatr Clin North Am* 1984; 31:1113–1131.

Mash E, Terdal L. *Behavioural Assessment of Childhood Disorders.* New York: Guilford Press, 1981.

McCormick ASM, Spargo PM. Parents in the anaesthetic room: a questionnaire survey of departments of anaesthesia. *Paediatr Anaesth* 1996; 6:183–186.

McEwen AW, Caldicott LD, Barker I. Parents in the anaesthetic room—parent's and anaesthetists' views. *Anaesthesia* 1994; 49:987–990.

Mehegan JE, Masek BJ, Harrison RH, Russo DC, Leviton A. A multicomponent behavioral treatment for pediatric migraine. *Clin J Pain* 1987; 2:191–196.

Merlijn VPBM, Hunfeld JAM, van der Wouden JC, et al. Psychosocial factors associated with chronic pain in adolescents. *Pain* 2003; 101:33–43.

Merskey H, Bogduk N (Eds). *Classification of Chronic Pain: Descriptions of Chronic Pain Syndromes and Definitions of Pain Terms,* 2nd ed. Seattle: IASP Press, 1994.

Miaskowski C, Zimmer EF, Barrett KM, Dibble SL, Wallhagen M. Differences in patients' and family caregivers' perceptions of the pain experience influence patient and caregiver outcomes. *Pain* 1997; 72:217–226.

Mikail SF, von Baeyer CL. Pain, somatic focus and emotional adjustment in children of chronic headache sufferers and controls. *Soc Sci Med* 1990; 31:51–59.

Miller AC, Johann-Murphy M, Zhelezniak V. Impact of the therapist-child dyad on children's pain and coping during medical procedures. *Dev Med Child Neurol* 2001; 43:118–123.

Miller D. Comparisons of pain ratings from postoperative children, their mothers and their nurses. *Pediatr Nurs* 1996; 22:145–149.

Minuchin S, Rosman BL, Baker L. *Psychosomatic Families*. Cambridge, MA: Harvard University Press, 1978.
Munro HM, Malviya S, Lauder GR, Voepel-Lewis T, Tait AR. Pain relief in children following outpatient surgery. *J Clin Anesth* 1999; 11:187–191.
Neill SJ. Parent participation 1: literature review and methodology. *Br J Nurs* 1996a; 5:34–40.
Neill SJ. Parent participation 2: findings and their implications for practice. *Br J Nurs* 1996b; 5:110–117.
O'Hara M, McGrath PJ, D'Astous J, Vair CA. Oral morphine versus injected meperidine (Demerol) pain relief in children after orthopedic surgery. *J Pediatr Orthop* 1987; 7:78–82.
Osborne RB, Hatcher JW, Richtsmeier AJ. The role of social modeling in unexplained pediatric pain. *J Pediatr Psychol* 1989; 14:43–61.
Palermo TM, Drotar DD, Tripi PA. Current status of psychosocial intervention research for pediatric outpatient surgery. *J Clin Psychol Med Settings* 1999; 6:405–426.
Palermo TM, Tripi PA, Burgess E. Parental presence during anaesthesia induction for outpatient surgery of the infant. *Paediatr Anaesth* 2000; 10:487–491.
Payne B, Norfleet MA. Chronic pain and the family: a review. *Pain* 1986; 26:1–22.
Peterson L, Oliver KK, Saldana L. Children's coping with stressful medical procedures. In: Wolchik SA, Sandler IN (Eds). *Handbook of Children's Coping: Linking Theory and Intervention*. New York: Plenum Press, 1997, pp. 333–360.
Powers SW. Empirically supported treatments in pediatric psychology: procedure-related pain. *J Pediatr Psychol* 1999; 24:131–145.
Powers KS, Rubenstein JS. Family presence during invasive procedures in the pediatric intensive care unit. *Arch Pediatr Adolesc Med* 1999; 153:955–958.
Powers SW, Blount RL, Bachanas PJ, Cotter MW, Swan SC. Helping preschool leukemia patients and parents cope during injections. *J Pediatr Psychol* 1993; 18:681–695.
Pringle B, Hilley L, Gelfand K, et al. Decreasing child distress during needle sticks and maintaining treatment gains over time. *J Clin Psychol Med Settings* 2001; 8:119–130.
Ramsden R, Friedman B, Williamson D. Treatment of childhood headache reports with contingency management procedures. *J Clin Child Psychol* 1983; 12:202–206.
Redinbaugh EM, Baum A, DeMoss C, Fello M, Arnold R. Factors associated with the accuracy of family caregiver estimates of patient pain. *J Pain Symptom Manage* 2002; 23:31–38.
Reid GJ, Hebb JPO, McGrath PJ, Finley GA, Forward SP. Cues parents use to assess postoperative pain in their children. *Clin J Pain* 1995; 11:229–235.
Reid GJ, Lang BA, McGrath PJ. Primary juvenile fibromyalgia: psychological adjustment, family functioning, coping, and functional disability. *Arthritis Rheum* 1997; 40:752–760.
Rickard K. The occurrence of maladaptive health-related behavior and teacher-rated conduct problems in children of chronic low back pain patients. *J Behav Med* 1988; 11:107–116.
Robinson JO, Alverez JH, Dodge JA. Life events and family history in children with recurrent abdominal pain. *J Psychosom Res* 1990; 34:171–181.
Roman DEM, Barker I, Reilly CS. Anaesthetists' attitudes to parental presence at induction of general anaesthesia in children. *Anaesthesia* 1993; 48:338–340.
Romsing J. Postoperative pain in children after day case surgery: children's and parent's ratings. *Eur Hosp Pharm* 1996; 2:21–23.
Romsing J, Walther-Larsen S. Postoperative pain in children: a survey of parents' expectations and perceptions of their children's pain experiences. *Paediatr Anaesth* 1996; 6:215–218.
Ross CK, Lavigne JV, Hayford JR, et al. Psychological factors affecting reported pain in juvenile rheumatoid arthritis. *J Pediatr Psychol* 1993; 18:561–573.
Routh DK, Ernst AR. Somatization disorders in relatives of children and adolescents with functional abdominal pain. *J Pediatr Psychol* 1984; 9:427–437.
Roy R. Annotation: chronic pain and the family: a review. *J Fam Ther* 1989; 11:197–204.
Roy R. Physical illness, chronic pain and family therapy. In: Roy R (Ed). *Chronic Pain: Psychosocial Factors in Rehabilitation*. Florida: Robert E. Krieger, 1990, pp 184–211.

Roy R, Thomas M, Mogilevsky I, Cook A. Influence of parental chronic pain on children: preliminary observations. *Headache Q* 1994; 5:20–26.

Royal College of Nursing. *The Recognition and Assessment of Acute Pain in Children: Recommendations: Clinical Practice Guidelines.* London: Royal College of Nursing, 1999.

Ryder IG, Spargo PM. Parents in the anaesthetic room: a questionnaire survey of parents' reactions. *Anaesthesia* 1991; 46:977–979.

Sacchetti A, Lichenstein R, Carraccio CA, Harris RH. Family member presence during pediatric emergency department procedures. *Pediatr Emerg Care* 1996; 12:268–271.

Salmon K, Pereira JK. Predicting children's response to an invasive medical investigation: the influence of effortful control and parent behaviour. *J Pediatr Psychol* 2002; 27:227–233.

Sanders MR, Rebgetz M, Morrison M, et al. Cognitive-behavioral treatment of recurrent nonspecific abdominal pain in children: an analysis of generalization, maintenance, and side effects. *J Consult Clin Psychol* 1989; 57:294–300.

Sanders MR, Shepherd RW, Cleghorn G, Woolford H. The treatment of recurrent abdominal pain in children: a controlled comparison of cognitive-behavioral family intervention and standard pediatric care. *J Consult Clin Psychol* 1994; 62:306–314.

Sanders MR, Cleghorn G, Shepherd RW, Patrick M. Predictors of clinical improvement in children with recurrent abdominal pain. *Behav Cognit Psychother* 1996; 24:27–38.

Schanberg LE, Keefe FJ, Lefebvre JC, Kredich DW, Gil KM. Social context of pain in children with juvenile primary fibromyalgia syndrome: parental pain history and family environment. *Clin J Pain* 1998; 14:107–115.

Schulman JL, Foley JM, Vernon DTA, Allan DA. A study of the effect of the mother's presence during anesthesia induction. *Pediatrics* 1967; 39:111–114.

Seid M, Varni JW. Pediatric day surgery outcomes management: the role of preoperative anxiety and a home pain management protocol. *J Clin Outcomes Manage* 1999; 6:24–30.

Shaw EG, Routh DK. Effect of mother presence on children's reaction to aversive procedures. *J Pediatr Psychol* 1982; 7:33–42.

Shin HS, Jung YY. A study on the preliminary validation of a postoperative pain measure for parents for children's pain assessment after surgery. *J Korean Acad Nurs* 2000; 30:847–856.

Simons J, Franck L, Roberson E. Parent involvement in children's pain care: views of parents and nurses. *J Adv Nurs* 2001; 36:591–599.

Snelling J. The role of the family in relation to chronic pain: review of the literature. *J Adv Nurs* 1990; 15:771–776.

Sutters KA, Miaskowski C. Inadequate pain management and associated morbidity in children at home after tonsillectomy. *J Pediatr Nurs* 1997; 12:178–185.

Sweet SD, McGrath PJ. Relative importance of mothers' versus medical staffs' behavior in the prediction of infant immunization pain behaviour. *J Pediatr Psychol* 1998; 23:249–256.

Terre L, Ghiselli W. A developmental perspective on family risk factors in somatization. *J Psych Res* 1997; 42:197–208.

Thastum M, Zachariae R, Scholer M, Bjerring P, Herlin T. Cold pressor pain: comparing responses of juvenile arthritis patients and their parents. *Scand J Rheumatol* 1997; 26:272–279.

Turk DC, Flor H, Rudy TE. Pain and families. I. Etiology, maintenance and psychosocial impact. *Pain* 1987; 30:3–27.

Turkat ID. An investigation of parental modeling in the etiology of diabetic illness behaviour. *Behav Res Ther* 1982; 20:547–552.

Turkat ID, Kuczmierczyk AR, Adams HE. An investigation of the aetiology of chronic headache: the role of headache models. *Br J Psychiatry* 1984; 145:665–666.

Vernon DTA, Foley JM, Schulman JL. Effect of mother-child separation and birth order on young children's responses to two potentially stressful experiences. *J Pers Soc Psychol* 1967; 5:162–174.

Vessey JA, Bogetz MS, Caserza CL, Liu KR, Cassidy MD. Parental upset associated with participation in induction of anaesthesia in children. *Can J Anesth* 1994; 41:276–280.

Visintainer MA, Wolfer JA. Psychological preparation for surgical pediatric patients: the effect on children's and parent's stress responses and adjustment. *Pediatrics* 1975; 56:187–202.

von Baeyer C. Presence of parents during painful procedures. *Pediatr Pain Lett* 1997; 1:56–59.

Walco GA, Sterling CM, Conte PM, Engel RG. Empirically supported treatments in pediatric psychology: disease-related pain. *J Pediatr Psychol* 1999; 24:155–167.

Walker LS. The evolution of research on recurrent abdominal pain: history, assumptions, and a conceptual model. In: McGrath PJ, Finley GA (Eds). *Chronic and Recurrent Pain in Children and Adolescents,* Progress in Pain Research and Management, Vol. 13. Seattle: IASP Press, 1999, pp 141–172.

Walker LS, Van Slyke DA. Do parents excuse the misbehavior of children with physical or emotional symptoms? An investigation of the pediatric sick role. *J Pediatr Psychol* 1995; 20:329–345.

Walker LS, Zeman JL. Parental response to child illness behaviour. *J Pediatr Psychol* 1992; 17:49–71.

Walker LS, Garber J, Greene JW. Psychosocial correlates of recurrent childhood pain: a comparison of pediatric patients with recurrent abdominal pain, organic illness, and psychiatric disorders. *J Abnorm Psychol* 1993; 102:248–258.

Walker LS, Claar RL, Garber J. Social consequences of children's pain: when do they encourage symptom maintenance? *J Pediatr Psychol* 2002; 27:689–698.

Wall BA, Holden EW, Gladstein J. Parent responses to pediatric headache. *Headache* 1997; 37:65–70.

Wall BA, Holden EW, Gladstein J. Parental response in pediatric headache. *Headache Q* 1998; 9:331–337.

While A. Personal view. *BMJ* 1985; 291:343.

Wolfer JA, Visintainer MA. Prehospital psychological preparation for tonsillectomy patients: effects on children's and parents' adjustment. *Pediatrics* 1979; 64:646–655.

Wolfram RW, Turner ED. Effects of parental presence during children's venipuncture. *Acad Emerg Med* 1996; 3:58–64.

Wolfram RW, Turner ED, Philput C. Effects of parental presence during young children's venipuncture. *Pediatr Emerg Care* 1997; 13:325–328.

Wood B, Watkins JB, Boyle JT, et al. The "psychosomatic family" model: an empirical and theoretical analysis. *Fam Process* 1989; 28:399–417.

Zelikovsky N, Rodrigue JR, Gidycz CA, Davis MA. Cognitive behavioral and behavioral interventions help young children cope during a voiding cystourethrogram. *J Pediatr Psychol* 2000; 25:535–543.

Zuckerman B, Stevenson J, Bailey V. Stomachaches and headaches in a community sample of preschool children. *Pediatrics* 1987; 79:677–682.

Correspondence to: Christine T. Chambers, PhD, Pediatric Pain Research Laboratory, IWK Health Centre, 5850 University Avenue, Halifax, NS, Canada B3J 3G9. Tel: 902-470-7702; Fax: 902-470-7709.

6

Chronic Illness and Pain in Children: A Review with Special Emphasis on Cancer

Gustaf Ljungman

Department of Children's and Women's Health, Uppsala University, and Unit for Pediatric Hematology and Oncology, University Children's Hospital, Uppsala, Sweden

CANCER IN CHILDREN

Thirty years ago almost no children with cancer could be cured (Zuelze 1966; Hoff et al. 1988; Adami et al. 1992). Therefore, the main issue in pediatric oncology has been to increase survival. The refinement of doses and schedules and the proper timing of surgery and radiotherapy in combination with rigorous evaluation of results and rational planning of treatment have led to the present situation where more than two-thirds of these children survive (Kaatsch et al. 1995; Miller et al. 1995; Stiller et al. 1995; Gustafsson et al. 1998a,b).

In industrialized countries the annual incidence rates vary from 110 to 150 cases per million children under the age of 15 and account for less than 1% of all cancer cases (Stiller and Draper 1998). This means that 1 out of 450–625 children develops cancer before the age of 15. Among childhood cancer diagnoses, one in three cases involves leukemia and one in four cases involves tumors of the central nervous system (CNS); other cases involve lymphomas, sympathetic nerve tumors, soft tissue sarcomas, bone tumors, germ cell tumors, and retinoblastomas (Parkin et al. 1988; Gustafsson et al. 1998a). On average, the duration of childhood cancer treatment is 6 months to 3 years. Cancer causes more deaths among children in the developed countries than any other disease. After accidents, it is the most common cause of death in this age group (American Cancer Society 1992).

EPIDEMIOLOGY AND ETIOLOGY OF PAIN IN CHILDREN WITH CANCER

Pain is the symptom most feared by young children with cancer (Lansky et al. 1989; Enskär et al. 1997). Despite significant advances in pain management over the recent decades, numerous studies have found that pain is still common in pediatric oncology (Miser et al. 1987a,b; McGrath et al. 1990a; Elliott et al. 1991; Ljungman et al. 1996, 1999; Collins et al. 2000, 2002) and in pediatric patients in general (Anand et al. 1987; Schechter 1989; Walco et al. 1994; Cummings et al. 1996).

Children with cancer may experience treatment-related pain resulting from the side effects of chemotherapy, tumor surgery, and radiation. Procedures such as lumbar puncture (LP), bone marrow aspiration (BMA), and biopsies also can be painful, as can the cancer itself, usually due to tumor infiltration into various organs or tissues. Treatment- and procedure-related pain dominates in the pediatric population with cancer (Miser et al. 1987a,b; McGrath et al. 1990a; Elliott et al. 1991; Ljungman et al. 1996, 1999; Collins et al. 2000, 2002), while a preponderance of tumor-related pain is found among adult patients (Coyle et al. 1990; Rawal et al. 1993; Zech et al. 1995). This difference may partly be ascribed to the aggressive, multimodality therapy regimens generally used in pediatric oncology. Furthermore, childhood malignancies show a high initial rate of response to treatment, resulting in a rapid reduction, and often disappearance, of tumor-related pain. Finally, children with unresponsive or relapsing, refractory cancer often deteriorate rapidly (Miser et al. 1987a).

A number of important studies have examined pain in children with cancer. At the pediatric branch of the National Cancer Institute, Miser and colleagues (1987b) followed 92 children and adolescents (median age 16 years) with newly diagnosed malignancy over a 26-month period. At first evaluation, 78% experienced pain that had been present for a median duration of 74 days (range 3–821 days) prior to the start of treatment, and 62% had experienced pain as the first symptom of cancer. In a second study, Miser et al. (1987a) evaluated the pain experienced by 139 children and young adults (median age 16 years). Among these, 54% of inpatients and 26% of outpatients reported some degree of pain at the time of assessment. Patients and one of the investigators rated pain intensity on a 100-mm visual analogue scale (VAS); the median score was 22 mm for inpatients and 18.5 mm for outpatients. Treatment-related pain due to mucositis, surgery, neuropathy, and infection predominated in both groups, and 35% of inpatients and 18% of outpatients reported tumor-related pain. Of patients experiencing pain, 58% of inpatients and 36% of outpatients used opioid analgesics.

In a survey of 77 outpatients (aged 2–19 years) at a pediatric oncology clinic, McGrath and colleagues (1990a) found that the incidence of moderate to severe pain (30–100 mm on a VAS, mean 49 mm) was 78% following BMA. The corresponding values for lumbar puncture, venipuncture, finger prick, chemotherapy, and disease were 61% (45 mm), 28% (20 mm), 23% (18 mm), 41% (25 mm) and 37% (24 mm), respectively. Elliott et al. (1991) surveyed all 160 children (28 inpatients and 132 outpatients) in a cooperative group including both community-based and tertiary care institutions seen during a 1-week period. Pain was reported by 39% of inpatients and 13% of outpatients. Side effects of cancer treatment accounted for 58%, cancer-related pain for 21%, and unrelated pain for 21% of the reported pain.

Ljungman and colleagues (1996) conducted a pain survey in Sweden using a national questionnaire for nurses and physicians, followed by a second study based on a regional investigation utilizing structured interviews for children and parents (Ljungman et al. 1999). At diagnosis 60% of patients had at some point experienced cancer-related pain, and 36% of patients had been in pain frequently or very frequently. However, throughout the course of treatment, most of the pain the children experienced was iatrogenic, either treatment or procedure related. In a third study involving 66 children and their families, Ljungman et al. (2000a) found that 49% of the patients had experienced cancer-related pain at diagnosis, and that reports of pain varied during treatment. According to 65% of the families, intense pain was more common at the beginning of treatment (1–3 months after diagnosis), and both children and parents frequently believed that pain relief could have been better. The corresponding figures for the intermediate period (4–6 months) and the final period (>10 months) were 17% and 14%, respectively. Initially the major problems involved procedure- and treatment-related pain. Procedural pain gradually decreased, but treatment-related pain was constant and dominating. For some procedures pain was rated highest initially, lower during the second period, and higher again during the final phase of treatment.

Collins and colleagues have validated two symptom assessment scales, the Memorial Symptom Assessment Scale (MSAS) 10–18 for children 10–18 years of age (Collins et al. 2000) and the MSAS 7–12 for children 7–12 years of age (Collins et al. 2002). Both used a multidimensional approach to assess symptoms with regard to prevalence, intensity, frequency, and the distress they caused. In the first study, comprising 160 children and adolescents with cancer, the instrument was administered to 45 inpatients and 115 outpatients. Patients were asked to report symptoms prevalent during the week prior to completion of the questionnaire. Along with lack of energy, the group reported pain as the most prevalent symptom (49.1%). Of those reporting pain, 80.8% stated the intensity to be "moderate" to "very severe," 35.9% the frequency to be "a lot" to "almost always," and 39.1% distress to be "quite a bit" to "very much." Lack of energy and feeling sad were the most distressing symptoms. Pain was the most prevalent symptom for inpatients, present in 84.4%, and causing "quite a bit" to "very much" distress in 52.8%. Among outpatients, 35.1% reported pain and 26.3% "quite a bit" to "very much" distress.

The second study (Collins et al. 2002) comprised 149 younger children, 90 in the United Kingdom and 59 in Australia; it included 15 inpatients and 134 outpatients. Children were asked to report symptoms prevalent during the 48 hours prior to completing the questionnaire. Tiredness was the most common symptom (35.6%), followed by pain (32.4%). Among those reporting pain, 51% reported a lot of pain, 64% said that pain was present almost all the time, and 37% said that their pain caused "very much" distress. Inpatients described significantly more symptoms and distress than outpatients. Both studies clearly showed that the treatment setting must be taken into account when examining pain prevalence, a correlation that other authors have found to be true of both the prevalence and type of pain (Miser et al. 1987a; Elliott et al. 1991). Another important factor is type of malignancy. Patients with solid tumors are more likely to have severe pain that is difficult to control (Collins et al. 1995; Flogegård and Ljungman 2003).

The results and conclusions of these and other studies show that pain still poses a major problem in children with cancer. However, pain evaluation and treatment can be improved for this group through increased education of professionals, repeated information to families, cooperation of health care professionals with children and parents, use and documentation of pain analysis and measurement, establishment of explicit protocols and routines, and cooperation between nurses and physicians in the implementation of these routines. Future research on pain in children with cancer should shift from descriptive studies to interventional studies, preferably using randomized controlled trials.

TREATMENT-RELATED PAIN

Most children with a diagnosis of cancer undergo surgery to implant an intravenous (i.v.) injection port (Port-a-Cath) or a central line to assure i.v. access, and most experience postoperative pain. Children requiring surgical removal of a tumor commonly experience pain and discomfort afterward. Less common, but often resistant to treatment, is neuropathic phantom limb pain following amputation (Bach et al. 1988; Wilkins et al. 1998).

Mucositis is a common painful side effect of chemotherapy that is often difficult to alleviate; it causes significant nutritional problems due to oral and at times esophageal and gastric pain. Management of mucositis often requires high doses of systemic opioids together with topical analgesics (Mahon and DeGregorio 1985). Another problematic side effect is intestinal pain caused by vinca alkaloids such as vincristine (Bradely et al. 1970; Vainionpää 1993). This pain is primarily of neuropathic origin, but intestinal immotility also causes distension, constipation, and anal pain. Vinca alkaloids cause neuropathic pain in the extremities as well, mainly the legs and jaws. This condition is often unresponsive to treatment with opioids (Arnér and Meyerson 1991), and opioids may even exacerbate the problem because they tend to further decrease intestinal motility. Because the pain usually resolves spontaneously within 2–5 days, treatment with antidepressants is rarely started.

Protracted vomiting is another cause of abdominal pain, although this problem has decreased substantially due to modern treatment of nausea with steroids and 5-HT$_3$-receptor-blocking agents (Cunningham et al. 1989; Smith et al. 1991). Dyspepsia, a side effect of corticosteroids, readily responds to treatment with antacids or H$_2$-receptor antagonists (Thompson and Walker 1984; Paimela et al. 1990). Keratoconjunctivitis, a painful side effect of high-dose cytarabine (Ara-C) treatment, can be avoided or alleviated by prophylactic treatment with steroid eye drops or artificial tears every 4 hours (Higa et al. 1991; Gococo et al. 1992).

Infections due to neutropenia sometimes cause localized inflammation and edema that can be very painful. Prolonged postlumbar headaches and radiation dermatitis are other painful side effects of treatment.

PROCEDURE-RELATED PAIN

Pain during minor procedures and the anticipatory anxiety beforehand are major problems. Although some children might be helped by sedation, clinicians often overlook this option when i.v. access is lacking. The introduction of subcutaneous ports and central venous catheters therefore marked a revolution in the care of children with cancer, greatly facilitating venous access. A safe, effective method of conscious sedation without i.v. access is also necessary in pediatric oncology, so as to preserve the child's cooperation during lengthy treatment protocols involving repeated medical procedures. Traditionally, oral and rectal administration of chloral hydrate or diazepam has been used, but these drugs are not ideal due to slow onset of action, protracted effect, and variable uptake. An ideal sedative drug should provide rapid onset, short recovery time, and a minimum of side effects, and should be safe and easy to administer.

Midazolam is a benzodiazepine that can be administered orally, nasally, rectally, intramuscularly, or intravenously because of its water-soluble properties. It has a short onset time (Wahlberg et al. 1991), a relatively rapid redistribution phase, and a plasma half-life of about 2 hours in all age groups except neonates, where the half-life is longer (Jaqz-Aigrain et al. 1990; Rey et al. 1991). Respiratory and circulatory depression is unlikely when midazolam is used as a single drug, and usage is considered safe (Ljung and Andréasson 1996; Geldner et al. 1997). However, when midazolam is combined with opioids or other sedatives, the risk of respiratory depression increases (Payne et al. 1989; Yaster et al. 1990; Maxwell and Yaster 1996). Due to its pharmacokinetic properties and a wide therapeutic window, midazolam is well suited for use in children. Oral and rectal routes of administration are not ideal choices, mainly because uptake is quite variable, onset is slower, and recovery is delayed (Payne et al. 1989). Rectal administration is also limited because it is objectionable to many children (Lejus et al. 1997), and it should be avoided in neutropenic patients due to the risk of infection. Midazolam administered intranasally fulfills many criteria of an ideal sedative drug (Rey et al. 1991; Wahlberg et al. 1991; Ljung and Andréasson 1996; Ljungman et al. 2000b), the spray being preferable to drops (Ljung and Andréasson 1996). Nasal discomfort, however, reduces tolerability (Khazin et al. 1995; Lejus et al. 1997; Ljungman et al. 2000b). It is important to remember that midazolam has no analgesic effect and therefore must be combined with an analgesic if pain is expected.

Because repeated intrathecal chemotherapy is necessary to prevent relapses in the CNS, children with leukemia and non-Hodgkin's lymphoma undergo lumbar punctures 15 to 20 times throughout the course of treatment (Tubergen et al. 1993; Gustafsson et al. 1998b). Lumbar punctures can produce a high degree of pain, fear, and anxiety (Zeltzer and LeBaron 1982; Jay et al. 1983, 1995; Weekes and Savedra 1988; Zeltzer et al. 1990; McGrath et al. 1990a). In addition to the procedure-related short-term distress, survivors of childhood cancer may recall disturbing memories of procedures up to 12 years after treatment (Stuber et al. 1996). The trend has been toward the use of deep sedation or general anesthesia instead of conscious sedation when giving intrathecal treatment, in order to reduce distress for the child. Another reason for the shift toward deep sedation is that conscious sedation has been questioned, mainly with respect to safety (Payne et al. 1989; Yaster et al. 1990; Maxwell and Yaster 1996). A recent Swedish study (Ljungman et al. 2001) with a randomized crossover design found that distress, discomfort, pain, postprocedural well-being and security, and procedural difficulties were similar when conscious sedation and deep sedation were compared.

Bone marrow aspiration and bone marrow biopsy are also regular events in the diagnostic and treatment protocols for pediatric malignancies. Previously, both were often performed under conscious sedation, but deep sedation and general anesthesia are becoming increasingly common because the pain and discomfort that arises when suction is applied to retrieve bone marrow is difficult to prevent in a conscious child.

Proper nutrition is essential in children treated for cancer. Over the last 10 years we have become increasingly aware of the need for active nutritional care to prevent malnutrition. It is therefore becoming increasingly common in pediatric oncology to insert a feeding tube, which may cause discomfort and sometimes pain (Ljungman et al. 1996, 1999). Generally the feeding tube is inserted after preparation and minor sedation.

CANCER-RELATED PAIN

Causes of cancer-related pain are often multifactorial. Pain can be the result of compression or direct invasion of bone, of soft tissue with or without viscous obstruction, or of peripheral nerves, the spinal cord, or the brain. At diagnosis of acute leukemia, children often report pain from the entire body, but mostly from the bones of the extremities. This pain is caused mainly by leukemic cells occupying the bone marrow and disturbing the microenvironment (Riehm et al. 1992). CNS involvement of solid tumors, leukemia, or carcinomatosis is associated with specific pain syndromes, including headache and vomiting, with early morning exacerbation as a sign of increased intracranial pressure. Spinal cord compression or invasion causes localized spinal or radiating pain, with or without concomitant neurological changes.

Our knowledge of cancer-related pain in children is limited. One reason is that the number of children with cancer-related pain is seldom large enough to support thorough analysis at a single institution. Consequently, multicenter and perhaps multinational efforts will be needed to increase knowledge in this area.

ASSESSMENT OF PAIN IN CHILDREN WITH CANCER

Pain assessment is complicated because the experience of pain depends on many different factors. Because pain is a subjective experience composed of both physiological and psychological factors, the gold standard for measurement is self-report (McGrath 1987).

The VAS can be used from the age of seven (Price et al. 1983, 1994; Berde 1991); for longer-lasting or recurrent pain, a pain diary is often more appropriate (McGrath et al. 1990b). For younger children from about 3 to 4 years of age, several scales have been validated, including the Faces Pain Scale (Bieri et al. 1990), the poker chip scale (Hester et al. 1990), and the Oucher scale (Beyer and Wells 1989).

For children younger than 3 to 4 years, there are no self-report measures. For these children, several scales are used to systematically evaluate age-specific pain behaviors. Such scales have been validated for children of all ages, including premature infants. Examples are the Children's Hospital of Eastern Ontario Pain Scale (CHEOPS; McGrath et al. 1985), the Observational Scale of Behavioral Distress (OSBD; Jay et al. 1983), and the Objective Pain Scale (OPS; Hannallah et al. 1987; Broadman et al. 1988; Norden et al. 1991). The younger the child, the more complicated the measurement because pain behaviors become more subtle and nonspecific with decreasing age. Biological measures include heart rate, transcutaneous measurement of oxygenation, sweating, and sometimes electroencephalogram (EEG) readings.

The major drawback to both behavioral and biological measures is that they can not discriminate between physical responses to pain and other forms of stress to the body. Furthermore, adaptation takes place with attenuation of both types of signals after a short period of time, which makes them most appropriate for use in acute pain such as that caused by procedures. An observational scale with potential for assessment of longer-term pain has received preliminary validation in pediatric oncology (Gauvain-Piquard et al. 1987, 1999).

TREATMENT OF PAIN IN CHILDREN WITH CANCER

Previously, treatment often has been either pharmacological or psychological. Today, most clinicians and researchers agree that a combination of the two is often the most successful alternative (Kazak et al. 1998a; Liossi 2002), and that a multidisciplinary approach is essential. In a randomized, controlled, prospective study, Kazak and colleagues (1998a) evaluated a combined pharmacological and psychological intervention scheme relative to purely pharmacological intervention in reducing child distress during invasive procedures in childhood leukemia. Pharmacological and psychological interventions were effective in reducing child and parent distress, supporting integration of the two approaches.

In long-term or chronic pain a multidisciplinary approach is even more essential, and a team consisting of a physician, nurse, psychologist, and physical therapist, all specialized in pediatric pain management, is advisable. It is important that health professionals working in pediatric oncology take an active interest in pain management issues.

PHARMACOLOGICAL PAIN TREATMENT

Evidence from basic scientific studies confirms the widespread belief that the most efficient way to treat pain is to block it before it arises (Woolf 1983; Wall 1988), but the role of pre-emptive analgesia also has been questioned (McQuay 1995). However, the important issue is that treatment should occur at the outset and continue for as long as pain persists, in order to prevent unnecessary suffering. In addition, data support the view that inadequate analgesia during initial procedures in young children may diminish the effect of adequate analgesia during subsequent procedures (Weisman et al. 1998).

Local anesthetic agents can be used on the skin, including lidocaine-prilocaine cream (eutectic mixture of local anesthetics [EMLA; Astra]; Clarke and Radford 1986; Bjerring and Arendt-Nielsen 1990), lidocaine iontophoresis (Zempsky et al. 1998), and vapocoolant spray (Reis and Holubkov 1997), and on the mucous membranes, and local anesthetic agents also can be administered subcutaneously (s.c.).

For treatment of pain in patients with cancer, the World Health Organization (1986, 1996) has proposed the sequential use of analgesic drugs in a three-step analgesic ladder. Acetaminophen and nonsteroidal anti-inflammatory drugs (NSAIDs) are the first step, although the latter have had limited use in childhood cancer due to their effects on platelets. Acetaminophen has a wide therapeutic window and is often the drug of choice in children with cancer. NSAIDs are the drug of choice when pain is caused by inflammation, and because of their different mechanism of action, it is not illogical to combine them with acetaminophen (Lloyd-Thomas et al. 1995).

The second step in the analgesic ladder is to add opioids for weak to moderate pain, and the third is to change to the use of opioids for moderate to severe pain. Opioids can be administrated orally, s.c., i.v., epidurally, or intrathecally. Intravenous administration offers the choice of injection, nurse-controlled infusion, and patient-controlled analgesia (Gaukroger et al. 1989; Collins et al. 1995; Flogegård and Ljungman 2003). Attitudes, myths, and side effects—mainly the risk of respiratory depression—have previously hampered the adequate use of opioids.

Neuropathic pain is often difficult to treat. Some researchers have reported an effect of opioids (Portenoy et al. 1990; Rowbotham et al. 1991), while others have found that chronic peripheral neuropathic pain is insensitive to this group of drugs (Arnér and Meyerson 1991). Although transcutaneous electrical nerve stimulation (TENS) often is ineffective in neuropathic pain, it should always be tried initially when the pain is moderate because it has few side effects (Lander and Fowler-Kerry 1991; Woolf and Thompson 1994). Medications often tried include tricyclic antidepressants (Walsh 1983; Rogers 1989; Epstein et al. 1991), carbamazepine (Swerdlow 1986; Leijon and Boivie 1989), and gabapentin (Terrence et al. 1985). Regional blocks employing local anesthetic, opioids, or both can sometimes be used (Jones et al. 1984; Desparmet et al. 1987; Collins et al. 1996), and neurosurgery may be indicated for palliative care in extreme cases (Rossitch and Madsen 1993).

A general problem in pediatrics is the lack of pharmacological data for different substances, and this is also true of pain treatment. Although the reasons for this inadequacy are many, the main one may be that the pediatric market represents limited profitability for pharmaceutical companies. Berde (1991) provides additional reasons for the paucity of controlled clinical trials of analgesic agents in children, including difficulty obtaining informed consent, age-related differences in pharmacokinetics and pharmacodynamics, and difficulties in venous sampling. Morphine is the preferred opioid in pediatric cancer pain due to extensive clinical experience and significant pharmacological data (Olkkola et al. 1988; Goldman and Bowman 1990; Goldman et al. 1990; Babul and Darke 1993). However, randomized controlled trials in children are needed to evaluate other opioids, as well as adjuvant analgesics including tricyclic antidepressants, anticonvulsants, and antiarrhythmics for neuropathic pain and corticosteroids and diphosphonates for bone pain (Babul and Darke 1993).

Methods of pain management in children with cancer are mostly the same as those used for children with noncancer pain. However, pediatric oncology employs specific treatment modalities as well. Steroids reduce inflammatory swelling, thereby decreasing pain (Bruera et al. 1985). In addition, steroids have an antineoplastic effect on lymphatic malignant cells in acute lymphoblastic leukemia and certain lymphomas. Chemotherapy and radiation can be given as palliation to reduce tumor volume and thus decrease compression and distension (Blitzer 1985; Zelefsky et al. 1989; MacDonald 1993). A new modality of palliative treatment is injection of radioactive particles that selectively find sites of tumor or metastases and exert a local radiation effect (Westlin et al. 1995; Charron et al. 1996).

PSYCHOLOGICAL TREATMENTS

Psychological methods that can be applied in pain treatment include preparation, deep breathing, relaxation (Richter et al. 1986), distraction (Fowler-Kerry and Lander 1987), play therapy (Linn et al. 1989; Walker 1989), cognitive therapy (Jay 1985; Jay et al. 1987, 1991, 1995; Kazak et al. 1996, 1998a), guided imagery (Brown 1984), and hypnosis (Katz et al. 1980, 1987; Zeltzer and LeBaron 1982). Of these, cognitive behavioral therapy and hypnosis have the best evidence base and have achieved the status of empirically validated interventions in pediatric procedure-related pain management (Liossi 2002).

Information and psychological preparation are central aspects of pain treatment. Children who are well prepared feel more secure and therefore have reduced requirements for analgesics (Wolfner and Visintainer 1975; Broome 1990; Harrison 1991; Edwinson-Månsson 1992).

Despite the above-mentioned trend toward deeper levels of sedation during procedures, the notion that general anesthesia is always less distressing has been challenged. Cognitive behavioral therapy (CBT) has been compared with general anesthesia in an interesting randomized crossover study among children undergoing BMA (Jay et al. 1995). Children exhibited more behavioral distress during the first minute of lying down on the treatment table when receiving CBT, compared with general anesthesia. No differences were found in self-reported pain and fear, pulse rate, or anticipation of the next BMA. Nor did any differences emerge in parental stress and coping or in children's or parents' preference for CBT versus general anesthesia. However, parents rated significantly more behavioral adjustment symptoms in their children 24 hours after the BMA under general anesthesia.

Again, psychological and pharmacological approaches are not alternatives to one another, but rather are complementary, because each can address several aspects of the complex and multidimensional experience of pain. Fanurik et al. (1993) have shown that some children, termed "attenders," prefer to handle acute pain through focusing on the pain, while others known as "distractors" turn away from the pain. Therefore, there can probably be no single method of choice. Some children prefer to handle procedural pain and discomfort through behavioral techniques, rather than undergoing deep sedation or general anesthesia, because it gives them a sense of control over the situation. One of the great advantages for children in learning different psychological techniques is the knowledge they gain on how to cope with difficult situations, not only for the present treatment, but for life in general. These methods also allow the child to be an active participant instead of a passive recipient. However, children should never be allowed to experience unnecessary pain simply because they have learned how to cope with it, or because skillful practitioners can minimize the long-term sequelae.

IMPACT OF CHRONIC ILLNESS AND PAIN IN CHILDREN

IMPACT OF CHRONIC ILLNESS AND PAIN IN GENERAL

Having a chronic illness that causes pain is unpleasant and disturbing. The negative effects cause disability (loss of function and activities), handicap (altered social roles), and impaired quality of life. Awareness and assessment of these effects is essential, because they are often easier to treat successfully than the pain per se, especially in long-term pain. A multidisciplinary approach is vital for successful management of chronic pain, and all dimensions of pain should be assessed comprehensively.

The relationship between pain or disease severity and disability, handicap, and quality of life is not linear, and it is often astonishing to see how resilient some children and adolescents are compared to others who are more vulnerable. It is not uncommon for children in pain to show some degree of disability, while their social roles as family members, as friends, and in school are generally less affected. On the other hand, a few children are both severely disabled and handicapped, sometimes without experiencing more severe pain than others. This finding highlights the fact that relationships and mechanisms are very complex and often incompletely understood. One study (Schanberg et al. 2001) showed that family pain history predicts child health status in children with chronic rheumatic disease. This factor is probably important in most other chronic illnesses as well.

A major problem in discussing the impact of chronic illness and pain is that causality is difficult to establish due to the very complex relationships involved. Often it is impossible to differentiate the effects of chronic illness from those of pain on social role and quality of life. Pain is often included in measures of health-related quality of life, but measures that discriminate between pain-related quality of life and disease-related quality of life are scarce and may not be meaningful when the pain arises in the context of a disease that has various effects other than pain. Pain-related quality of life instruments have been developed to assess childhood conditions where pain is the only or dominating symptom but where no organic cause is known, for example recurrent headache, recurrent abdominal pain, and chronic musculoskeletal pain (Langeveld et al. 1996, 1997; Hunfeld et al. 2002).

Although disability assessment has become standard in evaluation of adult pain outcomes in pain management services, research is limited regarding the assessment of pain-related functional limitations, handicap, and quality of life among children with recurrent or chronic pain (Palermo 2000). The development of such instruments and performance of well-designed studies to map the scope of the problem are important areas of future research.

IMPACT OF CHRONIC ILLNESS AND PAIN IN CHILDREN WITH CANCER

As mentioned above, it is often impossible to differentiate the effects of chronic illness from those of pain on function, social role, quality of life, depression, anxiety, and post-traumatic stress disorder (PTSD) in pediatric oncology. In addition, children with cancer are a very diverse group. In a comprehensive analysis it is important to differentiate between diagnoses, high- and low-intensity treatments, time point in the treatment protocol, and other factors.

Most children with cancer and their families do not show frank psychopathology (Zeltzer 1993; Evans et al. 1992; Last and Grootenhuis 1998), but they suffer almost universally from severe stress and reduced quality of life. Certain subgroups are more at risk, such as children with CNS tumors (Barr et al. 1999), children who have undergone treatment for Hodgkin's disease (Van Schaik et al. 1999), and children who have received megatherapy with bone marrow rescue (Crom et al. 1999).

School functioning. In one study (Sawyer et al. 1986), leukemic children and adolescents had significantly more school problems and less social competence than normal controls. Cognitive dysfunction constitutes the greatest burden of morbidity after treatment for childhood CNS tumors and occurs in about two-thirds of such cases (Glaser et al. 1997; Barr et al. 1999). These children worried more than controls, but attended school willingly. In another study of survivors of childhood brain tumors (Kennedy and Leyland 1999), 38% had moderate to severe disability, which was closely associated with provision of special education.

Physical activities. In a Brazilian study of psychosocial consequences after amputation in adolescents with cancer (Tebbi et al. 1989), survivors had major problems with walking, pain, and social issues. Another study of children with soft tissue sarcomas (Lampert et al. 1984) showed that children with lesions in the lower extremities had significantly more difficulties in activities of daily living and mobility than did children with lesions in the upper extremities. Childhood survivors of CNS tumors had reduced mobility and a reluctance to participate in organized physical activities (Glaser et al. 1997).

Pain. No specific instrument exists to measure pain-related quality of life in children with cancer. One research group has explored the impact of pain on the families of children with cancer with quantitative methodology (Ferrell et al. 1994; Ferrell 1995) and found that pain affects all domains of quality of life.

In children receiving active treatment for cancer, epidemiological studies have shown high frequencies of disturbing symptoms including pain, nausea, lack of energy, and lack of appetite (Miser et al. 1987a,b; Ljungman et al. 1996, 1999; Collins et al. 2000).

In palliative end-of-life care, pain is a very common symptom. In an interview study (Wolfe et al. 2000), parents of 103 children who had died of cancer stated that 89% of the children suffered a great deal from at least one symptom in their last month of life, most commonly pain, fatigue, or dyspnea. Of the children treated for specific symptoms, treatment was successful in 27% of those with pain and in 16% in those with dyspnea.

Pain was a problem in about 30% of survivors after megatherapy with bone marrow rescue (Kanabar et al. 1995), and in about 30% of children recovering from CNS tumors (Glaser et al. 1997; Barr et al. 1999). In a sample of 33 survivors of childhood Hogkin's disease, Van Schaik et al. (1999) showed that the attributes most affected were pain, emotion, and cognition. In a study of 220 adult long-term survivors of pediatric solid tumors more than 15 years after treatment (Crom et al. 1999), pain accounted for 10% of the variability in health functioning, 13% of the variability in global health-related quality of life, and 18% of the variability in financial impact.

Social activities. During treatment for cancer, most children suffer from not being able to spend as much time with peers as they would have wanted because of long periods of hospitalization for chemotherapy and treatment of side effects, radiation, and surgery. In a study on children who had received treatment for CNS tumors (Glaser et al. 1997), interaction with peers was normal. However, the need is clear for greater examination of this issue with children who suffer varying degrees of deficit following treatment.

Impact on family. The diagnosis of cancer is a major stress for children (Sawyer et al. 2000). It also causes stress for parents (Dongen-Melman et al. 1995a) and siblings (Dongen-Melman et al. 1995b; Murray 1999). Families of children with cancer experience serious difficulties and are at risk of developing psychosocial problems (Schuler et al. 1985; Dongen-Melman and Sanders-Woudstra 1986). High levels of distress continue over time, and it is important to identify those at risk in order to provide support for this population at an early stage (Sloper 2000). The child's adjustment is related to parental support and distress (Koocher 1986), which increases the incentive for clinicians to work with the whole family.

Families of a child with cancer suffer the burden of lost personal time, financial obligations, and missed work time because of their child's need for medication and medical appointments (Ljungman et al. 2003). Studies of the impact of pain on the family in children with cancer (Ferrell et al. 1994; Ferrell 1995) have concluded that although it is a horrible experience to have a child diagnosed with cancer, it is even more devastating to have that child experience unrelieved pain. Parents often found the child's pain experience to be worse at home. Although parents made an attempt to maintain normalcy in the family, siblings were reported as expressing fears of their brother's or sister's death. Many expressed jealousy because of the attention that the sick child received.

Quality of life. Children with cancer and survivors of childhood cancer are very diverse groups, and generalizations are therefore not easy to make. In many studies, most children in these groups do not show frank psychopathology, but it appears that certain subgroups fare worse. Survivors of CNS tumors (Barr et al. 1999), survivors of Hodgkin's disease (Van Schaik et al. 1999), and children who have undergone high-intensity treatments such as bone marrow transplant (Calaminus and Kiebert 1999; Crom et al. 1999) demonstrate more negative psychosocial outcomes. In addition, survivors with substantial late effects, comorbidity, relapse, or cognitive problems demonstrate less favorable outcomes (Zeltzer 1993; Crom et al. 1999). Kennedy and Leyland (1999) found that 50% of survivors of childhood brain tumors had high scores on a questionnaire designed to determine which individuals had a high risk of an emotional or behavioral problem.

Anxiety, depression, and somatization. A study of 43 children being treated or within 3 years of completion of treatment for cancer (Challinor et al. 1999) concluded that although children with cancer are in many ways similar to their healthy peers, they are at increased risk for anxiety, depression, and somatization. These symptoms occurred at frequencies of 32%, 19%, and 31%, respectively. Other studies have shown that children under treatment for cancer are not at such high risk, probably because personal and community resources are mobilized at that time, while the period following termination of treatment is characterized by a higher risk of psychosocial problems (Hedstrom and von Essen 2001; von Essen et al. 2000). In a study of 51 children on and off treatment for cancer, 14% reported a high level of depression (von Essen et al. 2000). Anxiety related to the possibility of recurrence was a problem in 70% of survivors after megatherapy with bone marrow rescue (Kanabar et al. 1995).

Post-traumatic stress disorder. Although most survivors of childhood cancer do well, those who experienced severe side effects from their treatment may be more at risk for psychological problems (Greenberg et al. 1989). Some evidence indicates that children experience cancer treatment as a repeated trauma (Stuber et al. 1998), and PTSD has been described among children who have survived cancer (Kazak et al. 1998b; Rourke et al. 1999) as well as their parents (Kazak et al. 1998b). In fact, parents seem to be more at risk.

Long-term perspective. In a study of long-term survivors of pediatric solid tumors more than 15 years after treatment (Crom et al. 1999), health-related quality of life was better among those who had received low-intensity therapy. Dyspnea and fatigue were common in survivors of Hodgkin's disease. Most of the survivors were experiencing moderately good to excellent quality of life.

In a study of 176 long-term survivors of childhood cancer (Zebrack and Chesler 2002), protracted effects such as fatigue, aches, and pain remained salient aspects of these individuals' quality of life. However, the physical domain did not seem as relevant to their quality of life as did psychological and social aspects.

IMPACT OF CHRONIC ILLNESS AND PAIN IN OTHER DISEASES OR DISORDERS

School functioning. A number of studies have reported on the impact of chronic pain on school functioning. Children with frequent or severe headaches (Stang and Osterhaus 1993), sickle cell disease (Shapiro 1995; Fuggle et al. 1996), widespread musculoskeletal pain (Mikkelsson et al. 1997), and recurrent abdominal pain (Walker et al. 1998) are more frequently absent from school than are healthy controls.

Sleep. Quantity and quality of sleep are other areas in which pain often has a negative impact. This is true of children with sickle cell disease (Shapiro 1995; Shapiro et al. 1995), and was reported by half of children in a study group with chronic pain due to cancer, hemophilia, sickle cell anemia, and juvenile chronic arthritis (Walters and Williamson 1999).

Both school absenteeism and sleep disturbances due to pain increase dysfunction, causing increased disability and handicap. It is therefore essential to identify and treat these problems immediately to interrupt the potentially chronic vicious cycle of pain and disability.

Physical activities. Children with cancer, hemophilia, sickle cell anemia, and juvenile chronic arthritis have reported moderate degrees of restriction in physical activities (Walters and Williamson 1999). To some extent, the activity restriction itself mediated the association between chronic pain and depression in these children. In another study (Hunfeld et al. 2002), adolescents with chronic limb pain and back pain reported problems in physical activities, whereas those with chronic headache reported problems in cognitive activities.

Social activities. Chronic pain has social implications as well. Children with sickle cell disease (Fuggle et al. 1996) and adolescents with headache (Langeveld et al. 1997; Hunfeld et al. 2002) and back and limb pain (Hunfeld et al. 2002) have reported a more negative impact on leisure time spent with peers compared to controls.

Impact on family. As is true of childhood cancer, the families of children with chronic pain of other origin may suffer the burden of lost personal time, greater financial obligations, and loss of income (Palermo 2000). Studies of children with headache, back pain, and limb pain have shown that the adolescent's pain had a significant impact on the family. Mothers of adolescents with intense pain reported more restrictions in social life and problems dealing with the stress of the adolescent's pain than did mothers of adolescents with less severe chronic pain (Hunfeld et al. 2001).

Quality of life. Few studies have examined quality of life among adolescents with chronic pain. Some reports have shown that higher pain intensity corresponds to poorer quality of life, especially in terms of psychological, somatic, and functional status. This is true of children with headache (Langeveld et al. 1997; Hunfeld et al. 2001) and abdominal, limb, and back pain (Hunfeld et al. 2001, 2002).

Long-term perspective. Children with chronic pain may develop lifelong difficulties due to pain and its consequences. In a recent community study (Hunfeld et al. 2002), adolescents with at least 3 years' history of chronic headache or chronic limb or back pain of unknown origin reported no changes in intensity and frequency of pain, quality of life, and impact of pain on the family during the 3-year study period. There was no deterioration, which might have been expected by extrapolation from adult studies (Skevington 1998). In contrast, the adolescents had adapted to the continuing pain. Several adolescents used self-management strategies such as daily physical exercise. They appeared to be skillful in coping with their pain, and continued their usual activities for as long as possible. A clinic-based study of children with recurrent abdominal pain (Walker et al. 1998) revealed more school absences and higher levels of disability compared to control subjects up to 5 years after clinical presentation. The study showed that functional disability, as well as pain, continued for an extended period. Community samples might differ in this important respect from clinic samples.

ASSESSMENT OF IMPACT OF CHRONIC ILLNESS AND PAIN IN CHILDREN

MEASURES OF IMPACT OF CHRONIC ILLNESS AND PAIN IN CHILDREN IN GENERAL

One research group has explored the impact of pain on the family of children with cancer using quantitative methodology (Ferrell et al. 1994; Ferrell 1995), and claims that pain affects all domains of quality of life. A problematic issue in the measurement of quality of life is to decide when to use generic instruments that allow comparison with other groups and thereby generalization, and when to use disease-specific instruments because the generic measures are not sensitive enough to detect and address specific symptoms or problems of that particular disease or disorder.

Another problem is that proxy respondents tend to both under- and overestimate components of health-related quality of life, leading to low inter-observer agreement (Calaminus and Kiebert 1999). However, cancer afflicts children in a wide range of ages, each with its specific level of physical, cognitive, and emotional functioning.

EXAMPLES OF MEASURES OF IMPACT OF CHRONIC ILLNESS AND PAIN IN CHILDREN WITH CANCER

Well-validated population-specific (Varni et al. 1998; Goodwin et al. 2000) and generic instruments (Landgraf and Abetz 1996) are available to measure health-related quality of life in children and adolescents receiving active treatment for cancer. Well-validated instruments also exist to measure this outcome in childhood cancer survivors (Feeny et al. 1992; Ferrans and Powers 1992), but no such instrument has been developed for children with cancer.

The Pediatric Cancer Quality of Life Inventory (PCQL-32; Varni et al. 1998) child and parent form is a standardized assessment instrument incorporating patient self-report and parent proxy-report; it was designed to systematically assess pediatric cancer patients' health-related quality of life outcomes.

The Health Utilities Index Mark 2 (HUI 2) and HUI 3 classification systems (Feeny et al. 1992, 1995) include important attributes of health status. The HUI 2 system includes major sequelae identified from the childhood cancer "late effects" literature. It consists of seven attributes with three to five levels each. The HUI 3 system consists of eight attributes with five or six levels each.

The Child Health Questionnaire (CHQ; Landgraf and Abetz 1996) child and parent forms were constructed to measure the physical and social well-being of children. The child form (CHQ-CF87) has been validated for a large number of different chronic diseases and disorders, including children with cancer, and for a normal school-based population. Likewise, the parent form (CHQ-PF50) was constructed and validated for use among children with and without chronic conditions.

For symptom assessment, the Memorial Symptom Assessment Scale 10-18 (MSAS 10-18; Collins et al. 2000) can be used for children and adolescents aged 10 to 18 years, and the MSAS 7-12 (Collins et al. 2002) can be used for children aged 7 to 12 years. These measures give information about frequency, prevalence, and intensity of a specific symptom, and also about how much distress it causes.

EXAMPLES OF MEASURES OF PAIN-RELATED QUALITY OF LIFE IN CHILDREN WITH CHRONIC NONCANCER ILLNESS AND PAIN

Langeveld et al. (1996) have created a disease-specific measure for headache pain-related quality of life, called the Quality of Life Headache-Youth (QLH-Y) scale. This instrument was adapted for adolescents with chronic pain in general as the Quality of Life Pain-Youth (QLP-Y) scale (Hunfeld et al. 2002). Other validated measures for functional disability and health-related quality of life are available, but their use in samples of children with chronic pain is limited. Examples of these measures are the Functional Disability Inventory (Walker and Greene 1991), Functional Status II (R) (Stein and Jessop 1990), and the Child Health Questionnaire (Landgraf and Abetz 1996).

PSYCHOSOCIAL INTERVENTIONS TO REDUCE THE IMPACT OF CHRONIC ILLNESS AND PAIN IN CHILDREN WITH CANCER

In children receiving active treatment for cancer, epidemiological studies have shown a high prevalence of different disturbing symptoms including pain, nausea, lack of energy, and lack of appetite. Although improved pharmacological management may provide relief, these problems must be approached comprehensively, combining psychosocial and medical care.

Social skills training is important for children with newly diagnosed cancer (Katz and Varni 1993), and relaxation, imagery, and cognitive behavioral therapy are helpful against mucositis pain (Syrjala et al. 1995).

Pharmacological and psychological interventions are successful in helping children to cope with procedures, and evidence supports integration of the two modalities (Kazak et al. 1998a; Liossi 2002). Cognitive behavioral interventions have also been successful in treatment of PTSD and anxiety in survivors of childhood cancer and their families (Kazak et al. 1998b; Kazak 1999).

Studies on chronic illness have clearly demonstrated that medical intervention alone is insufficient to allow for successful outcome (Wober-Bingol et al. 1996). Medical intervention typically focuses exclusively on the disease and does not teach the family self-management skills to cope with the condition. In children with cancer and their families, novel treatment strategies such as telephone or Internet-based interventions could be acceptable ways to provide information, to enhance peer social support, and to support self-management therapy. This approach might reduce the risk of psychosocial problems (Ljungman et al. 2003).

CONCLUSIONS

In conclusion, the impact of chronic illness and pain in children is extensive. However, many areas remain uncharted, and research methodology needs to be improved. A major problem in discussing the impact of chronic illness and pain is that causality is difficult to establish because of the complex relationships of various factors. To differentiate the effects of chronic illness from those of pain on social role and quality of life is often impossible. Pain is often included in measures of health-related quality of life, but measures that discriminate between pain-related and disease-related quality of life are scarce. No pain-related quality of life instruments exist as yet for children with cancer. Instruments to specifically measure pain-related disability, handicap, and quality of life are needed that better describe the prevalence and severity of these problems in children.

REFERENCES

Adami HO, Glimelius B, Sparén P, et al. Trends in childhood and adolescent cancer survival in Sweden 1960 through 1984. *Acta Oncol* 1992; 31:1–10.
American Cancer Society. *1992 Cancer Facts & Figures.* Atlanta, GA: American Cancer Society, 1992.
Anand KJS, Phil D, Hickey PR. Pain and its effects in the human neonate and fetus. *N Engl J Med* 1987; 317:1321–1329.
Arnér S, Meyerson BA. Opioid sensitivity of neuropathic pain—a controversial issue. In: Besson JM, Guilbaud G (Eds). *Lesions of Primary Afferent Fibers as a Tool for the Study of Clinical Pain.* Amsterdam: Elsevier, 1991, pp 259–275.

Babul N, Darke AC. Evaluation and use of opioid analgesics in pediatric cancer pain. *J Palliat Care* 1993; 9:19–25.
Bach S, Noreg MF, Tjellden NU. Phantom limb pain in amputees during the first 12 months following amputation after preoperative lumbar epidural blockade. *Pain* 1988; 33:297–301.
Barr RD, Simpson T, Whitton A, et al. Health-related quality of life in survivors of tumours of the central nervous system in childhood—a preference-based approach to measurement in a cross-sectional study. *Eur J Cancer* 1999; 35:248–255.
Berde CB. *Pediatric Analgesic Trials,* Vol. 18. New York: Raven Press, 1991.
Beyer JE, Wells N. The assessment of pain in children. *Pediatr Clin North Am* 1989; 36:837–854.
Bieri D, Reeve RA, Champion GD, Addicoat L, Ziegler JB. The Faces Pain Scale for the self-assessment of the severity of pain experienced by children: development, initial validation, and preliminary investigation for ratio scale properties. *Pain* 1990; 41:139–150.
Bjerring P, Arendt-Nielsen L. Depth and duration of skin analgesia to needle insertion after topical application of EMLA cream. *Br J Anaesth* 1990; 64:173–177.
Blitzer PH. Reanalysis of the RTOG study of the palliation of symptomatic osseous metastases. *Cancer* 1985; 55:1468–1472.
Bradely WG, Lassman LP, Walton GPJ. The neuropathy of vincristine in man: clinical, electrophysiological, and pathological studies. *J Neurol Sci* 1970; 10:107–131.
Broadman LM, Rice LJ, Hannallah RS. Testing the validity of an objective pain scale for infants and children. *Anesthesiology* 1988; A:69.
Broome ME. Preparation of children for painful procedures. *Pediatr Nurs* 1990; 16:537–541.
Brown J. Imagery coping strategies in the treatment of migraine. *Pain* 1984; 18:157–167.
Bruera E, Roca E, Cedaro L, Carraro S, Chacon R. Action of oral methylprednisolone in terminal cancer patients: a prospective randomized double-blind study. *Cancer Treat Rep* 1985; 69:751–754.
Calaminus G, Kiebert G. Studies on health-related quality of life in childhood cancer in the European setting: an overview. *Int J Cancer Suppl* 1999; 12:83–86.
Challinor JM, Miaskowski CA, Franck LS, et al. Somatization, anxiety and depression as measures of health-related quality of life of children/adolescents with cancer. *Int J Cancer Suppl* 1999; 12:52–57.
Charron M, Brown M, Rowland P, Mirro J. Pain palliation with strontium-89 in children with metastatic disease. *Med Pediatr Oncol* 1996; 26:393–396.
Clarke S, Radford M. Topical anesthesia for venepuncture. *Arch Dis Child* 1986; 61:1132–1134.
Collins JJ, Grier HE, Kinney HC, Berde CB. Control of severe pain in children with terminal malignancy. *J Pediatr* 1995; 126:653–657.
Collins JJ, Grier HE, Sethna NF, Wilder RT, Berde CB. Regional anesthesia for pain associated with terminal pediatric malignancy. *Pain* 1996; 65:63–69.
Collins JJ, Byrnes ME, Dunkel IJ, et al. The measurement of symptoms in children with cancer. *J Pain Symptom Manage* 2000; 19:363–377.
Collins JJ, Devine TD, Dick GS, et al. The measurement of symptoms in young children with cancer: the validation of the Memorial Symptom Assessment Scale in Children Aged 7-12. *J Pain Symptom Manage* 2002; 23:10–16.
Coyle N, Adelhart J, Foley KM, Portenoy RK. Character of terminal illness in the advanced cancer patient: pain and other symptoms in the last four weeks of life. *J Pain Symptom Manage* 1990; 5:83–93.
Crom DB, Chathaway DK, Tolley EA, Mulhern RK, Hudson MM. Health status and health-related quality of life in long-term adult survivors of pediatric solid tumors. *Int J Cancer Suppl* 1999; 12:25–31.
Cummings EA, Reid GJ, Finley GA, McGrath PJ, Ritchie JA. Prevalence and source of pain in pediatric inpatients. *Pain* 1996; 68:25–31.

Cunningham D, Turner A, Hawthorn J, Rosin RD. Ondansetron with and without dexamethasone to treat chemotherapy-induced emesis. *Lancet* 1989; i:1323.

Desparmet J, Meistelman C, Barre J, Saint-Maurice C. Continuous epidural bupivacaine for postoperative pain relief in children. *Anesthesiology* 1987; 67:108–112.

Dongen-Melman JE, Sanders-Woudstra JA. Psychosocial aspects of childhood cancer: a review of the literature [published erratum appears in *J Child Psychol Psychiatry* 1986; 27(5):713]. *J Child Psychol Psychiatry* 1986; 27:145–180.

Dongen-Melman JE, Pruyn JF, De Groot A, et al. Late psychosocial consequences for parents of children who survived cancer. *J Pediatr Psychol* 1995a; 20:567–586.

Dongen-Melman JE, De Groot A, Hahlen K. Verhulst FC. Siblings of childhood cancer survivors: how does this "forgotten" group of children adjust after cessation of successful cancer treatment? *Eur J Cancer* 1995b; 31A:2277–2283.

Edwinson-Månsson ME. The value of informing children prior to investigations and procedures. Dissertation. Lund University, Sweden, 1992.

Elliott SC, Miser AW, Dose AM, et al. Epidemiologic features of pain in pediatric cancer patients: a co-operative community-based study. *Clin J Pain* 1991; 7:263–268.

Enskär K, Carlsson M, Golsäter M, Hamrin E, Kreuger A. Life situation and problems as reported by children with cancer and their parents. *J Pediatr Oncol Nurs* 1997; 14:18-26.

Epstein JB, Schubert MM, Scully C. Evaluation and treatment of pain in patients with orofacial cancer: a review. *Pain Clin* 1991; 4:3–20.

Evans CA, Stevens M, Cushway D, Houghton J. Sibling response to childhood cancer: a new approach. *Child Care Health Dev* 1992; 18:229–244.

Fanurik D, Zeltzer L, Roberts M, Blount RL. The relationship between children's coping styles and psychological interventions for cold pressor pain. *Pain* 1993; 53:213–222.

Feeny DH, Furlong W, Barr RD, et al. A comprehensive multiattribute system for classifying the health status of survivors of childhood cancer. *J Clin Oncol* 1992; 10:923–928.

Feeny DH, Furlong W, Boyle M, Torrance GW. Multi-attribute health status classification systems: health utilities index. *PharmacoEconomics* 1995; 7:490–502.

Ferrans CE, Powers MJ. Psychometric assessment of the quality of life index. *Res Nurs Health* 1992; 15:29–38.

Ferrell BR. The impact of pain on quality of life: a decade of research. *Nurs Clin North Am* 1995; 30:609–624.

Ferrell BR, Rhiner M, Shapiro B, Dierkes M. The experience of pediatric cancer pain. Part I: Impact of pain on the family. *J Pediatr Nurs* 1994; 9:368–379.

Flogegård H, Ljungman G. Characteristics and adequacy of intravenous morphine infusions in children in a paediatric oncology setting. *Med Pediatr Oncol* 2003; 40:233–238.

Fowler-Kerry SE, Lander J. Management of injection pain in children. *Pain* 1987; 30:169–175.

Fuggle P, Shand PA, Gill LJ, Davies SC. Pain, quality of life, and coping in sickle cell disease. *Arch Dis Child* 1996; 75:199–203.

Gaukroger PB, Tomkins DP, van Der Walt J. Patient-controlled analgesia in children. *Anaesth Intensive Care* 1989; 17:264–268.

Gauvain-Piquard A, Rodary C, Rezvani A, Lemerle J. Pain in children aged 2–6 years: a new observational rating scale elaborated in a pediatric oncology unit—preliminary report. *Pain* 1987; 31(2):177–188.

Gauvain-Piquard A, Rodary C, Rezvani A, Serbouti S. The development of the DEGR: a scale to assess pain in young children with cancer. *Eur J Pain* 1999; 3:165-176.

Geldner G, Hubmann M, Knoll R, Jacobi K. Comparison between three transmucosal routes of administration of midazolam in children. *Paediatr Anaesth* 1997; 7(2):103-109.

Glaser AW, Abdul Rashid NF, U CL, Walker DA. School behavior and health status after central nervous system tumors in childhood. *Br J Cancer* 1997; 76:643-650.

Gococo KO, Lazarus HM, Lass JH. The use of prophylactic eye drops during high-dose cytosine arabinoside therapy. *Cancer* 1992; 69:2866-2867.

Goldman A, Bowman A. The role of oral controlled-release morphine for pain relief in children with cancer. *Palliat Med* 1990; 4:279-285.
Goldman A, Beardmore S, Hunt J. Palliative care for children with cancer. *Arch Dis Child* 1990; 65:641-643.
Goodwin DA, Boggs SR, Graham-Pole J. Development and validation of the Pediatric Oncology Quality of Life Scale. *Psychol Assess* 2000; 6:321-328.
Greenberg HS, Kazak AE, Meadows AT. Psychologic functioning. *J Pediatr* 1989; 114:488-493.
Gustafsson G, Langmark F, Pihkala U, Verdier BD, Lilleaas IJ. *Childhood Cancer in the Nordic Countries: Report on Epidemiologic and Therapeutic Results*. Reykjavik: Nordic Society of Pediatric Haematology and Oncology, 1998a.
Gustafsson G, Kreuger A, Clausen N, et al. Intensified treatment of acute childhood lymphoblastic leukaemia has improved prognosis, especially in non-high-risk patients: the Nordic experience of 2648 patients diagnosed between 1981 and 1996. *Acta Paediatr* 1998b; 87:1151-1161.
Hannallah RS, Broadman LM, Belman AS, Abramowitz MD, Epstein BS. Comparison of caudal and ilioinguinal/iliohypogastric nerve blocks for control of post-orchidopexy pain in pediatric ambulatory surgery. *Anesthesiology* 1987; 66:832-834.
Harrison A. Preparing children for venous blood sampling. *Pain* 1991; 45:299–306.
Hedstrom M, von Essen L. Disease and treatment related distress among children 4–7 years on or off treatment for cancer: parent and nurse perceptions. In: Gibson F, Soanes L, Sepion B (Eds). *Current Perspectives in Pediatric Oncology Nursing*. London: Whurr, 2001.
Hester NO, Foster R, Kristensen K. *Measurement of Pain in Children: Generalizability and Validity of the Pain Ladder and the Poker-Chip Tool*. New York: Raven Press, 1990.
Higa GM, Gockerman JP, Hunt AL, Jones MR, Horne BJ. The use of prophylactic eye drops during high-dose cytosine arabinoside therapy. *Cancer* 1991; 68:1691–1693.
Hoff JV, Schymura MJ, Curnen MM. Trends in the incidence of childhood and adolescent cancer in Connecticut. *Med Pediatr Oncol* 1988; 16:78–87.
Hunfeld JA, Passchier J, Perquin CW, van Suijlekom-Smit LW, van der Wouden JC. Quality of life in adolescents with chronic pain in the head or at other locations. *Cephalalgia* 2001; 21:201–206.
Hunfeld JA, Perquin CW, Bertina W, et al. Stability of pain parameters and pain-related quality of life in adolescents with persistent pain: a three-year follow-up. *Clin J Pain* 2002; 18:99–106.
Jaqz-Aigrain E, Wood E, Robieux I. Pharmacokinetics of midazolam in critically ill neonates. *Eur J Clin Pharmacol* 1990; 39:191–192.
Jay SM. Behavioral management of children's distress during painful medical procedures. *Behav Res Ther* 1985; 23:513–520.
Jay SM, Ozolins M, Elliott C, Caldwell S. Assessment of children's distress during painful procedures: developmental considerations. *J Health Psychol* 1983; 2:133–147.
Jay SM, Elliott CH, Katz ER, Siegel SE. Cognitive-behavioral and pharmacologic interventions for children's' distress during painful medical procedures. *J Consult Clin Psychol* 1987; 55:860–865.
Jay SM, Elliott CH, Woody PD, Siegel S. An investigation of cognitive-behavior therapy combined with oral Valium for children undergoing painful medical procedures. *Health Psychol* 1991; 10:317–322.
Jay S, Elliott CH, Fitzgibbons I, Woody P, Siegel S. A comparative study of cognitive behavior therapy versus general anesthesia for painful medical procedures in children. *Pain* 1995; 62:3–9.
Jones SEF, Beasly JM, McFarlane DWR, Davies JM, Hall-Davies G. Intrathecal morphine for postoperative pain relief in children. *Br J Anaesth* 1984; 56:137–139.
Kaatsch P, Haaf G, Michaelis J. Childhood malignancies in Germany—methods and results of a nationwide registry. *Eur J Cancer* 1995; 31A(6):993–999.

Kanabar DJ, Attard-Montalto S, Saha V, Eden OB. Quality of life in survivors of childhood cancer after megatherapy with autologous bone marrow rescue. *Pediatr Hematol Oncol* 1995; 12:29–36.

Katz ER, Varni JW. Social support and social cognitive problem-solving in children with newly diagnosed cancer. *Cancer* 1993; 71:3314–3319.

Katz ER, Kellerman J, Siegel SE. Distress behavior in children with cancer undergoing medical procedures: developmental considerations. *J Consult Clin Psychol* 1980; 48:356–365.

Katz ER, Kellerman J, Ellenberg L. Hypnosis in the reduction of acute pain and distress in children with cancer. *J Pediatr Psychol* 1987; 12:379–394.

Kazak AE. Effective psychosocial intervention for children with cancer and their families. *Med Pediatr Oncol* 1999; 32:292–293.

Kazak AE, Penati B, Boyer BA, et al. A randomized controlled prospective outcome study of a psychological and pharmacological intervention protocol for procedural distress in pediatric leukemia. *J Pediatr Psychol* 1996; 21:615–631.

Kazak AE, Penati B, Brophy P, Himelstein B. Pharmacologic and psychologic interventions for procedural pain. *Pediatrics* 1998a; 102:59–66.

Kazak AE, Stuber ML, Barakat LP, et al. Predicting posttraumatic stress symptoms in mothers and fathers of survivors of childhood cancers. *J Am Acad Child Adolesc Psychiatry* 1998b; 37:823–831.

Kennedy CR, Leyland K. Comparison of screening instruments for disability and emotional/behavioral disorders with a generic measure of health-related quality of life in survivors of childhood brain tumors. *Int J Cancer Suppl* 1999; 12:106–111.

Khazin V, Ezra S, Cohen A. Comparison of rectal to intranasal administration of midazolam for premedication of children. *Mil Med* 1995; 160(11):579–581.

Koocher GP. Psychosocial issues during the acute treatment of pediatric cancer. *Cancer* 1986; 58:468–472.

Lampert MH, Gerber LH, Glatstein E, Rosenberg SA, Danoff JV. Soft tissue sarcoma: functional outcome after wide local excision and radiation therapy. *Arch Phys Med Rehabil* 1984; 65:477–480.

Lander JR, Fowler-Kerry S. Age differences in children's pain. *Percept Mot Skills* 1991; 73:415–418.

Landgraf JM, Abetz LN. Measuring health outcomes in pediatric populations: issues in psychometrics and application. In: Spilker B (Ed). *Quality of Life and Pharmacoeconomics in Clinical Trials*. Philadelphia: Lippincott-Raven, 1996, pp 785–791.

Langeveld JH, Koot HM, Loonen MC, Hazebroek AAJM, Passchier J. A quality of life instrument for adolescents with chronic headache. *Cephalalgia* 1996; 16:183–196.

Langeveld JH, Koot HM, Passchier J. Headache intensity and quality of life in adolescents: how are changes in headache intensity in adolescents related to changes in experienced quality of life? *Headache* 1997; 37:37–42.

Lansky SB, Ritter-Sterr C, List MA, Hart MJ. Psychiatric and psychological support of the child and adolescent with cancer. In: Pizzo PA, Poplac DG (Eds). *Pediatric Oncology*. Philadelphia: Lippincott, 1989, pp 1127–1139.

Last BF, Grootenhuis MA. Emotions, coping and the need for support in families of children with cancer: a model for psychosocial care. *Patient Educ Couns* 1998; 33:169–179.

Leijon G, Boivie J. Central post-stroke pain—a controlled trial of amitriptyline and carbamazepine. *Pain* 1989; 36:27–36.

Lejus C, Renaudin M, Testa S, et al. Midazolam for premedication in children: nasal vs. rectal administration. *Eur J Anaesthesiol* 1997; 14:244–249.

Linn S, Beardslee W, Patenaude AF. Puppet therapy in pediatric bone marrow transplant patients. *J Pediatr Psychol* 1989; 11:37–46.

Liossi C. *Procedure-related Cancer Pain in Children*, Abingdon: Radcliff Medical Press, 2002.

Ljung B, Andréasson S. Comparison of midazolam nasal spray to nasal drops for the sedation of children. *J Nucl Med Technol* 1996; 24:32–34.

Ljungman G, Kreuger A, Gordh T, et al. Treatment of pain in pediatric oncology: a Swedish nationwide survey. *Pain* 1996; 68:385–394.

Ljungman G, Gordh T, Sorensen S, Kreuger A. Pain in paediatric oncology: interviews with children, adolescents and their parents. *Acta Paediatr* 1999; 88:623–630.

Ljungman G, Gordh T, Sörensen S, Kreuger A. Pain variations during cancer treatment in children: a descriptive survey. *Pediatr Hematol Oncol* 2000a; 17:211–221.

Ljungman G, Kreuger A, Andreasson S, Gordh T, Sorensen S. Midazolam nasal spray reduces procedural anxiety in children. *Pediatrics* 2000b; 105:73–78.

Ljungman G, Gordh T, Sörensen S, Kreuger A. Lumbar puncture in pediatric oncology: conscious sedation or general anesthesia. *Med Pediatr Oncol* 2001; 36:72–79.

Ljungman G, McGrath PJ, Cooper E, et al. Psychosocial needs of families with a child with cancer. *J Pediatr Hematol Oncol* 2003; 25:223–231.

Lloyd-Thomas AR, Howard RF, Llewellyn N. *The Management of Acute and Post-Operative Pain in Infancy and Childhood,* Vol. 3. London: Ballière Tindall, 1995.

MacDonald N. *Principles Governing the Use of Cancer Chemotherapy in Palliative Medicine.* Oxford: Oxford University Press, 1993.

Mahon WA, DeGregorio M. Benzydamine: a critical review of clinical data. *Int J Tissue React* 1985; 7:229–235.

Maxwell L, Yaster M. The myth of conscious sedation. *Arch Pediatr Adolesc Med* 1996; 150:665–667.

McGrath PA. An assessment of children's pain: a review of behavioral, physiological and direct scaling techniques. *Pain* 1987; 31:147–176.

McGrath PJ, Johnson G, Goodman JT, et al. *The CHEOPS: A Behavioral Scale to Measure Postoperative Pain in Children.* New York: Raven Press, 1985.

McGrath PJ, Hsu E, Cappelli M, Luke B. Pain from pediatric cancer: a survey of an outpatient oncology clinic. *J Psychosoc Oncol* 1990a; 8:109–124.

McGrath PJ, Cunningham SJ, Lascellis MA, Humphreys P. *Help Yourself: A Treatment for Migraine Headaches.* Ottawa: University of Ottawa Press, 1990b.

McQuay HJ. Pre-emptive analgesia: a systematic review of clinical studies. *Ann Med* 1995; 27:249–256.

Mikkelsson M, Sourander A, Piha J, Salminen JJ. Psychiatric symptoms in preadolescents with musculoskeletal pain and fibromyalgia. *Pediatrics* 1997; 100:220–227.

Miller RW, Young JL, Novakovic B. Childhood cancer. *Cancer* 1995; 75(Suppl 1):395–405.

Miser AW, Dothage JA, Wesley RA, Miser JS. The prevalence of pain in a pediatric and young adult cancer population. *Pain* 1987a; 29:73–83.

Miser AW, McCalla J, Dothage JA, Wesley M, Miser JS. Pain as a presenting symptom in children and young adults with newly diagnosed malignancy. *Pain* 1987b; 29:85–90.

Murray JS. Siblings of children with cancer: a review of the literature. *J Pediatr Oncol Nurs* 1999; 16:25–34.

Norden J, Hannallah RS, Getson P, et al. Reliability of an objective pain scale in children. *Anesth Analg* 1991; 72:S199.

Olkkola KT, Maunuksela EL, Korpela R. Kinetics and dynamics of postoperative intravenous morphine in children. *Clin Pharmacol Ther* 1988; 44:128–136.

Paimela H, Hockerstedt K, Numers HV, Ahonen J. Short-term high dose corticosteroids and gastroduodenal mucosa. A prospective clinical study on renal transplant recipients. *Transpl Int* 1990; 3:62–65.

Palermo TM. Impact of recurrent and chronic pain on child and family daily functioning: a critical review of the literature. *J Dev Behav Pediatr* 2000; 21:58–69.

Parkin DM, Stiller CA, Draper GJ, Bieber CA. The international incidence of childhood cancer. *Int J Cancer* 1988; 42:511–520.

Payne K, Mattheyse FJ, Liebenberg D, Dawes T. The pharmacokinetics of midazolam in pediatric patients. *Eur J Clin Pharmacol* 1989; 37:267–272.

Portenoy RK, Foley KM, Inturrisi CE. The nature of opioid responsiveness and its implications for neuropathic pain: new hypothesis derived from studies of opioid infusions. *Pain* 1990; 43:273–286.

Price D, McGrath PA, Raffii A, Buckingham B. The validation of the visual analogue scales as ratio scale measures for chronic and experimental pain. *Pain* 1983; 17:45–56.

Price DD, Bush FM, Long S, Harkins SW. A comparison of pain measurement characteristics of mechanical visual analogue and simple numerical rating scales. *Pain* 1994; 56:217–226.

Rawal N, Hylander J, Arnér S. Management of terminal cancer pain in Sweden: a nationwide survey. *Pain* 1993; 54:169–179.

Reis EC, Holubkov R. Vapocoolant spray is equally effective as EMLA cream in reducing immunization pain in school-aged children. *Pediatrics* 1997; 100:e5.

Rey E, Delaunay L, Pons G, et al. Pharmacokinetics of midazolam in children: comparative study of intranasal and intravenous administration. *Eur J Clin Pharmacol* 1991; 41:355–357.

Richter IL, McGrath PJ, Humphreys PJ, et al. Cognitive and relaxation treatment of pediatric migraine. *Pain* 1986; 25:195–203.

Riehm H, Ebell W, Feickert HJ, Reiter A. *Acute Lymphoblastic Leukaemia.* New York: Springer-Verlag, 1992.

Rogers AG. Use of amitriptyline (Elavil) for phantom limb pain in younger children. *J Pain Symptom Manage* 1989; 4:96.

Rossitch E, Madsen JR. *Neurosurgical Procedures for the Relief of Pain in Children and Adolescents.* Baltimore: Williams & Wilkins, 1993.

Rourke MT, Stuber ML, Hobbie WL, Kazak AE. Posttraumatic stress disorder: understanding the psychosocial impact of surviving childhood cancer into young adulthood. *J Pediatr Oncol Nurs* 1999; 16:126–135.

Rowbotham MC, Reisner-Keller LA, Fields HL. Both intravenous lidocaine and morphine reduce pain in postherpetic neuralgia. *Neurology* 1991; 41:1024–1028.

Sawyer M, Crettenden A, Toogood I. Psychological adjustment of families of children and adolescents treated for leukemia. *Am J Pediatr Hematol Oncol* 1986; 8:200–207.

Sawyer M, Antoniou G, Toogood I, Rice M, Baghurst P. Childhood cancer: a 4-year prospective study of the psychological adjustment of children and parents. *J Pediatr Hematol Oncol* 2000; 22:214–220.

Schanberg LE, Anthony KK, Gil KM, Lefebvre JC, Macharoni LM. Family pain history predicts child health status in children with chronic rheumatic disease. *Pediatrics* 2001; 108:E47.

Schechter NL. The undertreatment of pain in children: an overview. *Pediatr Clin North Am* 1989; 36:781–794.

Schuler D, Bakos M, Zsambor C, et al. Psychosocial problems in families of a child with cancer. *Med Pediatr Oncol* 1985; 13:173–179.

Shapiro BS. Treatment of chronic pain in children and adolescents. *Pediatr Ann* 1995; 24:148–156.

Shapiro BS, Dinges DF, Orne EC, et al. Home management of sickle cell-related pain in children and adolescents: natural history and impact on school attendance. *Pain* 1995; 61:139–144.

Skevington SM. Investigating the relationship between pain and discomfort and quality of life, using the WHOQOL. *Pain* 1998; 76:395–406.

Sloper P. Predictors of distress in parents of children with cancer: a prospective study. *J Pediatr Psychol* 2000; 25:79–91.

Smith DB, Newlands ES, Rustin GJ, et al. Comparison of ondansetron and ondansetron plus dexamethasone as anti-emetic prophylaxis during cisplatin-containing chemotherapy. *Lancet* 1991; 338:487–490.

Stang PE, Osterhaus JT. Impact of migraine in the United States: data from the National Health Interview Survey. *Headache* 1993; 33:29–35.

Stein REK, Jessop D. Functional Status II (R): a measure of child health status. *Med Care* 1990; 28:1041–1055.

Stiller CA, Draper GJ. *The Epidemiology of Cancer in Children.* Oxford: Oxford University Books, 1998.

Stiller CA, Allen MB, Eatock EM. Childhood cancer in Britain: The National Registry of Childhood Tumours and incidence rates 1978–1987. *Eur J Cancer* 1995; 31A(12):2028–2034.

Stuber M, Christakis D, Houskamp B, Kazak A. Post trauma symptoms in childhood leukemia survivors and their parents. *Psychosomatics* 1996; 37:254–261.

Stuber ML, Kazak AE, Meeske K, Barakat L. Is posttraumatic stress a viable model for understanding responses to childhood cancer? *Child Adolesc Psychiatr Clin N Am* 1998; 7:169–182.

Swerdlow M. Anticonvulsants in the neuralgic pain. *Pain Clin* 1986; 1:9–19.

Syrjala KL, Donaldson GW, Davis MW, Kippes ME, Carr JE. Relaxation and imagery and cognitive-behavioral training reduce pain during cancer treatment: a controlled clinical trial. *Pain* 1995; 63:189–198.

Tebbi CK, Petrilli AS, Richards ME. Adjustment to amputation among adolescent oncology patients. *Am J Pediatr Hematol Oncol* 1989; 11:276–280.

Terrence CF, Fromm GH, Tenicela R. Baclofen as an analgesic in chronic peripheral nerve disease. *Eur Neurol* 1985; 24:380–385.

Thompson JC, Walker JP. Indications for the use of parenteral H2-receptor antagonists. *Am J Med* 1984; 19:111–115.

Tubergen DG, Gilchrist GS, O'Brien RT, et al. Improved outcome with delayed intensification for children with acute lymphoblastic leukemia and intermediate presenting features: a Children's Cancer Group Phase III trial. *J Clin Oncol* 1993; 11:527–537.

Vainionpää L. Clinical neurological findings of children with acute lymphoblastic leukaemia at diagnosis and during treatment. *Eur J Pediatr* 1993; 152:115–119.

Van Schaik CS, Barr RD, Depauw S, Furlong W, Feeny D. Assessment of health status and health-related quality of life in survivors of Hodgkin's disease in childhood. *Int J Cancer Suppl* 1999; 12:32–38.

Varni JW, Katz ER, Seid M, Quiggins DJ, Friedman-Bender A. The pediatric cancer quality of life inventory-32 (PCQL-32): I. Reliability and validity. *Cancer* 1998; 82:1184–1196.

von Essen L, Enskar K, Kreuger A, Larsson B, Sjoden PO. Self-esteem, depression and anxiety among Swedish children and adolescents on and off cancer treatment. *Acta Paediatr* 2000; 89:229–236.

Wahlberg EJ, Wills RJ, Eckhert J. Plasma concentrations of midazolam in children following intranasal administration. *Anesthesiology* 1991; 74:233–235.

Walco GA, Cassidy RC, Schechter NL. Pain, hurt, and harm, the ethics of pain control in infants and children. *New Engl J Med* 1994; 331:541–544.

Walker C. Use of art and play therapy in pediatric oncology. *J Pediatr Oncol Nurs* 1989; 6:126.

Walker LS, Greene JW. The functional disability inventory: measuring a neglected dimension of child health status. *J Pediatr Psychol* 1991; 16:39–58.

Walker LS, Guite MS, Duke M, Barnard JA, Greene JW. Recurrent abdominal pain: a potential precursor of irritable bowel syndrome in adolescents and young adults. *J Pediatr* 1998; 132:110–115.

Wall PD. The prevention of postoperative pain. *Pain* 1988; 33:289–290.

Walsh TD. Antidepressants in chronic pain. *Clin Neuropharmacol* 1983; 6:271–295.

Walters AS, Williamson GM. The role of activity restriction in the association between pain and depression: a study of pediatric patients with chronic pain. *Children's Health Care* 1999; 28:33–50.

Weekes DP, Savedra M. Adolescent cancer: coping with treatment related pain. *J Pediatr Nurs* 1988; 3:318–328.

Weisman SJ, Bernstein B, Schechter NL. Consequences of inadequate analgesia during painful procedures in children. *Arch Pediatr Adolesc Med* 1998; 152:147–149.

Westlin JE, Letocha H, Jakobson Å, et al. Rapid, reproducible pain relief with [131I]iodine-meta-iodobenzylguanidine in a boy with disseminated neuroblastoma. *Pain* 1995; 60:11–114.

Wilkins C, McGrath PJ, Finley GA, Katz J. Phantom limb sensations and phantom limb pain in child and adolescent amputees. *Pain* 1998; 78:7–12.

Wolfe J, Grier HE, Klar N, et al. Symptoms and suffering at the end of life in children with cancer. *N Engl J Med* 2000; 342:326–333.

Wolfner JA, Visintainer MA. Pediatric surgical patient's stress responses and adjustment. *Nurs Res* 1975; 24:244–255.

Woolf CJ. Evidence for a central component of post-injury pain hypersensitivity. *Nature* 1983; 306:686–688.

Woolf CJ, Thompson JW. *Stimulation Induced Analgesia: Transcutaneous Electrical Nerve Stimulation (TENS) and Vibration.* Edinburgh: Churchill Livingstone, 1994.

World Health Organization. *Cancer Pain Relief.* Geneva: World Health Organization, 1986.

World Health Organization. *Cancer Pain Relief,* 2nd ed. Geneva: World Health Organization, 1996.

Yaster M, Nichols DG, Deshpande JK, Wetzel RC. Midazolam-fentanyl intravenous sedation in children: case report of respiratory arrest. *Pediatrics* 1990; 86:463–467.

Zebrack BJ, Chesler MA. Quality of life in childhood cancer survivors. *Psychooncology* 2002; 11:132–141.

Zech DFJ, Grond S, Lynch J, Hertel D, Lehmann KA. Validation of World Health Organization guidelines for cancer pain relief: a 10-year prospective study. *Pain* 1995; 63:65–76.

Zelefsky MJ, Scher HI, Forman JD et al. Palliative hemiskeletal irradiation for widespread metastatic prostate cancer: a comparison of single dose and fractionated regimens. *Int J Radiat Oncol Biol Phys* 1989; 17:1281–1285.

Zeltzer LK. Cancer in adolescents and young adults: psychosocial aspects: long-term survivors. *Cancer* 1993; 71:3463–3468.

Zeltzer L, LeBaron S. Hypnosis and non-hypnotic techniques for reduction of pain and anxiety during painful procedures in children and adolescents with cancer. *J Pediatr* 1982; 101:1032–1035.

Zeltzer LK, Altman A, Cohen D, et al. Report of the Subcommittee on the Management of Pain Associated with Procedures in Children with Cancer. *Pediatrics* 1990; 86:826–831.

Zempsky WT, Anand KJS, Sullivan KM, Fraser D, Cusina K. Lidocaine iontophoresis for topical anesthesia before intravenous line placement in children. *J Pediatr* 1998; 132:1061–1063.

Zuelze WW. Implications of long-term survival in acute stem cell leukaemia of childhood treated with composite cyclic therapy. *Blood* 1966; 24:477–494.

Correspondence to: Gustaf Ljungman, MD, PhD, Unit for Pediatric Hematology and Oncology, University Children's Hospital, SE-751 85 Uppsala, Sweden. Tel: 46-18-6115586; Fax: 46-18-500949; email: gustaf.ljungman@kbh.uu.se.

7

Social Influences, Culture, and Ethnicity

Kenneth D. Craig and Rebecca R. Pillai Riddell

Department of Psychology, University of British Columbia, Vancouver, British Columbia, Canada

Regardless of personal background, pain and suffering are inevitable human experiences. However, similar injuries and diseases can have a remarkably different effect on pain and illness behavior. These variations are heavily dependent upon the social contexts in which people live and have lived. This chapter describes differences among individuals that arise from their personal and cultural social heritage and proposes mechanisms responsible for the variation, devoting some attention to the necessity of cultural sensitivity in practice and research.

The emphasis of this chapter is on social processes rather than genetic variation responsible for phenotypic differences (see Smith and Mogil, this volume, for more detail on genetic variation in pain). It is clear that both biological factors (genetics, nutrition, injury, and disease) and socio-environmental factors (family, socio-economic status, community, and culture) must be elucidated in a comprehensive understanding of pain. Social and other environmental influences have an impact only through the biological systems that constitute the basis for all behavior. Nevertheless, these social factors represent defining features of human environments and are powerful sources of variation in how biological systems operate. Humans have a remarkable ability to learn, to understand their environments, to benefit from the experiences of others with whom they associate, and to develop socially constructed adaptive strategies for solving life's demands. A better appreciation of how different cultures approach the universal challenges of pain control allows for a more comprehensive understanding of pain and has the potential to contribute to novel preventive and treatment interventions.

In general, adaptation to environmental pressures represents a significant source of individual differences in observed pain behavior. Two major sources of variation can be identified. Some individual differences in pain and illness behavior are stable and reflect the individual's long-term personal history, beginning in early childhood. These enduring behavioral dispositions are the product of the person's unique social legacy, largely transmitted through his or her family in the course of development, with family patterns in turn echoing the local community, ethnic identities, and cultural history. Individual environments can be remarkably different, as witnessed by the dramatic variation even among siblings in the same family, but even then the collective wisdom of the community will be reflected. An anthropological perspective is required to appreciate broad sociocultural schemas and patterns of behavior as an ethnic group's best solution to the vexing and sometimes overwhelming challenges of collectively caring for members of its community.

Note, however, a second source of individual variation. The dispositions acquired during childhood, reflecting the shared values and attitudes of the community, are not entirely robust. Other context-driven variation reflects moment-to-moment problem-solving reactions to the individual's perception of immediate circumstances. Individuals display substantial sensitivity to social contexts, as evidenced by considerable plasticity in pain behavior. Situational demands can instigate behavior inconsistent with long-term dispositions. Humans can be characterized as a species by their range of adaptive responses to situational demands; adhering inflexibly to cultural strictures could represent maladaptive patterns that would reduce the likelihood of successful coping with novel circumstances. Thus, behavior that is out of keeping with common social scripts can be understood as the individual's utilization of his or her resources to provide an optimal solution to perceived demands.

This perspective on individual differences in human behavior has been systematized in the writings of Walter Mischel (1968, 1970), who succeeded in reorienting research that was preoccupied with personality traits and enduring childhood origins of adult behavior to an appreciation for interactions between enduring personal dispositions and situational determinants of behavior. By recognizing that behavior is the active and dynamic outcome of an interaction between the individual and his or her environment, Mischel emphasized that the individual is neither a slave to "personality" nor a capricious product of immediate environmental forces. To adequately appreciate the role of social influences on pain, one requires a dynamic, systems-based perspective. The experience of pain not only is influenced by this broad domain of variables, but also influences the social contexts of people's lives, thereby setting up continuously looping feedback systems.

KEY CONCEPTS

What is the suitable unit of analysis for best understanding the impact of social influences on pain? The possibilities range through different types and sizes of collectives, including the family, community, and ethnic identities. Anthropological perspectives might suggest bands, tribes, chiefdoms, and states (Diamond 1997). Bronfenbrenner (1979) observed that the "individual's ecological environment is akin to a set of nested structures, each inside the next, like a set of Russian dolls. At the inner-most level is the immediate setting containing the developing person." Each concentric layer represents a system or subsystem that plays a crucial role in the person's life. These systems can be seen to interact with each other, with some having a proximal influence and others being more distal. Ultimately, theoretical models incorporating social influences on pain will have to accommodate all levels of these factors. The following paragraphs represent some logical characterizations of collectives that are important, but the list is not all-inclusive.

The family. Elsewhere in this volume, Chambers examines origins of childhood pain experience and behavior in family interactions. Certain patterns of behavior are expected, modeled, and valued by parents and other family members, with conformity positively reinforced and nonconformity potentially subject to punishment. The family represents the most powerful common pathway whereby socialization has an impact on pain.

Ethnic identity. People are often classified through their association with large groups that have a common national, tribal, religious, linguistic, or cultural origin or background. Ethnic groups usually share a common culture or common values, world-views, and patterns of behavior. Lipton and Marbach (1984) observe that "ethnic group membership influences how one perceives, labels, responds to and communicates various symptoms, as well as from whom one selects to obtain care, when it is sought, and the types of treatment received." This view represents the adult outcome, but as noted below, there are few investigations of children's ethnicity and pain addressing how and when this influence takes place.

Religion. Religion provides an important example of a form of ethnic identity that is built upon strong belief systems. Religious instruction often addresses the value and meaning of pain and provides role models and expectations. The intensely personal meaning of pain and concomitant suffering is often determined by identification with religious beliefs and world views, with this conscious awareness and interpretation of the experience not presently reducible to neurophysiological mechanisms. Some major religions recognize pain and resultant suffering as beneficial or as a means of purifying the soul, and many acts of martyrdom, penitence, and self-injury have their origins in these beliefs (Tu 1980; Glucklich 2001). Devout religiosity of any type may result in an underreporting of pain.

The community. When considering social influences on pain, we need a concept that addresses the local social environments to which children are exposed intermediate to family and ethnicity. Participation in school, friendship groups, extracurricular activities (e.g., sports, music, volunteer work), and other interactions in the community heavily influences children outside the family. In the developed world, adolescence has become a time of life when family controls and influence are relaxed, or opposed, and peer influences exert a more powerful impact (Harris 1995). While highly structured ethnic communities certainly exist, and families can identify strongly with a specific ethnic heritage, complex pluralistic and multicultural communities and societies often lead to diverse exposures, and children often can be identified as belonging to multiple ethnicities. For example, a Protestant Scottish Anglophone, an Irish Jew, or a Catholic Inuit would not be unusual in Canada. Communities that respect multicultural diversity are less likely to be ethnocentric, believing that only one's own ethnic group is superior. Cultural relativism as an alternative position is more likely to lead to tolerance of diversity and to incorporate good ideas from other communities (Cauce et al. 1998). The community also may heavily reflect socioeconomic circumstances. With few exceptions, income dictates the amount the family can afford to pay for a house, the schools the children attend, the organizations the family joins, the church where they worship, and their access to a social network.

Culture. These differing groups all operate through transmission of culture-specific patterns of ways of thinking, feeling, and behaving. The concept of *culture* refers to belief systems and patterns of learned behavior that are shared and transmitted within a group across generations or to new members. These would be acquired either in the course of socialization within families identifying with the ethnic group or by acculturation in a different ethnic group through exposure to its practices, values, and standards, perhaps as a consequence of immigration or as a result of choosing to join a different religious group. To a considerable extent, human cultures emerge because communal living affords advantages of shared resources, including food production, personal safety, and improved health (Diamond 1997). Failure to provide the requisite resources, as in the case of famine, disease epidemics, and war, represents the breakdown of the community and an increased likelihood of pain and suffering.

Race. The concept of *race* presumes a basis for broad biological classification of groups of people based on physical and genetic characteristics, but it now is recognized as having limited application because it implies more consistency than is warranted. Three primary races typically are identified: Caucasoid, Mongoloid, and Negroid. Major biological differences among these groups cannot be identified at either the anatomical or genetic level (Goodman 2000). These distinctions are too crude to capture the complexities of biological dispositions. The history of *Homo sapiens* reflects high levels of sexual interaction among races, leading to greater genetic heterogeneity than these three categories suggest. The distinctions seem at best to refer to variation in minor anatomical features, such as skin pigmentation, rather than major physiological variation. Contrasts of those representing prototypical representatives of the presumed races do not show major differentiating commonalities in DNA structure. When behavioral commonalities can be observed, these can better be understood to represent the product of ethnicity. While visible inherited characteristics might distinguish minority groups from dominant people in a culture, it appears wrong to assume that behavioral differences are attributable to genetic variation. The visible differences also lead to differences in the way people are treated or socialized, and these must be respected as a probable major cause of behavioral variation (Kaplan and Bennett 2003).

INTRAPERSONAL AND INTERPERSONAL MODELS OF PAIN

Appreciating and endorsing the importance of social influences on pain requires a different perspective on the nature of pain than that which dominates most ways of thinking. The overwhelming focus for those conceptualizing pain has been its intrapersonal features. This is not difficult to illustrate. The widely accepted definition of pain developed and promulgated by the International Association for the Study of Pain (Merskey and Bogduk 1994) is oriented toward intrapersonal aspects of the phenomenon. It describes pain as "an unpleasant sensory and emotional experience associated with actual or potential tissue damage, or described in terms of such damage. … Pain is always subjective." Other definitions of pain also focus upon its internal features. Efforts to articulate why people suffer from pain almost invariably describe it as an inherent biological mechanism serving to protect the individual from physical harm by warning of tissue damage or stress and motivating escape, avoidance, or recuperative efforts. The biological sciences are preoccupied with efforts to understand the underlying internal regulatory mechanisms. Medical approaches to understanding pain focus upon internal biological mechanisms and somatosensory features of the experience. Accordingly, medical treatment in the first instance invariably involves pharmaceutical and surgical management oriented toward transforming biological sources of pain, and only when these fail do we consider psychological and social mechanisms. The rigid model that pain must be proportional to tissue damage becomes problematic when one considers chronic pain or pain in the absence of a medical explanation. Regrettably, this pervasive perspective also tends to ignore social and psychological variables that affect both pain experience and expression.

It takes some effort to reorient oneself toward interpersonal aspects of pain because the considerations outlined above overwhelm our thinking. Nevertheless, some basic reflection leads to the discovery of many key features. Our species has proliferated because we are social animals (Craig and Badali, in press). Extraordinary transformations in hominid evolution took place over perhaps a million years when humans began to band together and enjoyed the fruits of collective enterprise, including the development of language and the ability to transmit complex culture from generation to generation. Our brains evolved to permit engagement with others in complex social interactions and organizations. While newborns of some nonhuman species require and receive care following birth, in humans the maturation period is protracted for many years, in order to protect children and to introduce them to intricate social complexities, including language and other forms of communication.

Pain reflects this evolutionary transformation. From the evolutionary biology perspective, the model of pain proposed here is fundamentally human. In humans, the functions of pain transcend personal safety. Pain is rarely fully private and is always embedded in highly complex social contexts. A person's experience of pain usually is of profound importance to others and has automatic overt features that serve social communication functions (Hadjistavropoulos and Craig 2002; Hill and Craig 2002). Expressions of pain usually are highly salient crises that command attention and instigate in observers automatic, involuntary concern for personal safety (Ohman 2002). They can serve in both nonhuman species and humans to alarm others about dangerous situations. They also can serve to trigger intense concern for the welfare of the one in pain and are likely to instigate efforts to assist the one in distress (Craig et al. 1986). Humans are relatively unique in their capacity to use language and facial expression as forms of communication to influence others. Nonhuman primates and some other species use limited forms of oral communication or utilize the face to display social signals, but human language capabilities greatly exceed those of even our closest primate relatives, and the human face has a more complex musculature and more versatile neural innervation than that of other primates (Ohman 2002). Natural selection has adapted humans to very sophisticated forms of social communication during pain.

The interaction between a person in pain and an observer during an acute painful crisis can have a sustained impact. During childhood, when children face challenges of establishing secure attachments to primary caregivers (Ainsworth and Bell 1974; Bowlby 1980), pain could influence bonding, feelings of security, and trust in others. Exposing children to repeated, prolonged, or recurrent pain could risk affecting these relationships. In the long run, the person suffering from persistent pain, at any age, probably will experience social isolation, diminished opportunities to interact with others, loss of skills, and even a risk of becoming stigmatized. Elsewhere in this volume, von Baeyer and Spagrud describe the importance of social factors in human development and their role in pain expression and experience. At the level of subjective experience, the interpersonal implications of pain tend to be a focus during both acute and chronic pain, and people in pain are aware that their role in complex social systems is likely to be diminished. Caring, compassionate communities offer institutions designed to help parents and others prevent and control pain in infants and children. While they may be less effective than we could wish (Ellis et al. 2002), these institutions reflect social concern for children's pain.

These social parameters of pain become more meaningful when one considers pain in infants and young children. Neonatal pain is intensely public. The newborn usually reacts vigorously with crying, facial grimaces, and body language. The magnitude of these behavioral reactions no doubt reflects severe subjective distress in the child, but the more prominent adaptive function would seem to be that they command the mother's attention and protection, prompting intense concern and preoccupation that may be shared by others (Craig et al. 2002). Mothers' reactions to pain in their infants include substantial physiological arousal (Murray 1979), and mothers and nurses report identical cues as especially salient, despite substantial variations in background and experience when responding to an infant's pain (Pillai et al. 2002). Early humans, who were often subject to attacks of efficient predators, might have reacted to a baby's cry with fear for their own safety (Craig et al. 2000). This risk of imminent physical danger is less likely today, but in ancestral human and nonhuman species, as with many nonhuman species today, pain and panic reactions in others served as important safeguards (Barr 1998).

DIVERSE IMPACTS OF SOCIAL INFLUENCES ON PAIN

Numerous parameters of children's pain are subject to social influence. The sociocommunications model of children's pain (Craig et al. 1996, 2002) provides a perspective for appreciating the extent of these influences, because it is inclusive of important variables that traditional concepts of pain ignore. Any given incident of childhood pain is likely to include a sequence of tissue stress or trauma, the experience of pain, expression of pain, caregivers' observations and assessments of the event, and subsequent interventions. All represent potential targets for social influences on children's pain, as depicted in the model in Fig. 1.

This model characterizes the relationships among the experiences and roles of children and caregivers within the context of acute pediatric pain. Thick arrows down the center delineate over time the sequence of events, described above. Given that the interactions between the child and caregiver will continue over time, curved arrows highlight reciprocal feedback loops. The concentric ellipses illustrate the varying layers of social influences on both children and their caregivers. Identical labeling of social factors influencing both the child and the caregiver acknowledge the common interests of the community in the child. The bidirectional arrows and the dotted lines used for the concentric ellipses direct attention to the interactive nature of the social influences. Each layer influences every other layer,

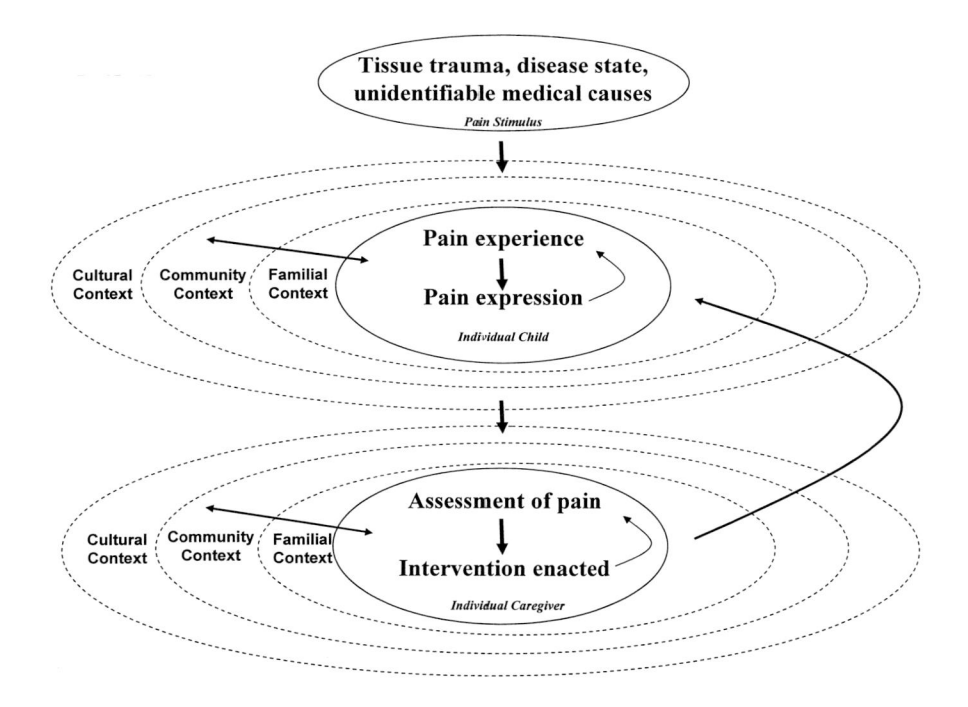

Fig. 1. Social influences on childhood pain.

either directly or indirectly. The solid lines around the child and the caregiver represent the unique synthesis of social influences created in all individuals because of their relatively idiosyncratic biological makeup and their niche in their family, community, and ethnic group. The cultural context layers refer not only to mainstream cultural influences but also to the complexities of living in a mainstream culture after coming from a different cultural heritage. The following sections provide a more in-depth discussion of social influences on the sequence of events following acute tissue insult in a child.

Tissue stress or trauma. Variation is substantial in the extent to which families, communities, and societies unintentionally or purposefully expose children to danger. The epidemiological literature on children's pain reflects sources and risk factors (Goodman and McGrath 1991; McGrath 1999); hence, it provides a sense of vulnerabilities and potential targets for prevention. Lifestyle factors can be recognized as important in most injuries and illnesses. For example, automobile seat belts, safe playgrounds, immunization programs, vigilance regarding neglect and child abuse, and hygienic environments play important roles in the prevention of pain in children. Flores et al. (2000) provide evidence that socioeconomic and minority group status are related to access to pediatric care, adherence to recommended health care protocols, health status, continuity of care, preventive screening, doctor-patient communication, adequacy of analgesia, likelihood of regular care, avoidance of harmful remedies, immunization rates, and prescription practices. Bonham (2001) found different and less than optimal management of health care for children of minority and ethnic families compared to children of mainstream American families. The authors attributed the differences to stereotypes, language barriers, ineffective communication, failure to understand the patient's expressions of pain and distress, and socioeconomic factors.

Garg and colleagues demonstrate in this volume that multiple exposures to unintended or culturally sanctioned pain may have a major impact on the biological systems that control pain, potentially dampening reactivity or producing hypersensitivity, among other possibilities. Grunau (this volume) also observes that repeated pain early in life affects how children interact with others. For example, children born early with low birth weights who are exposed frequently to pain in neonatal intensive care units become predisposed to increased somatization in interactions with their mothers.

Pain experience. Pain and suffering are appreciated by individuals as a synthesis of sensory and affective input modulated by personal experiences and beliefs learned in social contexts. Table I parses some of the domains of private pain experience influenced by social factors. There has been considerable microanalysis of these factors, mostly with adults, with the developmental transformations awaiting exploration. It is difficult to analyze these qualities in children because of the challenges of effective communication with them. The distinction between internal and external features of pain is particularly problematic, because we have no means of inferring private experience other than through public manifestations (Prkachin and Craig 1985). The role of social factors is conceivably more important in younger children because they have fewer self-management skills and remain dependent upon adults for care. The pain experiences of infants are dominated by sensory and affective qualities, without memory or understanding to provide a sense that pain will not be of infinite duration or that they can control their experiences (R.R. Pillai Riddell, M.A. Badali, and K.D. Craig, unpublished manuscript).

Pain expression. Typically researchers categorize the various sources of information available from children as self-report, nonverbal expression, and physiological activity (Table II). These kinds of expression could also be categorized as intentional and unintentional (Hadjistavropoulos and Craig 2002). The former would include self-report and certain nonverbal actions under the control of higher executive cognitive functions. Involuntary actions would include reflexive features of nonverbal display and physiological activity. The involuntary and public nature of certain nonverbal display features is illustrated by evidence that the facial grimace of pain cannot be wholly suppressed (Hadjistavropoulos and Craig 1994; Hill and Craig 2002). Note that pain expression not only reflects internal experience and processes, but also appears to be socially motivated. It is predicated upon its impact on others. Operant psychology has made it clear that even involuntary behaviors are subject to reinforcement control. Family members and others can unwittingly increase the likelihood of pain behaviors through social reinforcement (Caudhill 2001).

Observers' assessment or attribution of pain to the child. With some exceptions, those observing a child in pain appear to have involuntary

Table I
Features of pain experience subject to social influence

Perception of somatic events as symptoms
Perceived severity of somatic events
Pain thresholds and severity
Meaning of the event
Health-related schemas and representations
Personal and interpersonal motivations
Coping strategies (e.g., catatrophizing)
Emotional distress (fear, generalized anxiety, depression, anger)

Table II
Pain expression (public)

Complaints and accounts of qualities and intensity
Paralinguistic vocalization
Nonverbal actions including facial grimaces and body language
Pain intolerance
Illness behavior
Pain-related disability

sympathetic reactions (Murray 1979), but it is also clear that experience with children and socialized belief systems determine the nature of the observer's reaction. The task of understanding pain in children can be complex and difficult. There is a general propensity for parents and nurses to underestimate the severity of pain in children (Chambers et al. 1998). Furthermore, substantial evidence of neglect of children's pain suggests that false beliefs and inappropriate attitudes often lead to misunderstandings (Gedaly-Duff and Ziebarth 1994; Finley et al. 1996; Forward et al. 1996). In the infant literature, recent trends indicate increasing willingness to believe that infants experience pain, but practitioners remain reluctant to provide adequate analgesia (McIntosh 1997; Stevens and Koren 1998). In recent studies examining the willingness of parents, nurses, and pediatricians to attribute pain to infants during routine immunization, all three groups roughly estimated that an adult would experience half the amount of pain as would an infant undergoing the same needle stick (R.R. Pillai Riddell and K.D. Craig, unpublished manuscript).

Interventions. Finally, social factors influence how the child is treated once pain has been recognized. One can construe pain as desirable (e.g., "spare the rod and spoil the child") or character building and elect not to intervene, as in the case of various religious perspectives and for adults electing to use corporal punishment in child discipline. Social factors can determine which strategies are utilized. Professional training determines the use of interventions. Traditional Chinese medicine, for example, calls for substantially different interventions than would be used in contemporary Western medicine (Kleinman 1982). In North America, use of pharmaceuticals for pain control in infants is yielding to a more inclusive approach incorporating environmental and comfort measures, such as kangaroo care, rocking, use of pacifiers, and dim lights (Stevens 2002). The treatment strategies selected by a given caregiver are also greatly influenced by pain coping schemas reflecting familial, community, and cultural contexts. These contexts can determine whether the coping strategy is active or passive, emotion-focused or problem-focused, and independent or interdependent coping (Flores et al. 2000).

EXAMPLES OF ETHNIC VARIABILITY

The distinction between disease states and illness behavior is important. The pathophysiological mechanisms are common across people in different cultures, but the patterns of illness behavior, including personal, interpersonal, and cultural reactions to disease, can vary substantially (Kleinman 1980). Mechanic (1962) observed that individuals perceive, evaluate, and act upon physical symptoms in different ways depending upon the cultures or sectors of society to which they belong.

There is considerable scope for ethnic variation, but caution is needed in interpreting this literature. First, it is difficult to escape value judgments when characterizing other people's pain and illness behavior. One community may prize high levels of pain tolerance, characterizing it as reflecting strength of character and great fortitude, whereas another may describe it as foolhardy and reckless to endure severe pain, particularly if pain control is available. Ethnocentrism is likely to lead to condemnation of others' practices. Second, as a general principle, there will be greater variability in pain behavior within an ethnic community than there will be differences between communities. This also will be reflected in overlap in the distributions between communities being contrasted. Researchers must exercise caution not to stereotype representatives of ethnic groups. Group stereotypes cannot be seen to characterize individuals, just as the behavior of individuals must not be looked upon as representative of ethnic groups to which they belong.

The classic studies of ethnic variation were conducted by Zborowski (1969), who contrasted "Old Americans" with Jews, Italians, and Irish immigrants and their descendants living in New York city. The participants in his studies were all male World War II veterans residing in a large hospital. The characterizations were nonsystematic and impressionistic descriptions rich in language and detail. Other investigators subsequently studied these groups more systematically (e.g., Zola 1966; Tursky and Sternbach 1967), providing a legacy of belief that people of Mediterranean cultural extraction were more likely to be aware of and to communicate symptoms of physical discomfort than were Northern European peoples. Similar general descriptions of other ethnic groups are available (e.g., Weisenberg 1982; Meinhart and McCaffery 1983), but there is presently a concern about the risks of overly general stereotyping.

Situational adaptations superimposed on ethnic training have been demonstrated. Pilowsky and Spence (1977) observed that ethnic Greek patients consulting a general practitioner in Australia displayed more hypochondriacal attitudes, greater disease conviction, and a preference for somatic rather than psychological explanations of their symptoms, relative to patients of Anglo-Saxon origins. However, ethnic Greek patients who had become acculturated to Australian customs provided evidence of transformations in their values and beliefs toward those of the more dominant Anglo-Saxon culture. Zborowski (1969) had observed that successive generations of immigrant families increasingly resemble their host culture. These changes represent appropriate and adaptive reactions to social demands, which are heavily contributory to acculturation.

More immediate adaptations can be observed. Lambert and colleagues (1960) found that students at McGill University in Montreal, Canada, identifying with Jewish and Protestant faiths, did not differ on baseline pain reports, nor did these reports differ following an assertion by a researcher that members of their faith were less tolerant of pain than were adherents of the other faith. However, after hearing this assertion both groups dramatically increased their pain tolerance.

Ethnic variation can be observed in studies of children. Abu-Saad (1984) contrasted children living in California in the United States who had Arab-American, Asian-American, and Latin-American family backgrounds. This study compared 24 children per group, aged 9 to 12 years, using semi-structured interviews in homes, schools, and recreational facilities. The following illustrates some of the complex findings. The children identified both physical and psychological causes of their painful distress, noting that falls were the most common sources of pain, but also including death and divorce, indicating an appreciation of the complexity of the phenomenon. The Latin-American children favored physical causes, for example, headaches, ear aches, and stomach aches, while the Asian-American children were more likely to include psychological causes, for example "people making fun of me" or "people calling me names." The children were able to use diverse descriptors across sensory, affective, and evaluative categories to describe pain. In describing affective discomfort, the Arab-American children were more inclined to report "feeling sick to my stomach" whereas the Latin-American children frequently described themselves as "feeling bad" or feeling "like not doing anything." There was similar diversity in how the children reported coping with pain.

Most children gave no answer to the question "What is good about pain?" However, some children recognized advantages. Trends were different across the ethnic groups: a few Arab-American children noted that pain might involve "missing school," "getting sympathy," and "learning from the experience," and that "pain prepares you for life," while Asian-American children observed that "pain lets you know what's wrong with your body," "it shows if your friends are helpful," and "when I'm in pain, no one pushes me around." Latin-American children were described as favoring "friends visit you," "Mom calms you down," and "you don't die from it." These brief comments also illustrate the social importance and significance of pain to these children.

There also have been interesting behavioral observations. Rosmus et al. (2000) used facial activity and crying to characterize Canadian-born Chinese and non-Chinese babies receiving immunization injections at 2 months of age. The Chinese babies were more responsive to pain. The findings invite speculation on biological, socialization, and situational determinants. The authors favored the latter because the Chinese mothers were more interactive with their babies prior to the injection, suggesting a likelihood that these babies would be more responsive during the injection procedure.

The complexities of measuring differences across culture become evident in a study by Litcher et al. (2000), who attempted to contrast somatization behavior in children in Nashville, Tennessee, in the United States with that of children in Kyiv, in the Ukraine. Many of the Ukrainian children had been exposed to nuclear radiation during the Chernobyl disaster and had been evacuated. Both the children and mothers reporting on their behalf completed the Children's Somatization Inventory. While the Ukrainian children reported fewer symptoms than did the children in the United States, the mothers of the Ukrainian children reported fully three times as many symptoms. It seemed likely that the mothers of the Ukrainian children had been sensitized to their children's health.

The history of systematic research on ethnic variation in pain in children is relatively brief. The usual challenges of access and assessment in conducting studies with children perhaps are complicated in attempts to work with diverse cultures where communication challenges are encountered and there must be sensitivity to different value systems.

ORIGINS OF ETHNIC VARIATION

A very long-term historical perspective is required to understand the origins of ethnic and cultural variation in pain and illness behavior. Humans are a prolific, nomadic species, with *Homo sapiens* migrating out of Africa and in the span of perhaps 150,000 years inhabiting almost all regions of our planet, including some that are harsh and hostile, from the frozen Arctic to searing deserts. The evidence indicates that modern human behavior could be recognized 40,000 to 50,000 years ago, if artifacts suggestive of tools, decorative arts, and funerary customs are accepted (Diamond 1997). We have had a long time to evolve patterns of caring for one another. In all settings, including those that could be construed as more benign, painful injuries and diseases were inevitable, as were inventive, culture-specific efforts to devise solutions to the challenges of pain.

No culture can lay claim to a universally effective form of treating pain. Neither the technologically sophisticated approaches to be found in the developed world nor alternative interventions employed in other cultures have proven wholly successful. Thus, all variations represent imperfect attempts at solving the challenges of pain emerging among groups of people living in relatively isolated locations and confronting the challenges of dangerous environments. Their attempts were evidence-based (based on trial and error and subject to corrective contingencies), but variable in application of the methodological tools of science that are recognized as necessary to establish the credibility and validity of assertions. As isolated communities came into contact, there would have been cultural diffusion of concepts and treatments, much as other human inventions including language, writing, modes of transportation, and other technologies were distributed (Diamond 1997). In recent decades the developed world has become more receptive to exploring the use of alternative and complementary medicine, in part because of frustration with inadequacies of care for chronic conditions and terminal illnesses. This modern trend very effectively illustrates the role of cultural diffusion. Similarly, effective pain control strategies developed in the Western world are being introduced in other countries, but resource limitations and other barriers slow the process.

Different culturally based solutions would have evolved slowly and erratically, but progressively, over time as a result of individuals and those who cared for them confronting pain and attempting the use of a broad range of palliatives. Some would be time-honored, hence inevitable in a particular ethnic setting, and others experimental if the traditional remedies proved ineffective. These nostrums became recognized as useless and were discarded, whereas other interventions would prove effective, sometimes because very specific factors were operating, for example, the availability of salicylates from willow bark. In other cases, there would have been no specific effect, but the intervention could have appeared effective as a result of nonspecific effects. For example, hypnotically induced analgesia can control pain, but not for the reasons proposed by many of its advocates. For example, Anton Mesmer proposed concepts of animal magnetism, but these were rejected by his contemporaries who favored explanations now rooted in social psychology (Binet and Féré 1888). Sorting out the underlying mechanism is complex, in part, because diseases and injuries remit and relapse, frequently unpredictably, and hindsight analyses often dominate interpretations of events. Different culturally based perspectives on pain and its management would have emerged piecemeal in different regions of the world as a result of the accumulation over time of very large numbers of individual decisions about how one should understand and control pain.

TRANSFORMATIONS WITHIN A CULTURE

We best know the transformations in understanding and practice that took place in Western cultures. The history of concepts of pain in childhood dramatically illustrates the types of transformations that can emerge over time. Unruh (1992) provides an account based upon a review of ancient and contemporary writings. Remarkably, these indicate that until roughly the 20th century physicians believed children experienced more pain than adults. During the ancient age of medicine, pain was attributed to many metaphysical causes, including poor alignment of the constellations, the afflictions of demons, punishment from enraged deities, or humoral imbalances.

More unified and scientific concepts began with Descartes (1664), who postulated pathways in the body that one could find and see. This turning point initiated the remarkable biological research traditions that led to contemporary neuroscientific approaches to understanding pain. Unfortunately, it also created the Cartesian dualism that relegated our understanding of psychological mechanisms in pain to the study of mind, rather than to study of the psychological functions of biological mechanisms. The late 19th century saw a flowering of psychophysical research investigating pain as a somatosensory experience. This concept was questioned by Melzack and Wall (1965) in their remarkable gate control theory of pain. This theory permitted investigation of the intricate interactions between neurobiological mechanisms implicated in pain and the complexities of thoughts and feelings, as well as sensory input, during painful experiences. Now we can add the importance of social constructs to this mixture and hope for a truly biopsychosocial perspective on children's pain.

Regrettably, the study of pain in children was largely ignored until the decades of the late 20th century. This omission may have reflected beliefs that understanding pain in adults would inevitably help us understand pain in children. More insidiously, the concept emerged that the biological systems necessary to experience pain needed to be fully developed before pain could be felt. Infants were seen as "decorticate" (McGraw 1943), and the protracted time required for postnatal myelinization of nociceptive afferent fibers was seen inappropriately as an impediment to the true experience of pain. Moreover, preoccupation with a false sense of the importance of self-report measures of pain meant that serious investigation of pain in infants and young children was ignored. After all, the Latin root *infans* means "incapable of speech." McGrath and Unruh quote Hess (1849), a 19th-century physician who described working with children as the "most arduous branch of medical art" due to the "inability or the unwillingness of children to give a proper description of their feelings" (McGrath and Unruh 1987). Failure to mount the necessary observational studies of pain in children no doubt contributed to a large number of myths and inappropriate attitudes toward the nature of pain in children and its management, some of which continue to the present time.

While infants and young children clearly have the capacity to experience pain (Anand and Hickey 1987; Fitzgerald 1993), rampant evidence testifies to the undermanagement of pain in children. Continuing beliefs appear to sustain inadequate care. For example, it has been argued that children do not have a capacity to remember pain and that only after about 12 months of life do the requisite capacities for understanding and remembering pain emerge (Leventhal and Sherer 1987; Derbyshire 1996, 1999). Fortunately, these academic arguments do not sustain parents' interpretations of infant pain reactions. R.R. Pillai Riddell, M.A. Badali, and K.D. Craig (unpublished manuscript) reported that parents recognize that the cognitive capacity for appreciating the meaning of pain and explicit memory emerges only slowly over the first years of life. However, parents had little difficulty attributing pain to the reactions of infants aged 2, 4, 6, 12, and 18 months to immunization needle sticks. Infants' capacity for conscious experience of pain may not be as differentiated and complex as that of older children and adults, but some core of conscious experience was recognized. If cortical development must be complete for pain to be experienced, it could be argued that any healthy child or adolescent could not experience pain.

ORIGINS OF INDIVIDUAL VARIATION: CULTURAL TRANSMISSION TO THE INDIVIDUAL

Children largely learn about pain through their families, and thus culture shapes pain experience and behavior. Families provide relatively unique mini-cultures, allowing children opportunities to learn what is likely to be painful, how they are likely to react and feel, the meaning of the experience, and what types of behaviors will prove useful or effective as they endeavor to cope with the challenges. Children are strongly motivated to learn and benefit from the social models of pain experience and behavior provided by family members. Direction can be provided through opportunities to learn by direct observation or through verbal symbolic modeling, verbal guidance, and physical restraint. Parents and other adult family members usually accept responsibility for the safety and well-being of children and can be expected to constrain activities, supervise, provide physical and verbal directions, and reinforce and punish adherence to their expectations (Craig 1986). Through these mechanisms, children learn familial/ethnic behavioral patterns, and these behaviors are maintained through positive reinforcement of conformity, with deviance considered a threat to personal safety and hence subject to punishment. Parents tend to be very conservative when danger to their children is implicated. Sargent (1984) provides a fascinating illustration of these mechanisms in an anthropological study of the Bariba culture in northern Benin and Nigeria. These people idealize stoicism in response to pain, with their socialization processes demanding courage and honor as crucial values in such practices as circumcision and clitoridectomy. Family, peer groups, and others model an "absence of manifest behavior" when confronted with apparently painful events such as childbirth, wounds, or initiation ordeals. Great honor is associated with conformity to cultural ideals, and humiliation and shame are accorded to those who fail to meet the standards, along with their families.

But children also learn about pain outside the family context, particularly where the family's expectations and patterns deviate from those of the broader culture within which it resides. Age peers, public media, health care practitioners, and others provide the opportunities for learning alternative practices. The relative impact of multiple sources will also depend upon cognitive and affective development. For these reasons, the impact of culture on any given individual's behavior will differ depending upon development and life circumstances (Weisz et al. 1997).

SENSITIVITY IN INTERPRETING AND COMMUNICATING CULTURAL FINDINGS

The potential for misunderstandings and errors in pain assessment and management because of insensitivity to cultural norms is considerable. Practitioners have a duty to be responsive to ethnic variation in pain and illness behaviors. Similarly, researchers have an ethical obligation to examine and develop an understanding of the differences and their origins. One cannot assume that one's own cultural standards apply to others. Moreover, stereotypic conceptions of other cultures do not apply to individual representatives of those cultures. The stereotypes are often based on unsubstantiated social anecdotes and clinical impressions. Treatment based on these impressions should be undertaken with considerable caution. If a child came from an ethnic group usually described as prone to exaggeration and this child were to vigorously complain, there would be a risk of discounting the complaints and neglecting real, important problems.

Clinicians need to be particularly sensitivity to the risks of inappropriate treatment with people in minority groups (Korol and Craig 2001). There are risks of patient compliance in the absence of fully informed consent, misperceptions of patients' needs, or inadvertent coercion. Patients' perceptions of personal needs can be very important. Different cultures perceive the power differential between patient and professional in varying ways. Some ill patients may be particularly reluctant to react in a manner discordant with their perception of how one should behave in the presence of authority figures.

Fisher (1993) discusses this duty to understand the impact of culture in terms of three overarching moral principles: *beneficence, respect,* and *justice.* She argues that the first two values usually are evident in practice, but the third is least often accomplished. The principle of justice concerns the importance of equitable distribution of social benefits and costs. In a just society, there would be nondiscriminatory distribution of resources and understanding of individuals varying in ethnic background across, for example, nationality, religion, age, sex, or social status. It is this sensitivity to cultural diversity that we are seeking.

METHODOLOGICAL CONSIDERATIONS IN STUDYING ETHNIC AND CULTURAL FACTORS IN CHILDREN'S PAIN

The principle of justice (Fisher 1993) applies directly to the study of pain in children with different backgrounds. Only recently have we recognized the importance of the study of pain in children with cognitive impairment and developmental disabilities (McGrath et al. 1998; Hadjistavropoulos et al. 2001), and likewise it is imperative to strive for equitable selection and treatment of research participants of various ethnic backgrounds. We must prioritize the inclusion of disadvantaged and minority populations in developmental pain research. Not doing so runs the risk of an inadequate knowledge base for suitable and effective services. Given that ethnic minorities often lack adequate health maintenance and seek medical care only during a crisis or after a disease has progressed (Canino and Spurlock 1994), efforts should be redoubled to include these populations in pediatric pain research.

One constant challenge concerns definition and operationalization of the population of interest. Allowing participants to self-identify through checking a box to indicate ethnicity is not enough (Kaplan and Bennett 2003). Identifying ethnic background requires an understanding of the many interacting cultural influences on any given individual. Declared ethnicity (e.g., Asian, Protestant, Native) does not identify how intensely a declared ethnic identity penetrates beliefs, values, or behavior. Representatives of minority groups are particularly problematic because they are in a process of acculturation into mainstream culture. At a minimum one would be interested in information from these individuals concerning how strongly they identify with heritage and mainstream cultures and how well they were assimilated into the mainstream culture (Berry 1988). Relevant information might include number of familial generations and number of years in a country, language fluency, degree of individualistic or collectivist beliefs, level of education, level of income, change in social status as a result of emigration, current social status, sociopolitical affiliation, and gender (APA Office of Ethnic Minority Affairs 1993).

Study design also poses major problems. Experimental designs are not possible; participants cannot be randomly assigned to enculturation groups. Hence, quasi-experimental designs must be used, but they are limited in their usefulness in inferring causal factors. The complexities of the factors impinging upon any given individual also are considerable, depending upon the level of detail required, leading researchers to consider multivariate designs that identify key operative factors.

Selection of measures is also demanding. Helms (1992) argues for consideration of four criteria to ensure that measures have the same internal structure and hold similar meaning across cultural groups: functional, conceptual, linguistic, and psychometric/scalar equivalence. Cauce and colleagues (1998) offer a range of additional recommendations to ensure sensitive conduct of studies, including ensuring prior consultation with members of the ethnic group, using focus groups during piloting of the study, and providing at all stages someone fluent in the language of the culture to facilitate culturally unbiased research.

Location and time of studies also should be carefully considered. Willis (2002) cites data from the U.S. National Institute of Child Health and Human Development reporting that in the United States African-American and Hispanic children have a poverty rate four times that of white children. Low socioeconomic status in these minority groups can be attributed to a high proportion of single-parent households. These several factors would add barriers to feasibility, recruitment, and implementation. Researchers must make culturally appropriate attempts to remove barriers preventing individuals of minority background from participating in studies. It may be necessary to collect data within the community or after already scheduled medical appointments rather than asking subjects to make a special trip to a location that could be hours away by public transportation. One might offer day care for other children within the family so that a single parent would not perceive time spent away from home to participate in the study to be a barrier. Collecting data in early mornings, late evenings, or on weekends would help facilitate the participation of families that have parents doing shift work or families unwilling to lose money to participate in a research study. The complexities are considerable. Researcher and technician ethnicity may influence results. It may not be possible for researchers to remain blind as to participants' ethnic identity; this limitation could introduce observer bias into collection and treatment of data.

Having a culturally informed study does not stop with methodology. How a researcher interprets and disseminates findings is of key importance (Cauce et al. 1998). As a rule of thumb, one should always know the demographic breakdown of the standardization sample used to create the norms for all measures used (instrument validity). One should be wary of interpreting clinical elevations without an appropriate normative sample for reference. Researchers should always strive to contemplate how their own cultural values and beliefs influence research design, intervention protocols, and interpretation of results. Collaboratively written discussion sections with input from individuals of different cultural perspectives may help prevent value-laden judgments. When statistical analysis suggests retention of the null hypothesis, it is always important to provide a power analysis to ensure that the sample was large enough, thereby avoiding a Type II error. When one rejects the null hypothesis it is good practice to report effect sizes. Cultural similarities and differences tend to make sensationalist copy for the popular media. Effect sizes and power analyses are not generally accessible to the public, but they ensure that journal findings are properly couched in terms that should encourage lay journalists and others to avoid overinterpretation of cultural differences and similarities. It is also a reasonable expectation that investigators in this field should endeavor to translate their findings for public knowledge. Fisher (1993) argues for responsible dissemination of findings by suggesting that "all investigators should examine the potential real world implications of their findings and clarify in their writings and public presentations the extent, as well as the limits, of the applications of their findings to practice or social policy."

ACKNOWLEDGMENTS

The authors and their research reported here were supported by fellowships and operating grants from the Canadian Institutes of Health Research, the Michael Smith Foundation for Health Research, and the Social Sciences and Humanities Research Council of Canada.

REFERENCES

Abu-Saad H. Cultural group indicators of pain in children. *Maternal Nurs J* 1984; 187–196.
Ainsworth MDS, Bell SM. Mother-infant interaction and the development of competence. In: Connolly K, Bruner J (Eds). *The Growth of Competence*. London: Academic Press, 1974.
Anand KJS, Hickey PR. Pain and its effects in the human neonate and fetus. *N Engl J Med* 1987; 317:1321–1347.
APA Office of Ethnic Minority Affairs. Guidelines for providers of psychological services to ethnic, linguistic, and culturally diverse populations. *Am Psychol* 1993; 48(1):45–48.
Barr RG. Reflections on measuring pain in infants: dissociation in responsive systems and "honest signalling." *Arch Dis Child* 1998; 79:F152–F156.
Bates MS. Ethnicity and pain: a biocultural model. *Soc Sci Med* 1987; 24:47–50.
Berry JW. Acculturation and mental health. In: Dasen PR, Berry JW, Sartorius N (Eds). *Health and Cross-Cultural Psychology*. Newbury Park, CA: Sage, 1988.
Binet A, Féré C. *Animal Magnetism*. New York: Appleton, 1888.
Bonham VL. Race, ethnicity, and pain treatment: striving to understand the causes and solutions to the disparities in pain treatment. *J Law Med Ethics* 2001, 29:52–68.
Bowlby J. *Attachment and Loss*, Vol. 3. New York: Basic Books, 1980.
Bronfenbrenner U. *The Ecology of Human Development: Experiments by Nature and Design*. Cambridge, MA: Harvard University Press, 1979.
Canino IA, Spurlock J. *Culturally Diverse Children and Adolescents: Assessment, Diagnosis and Treatment*. New York: Guilford Press, 1994.
Cauce AM, Coronado N, Watson J. Conceptual, methodological, and statistical issues in culturally competent research. In: Hernadez M, Issacs M (Eds). *Promoting Cultural Competence in Children's Mental Health*. Baltimore: Paul H. Brookes, 1998.
Caudhill M. *Managing Pain Before It Manages You*. New York: Guilford Press, 2001.
Chambers CT, Reid GJ, Craig KD, McGrath PJ, Finley GA. Agreement between child and parent reports of pain. *Clin J Pain* 1998; 142:336–342.
Craig KD. Social modeling influences: pain in context. In: Sternbach RA (Ed). *The Psychology of Pain*, 2nd ed. New York: Raven Press, 1986.
Craig KD, Badali MA. Pain in the social animal. Commentary for: Williams, AC de C. Facial expression of pain: an evolutionary account. *Behav Brain Sci*; in press.
Craig KD, Gilbert-MacLeod C, Lilley CM. Cry as an indicator of pain in infants. In: Barr RG, Hopkins B, Green JA (Eds). *Crying as a Sign, a Symptom, and a Signal*. London: Mac Keith Press, 2000, pp 23–40.
Craig KD, Korol C, Pillai RR. Challenges of judging pain in vulnerable infants. *Clin Perinatol* 2002; 29:1–13.
Craig KD, Lilley CM, Gilbert CA. Social barriers to optimal pain management in infants and children. *Clin J Pain* 1996; 12:232–242.
Derbyshire SWG. Comment on editorial by Anand and Craig. *Pain* 1996; 67:210–211.
Derbyshire SWG. Locating the beginnings of pain. *Bioethics* 1999; 13(1):1–31.
Descartes R. *L'homme de René Descartes*. Paris: Charles Angot, 1664.
Diamond J. *Guns, Germs, and Steel*. New York: Norton, 1997.

Ellis JA, O'Connor BV, Cappelli M, et al. Pain in hospitalized pediatric patients: how are we doing? *Clin J Pain* 2002; 18:262–269.

Fisher CB. Integrating science and ethics in research with high-risk children and youth. *Soc Policy Rep* 1993; 7(4):1–28.

Finley GA, McGrath PJ, Forward SP, McNeill G, Fitzgerald P. Parents' management of children's pain following 'minor' surgery. *Pain* 1996; 64:83–87.

Fitzgerald M. Development of pain pathways and mechanisms. In: Anand KJS, McGrath PJ (Eds). *Pain in Neonates*. Amsterdam: Elsevier, 1993.

Flores G, Abreu M, Schwartz I, Hill M. The importance of language and culture in pediatric care: case studies from the Latino community. *J Pediatr* 2000; 137(6):842–848.

Forward SP, Brown TL, McGrath PJ. Mothers' attitudes and behavior toward medicating children's pain. *Pain* 1996; 67:469–474.

Gedaly-Duff, V, Ziebarth D. Mothers' management of adenoid-tonsillectomy pain in 4 to 8 year olds: a preliminary study. *Pain* 1994; 57:293–299.

Glucklich A. *Sacred Pain*. Oxford: Oxford University Press, 2001.

Goodman AH. Why genes don't count (for racial differences in health). *Am J Public Health* 2000; 90:1699–1703

Goodman JE, McGrath PJ. The epidemiology of pain in children and adolescents: a review. *Pain* 1991; 46:247–264.

Hadjistavropoulos HD, Craig KD. Acute and chronic low back pain: cognitive, affective and behavioral dimensions. *J Consult Clin Psychol* 1994; 62:341–349.

Hadjistavropoulos T, Craig KD. A theoretical framework for understanding self-report and observational measures of pain: a communications model. *Behav Res Ther* 2002; 40:551–570.

Hadjistavropoulos T, von Baeyer C, Craig, KD. Pain assessment in persons with limited ability to communicate. In: Turk DD, Melzack R (Eds). *Handbook of Pain Assessment,* 2nd ed. New York: Guilford Press, 2001.

Harris JR. Where is the child's environment? A group socialization theory of development. *Psychol Rev* 1995; 102:458–489.

Helms JF. Why is there no study of cultural equivalence in standardized cognitive ability testing? *Am Psychol* 1992; 47:1083–1101.

Hill ML, Craig KD. Detecting deception in pain expressions: the structure of genuine and deceptive facial displays. *Pain* 2002; 96:135–144.

Kaplan JB, Bennett T. Use of race and ethnicity in biomedical publication. *JAMA* 2003; 289:2709–2716.

Kleinman A. Neurasthenia and depression: a study of somatization and culture in China. *Cult Med Psychiatry* 1982, 6:117–190.

Korol CT, Craig KD. Pain from the perspectives of health psychology and culture. In: Evans D, Kazarian S (Eds). *Handbook of Cultural Health Psychology*. San Diego: Academic Press, 2001, pp 241–265.

Lambert WE, Libman E, Poser, EG. The effect of increased salience of a membership group on pain tolerance. *J Personality* 1960; 28:350–357.

Leventhal H, Sherer K. The relationship of emotion to cognition: a functional approach to a semantic controversy. *Cognition Emotion* 1987; 1:3–28.

Lipton JA, Marbach JJ. Ethnicity and the pain experience. *Soc Sci Med* 1984; 19(12):1279–1298.

Litcher L, Bromet E, Carlson G, et al. Ukrainian application of the children's somatization inventory: psychometric properties and associations with internalizing symptoms. *J Abnorm Child Psychol* 2000; 29(2):165–175.

McGrath PA. Pain in children. In: Crombie IK, Croft PR, Linton SJ, LeResche L, von Korff M (Eds). *Epidemiology of Pain*. Seattle: IASP Press, 1999.

McGrath PJ, Unruh AM. *Pain in Children and Adolescents*. Amsterdam: Elsevier, 1987.

McGrath PJ, Rosmus D, Camfield D, Campbell MA, Hennigar A. Behaviours caregivers use to determine pain in non-verbal cognitively impaired individuals. *Dev Med Child Neurol* 1998; 40:340–343.

McGraw M. *The Neuromuscular Development of the Human Infant.* New York: Columbia University Press, 1943.
McIntosh N. Pain in the newborn, a possible new starting point. *Eur J Pediatr* 1997; 156:173–177.
Mechanic D. The concept of illness behavior. *J Chronic Dis* 1962; 15:189–194.
Meinhart NT, McCaffery M. *Pain: A Nursing Approach to Assessment and Analysis.* Norwalk, CN: Appleton-Century-Croft, 1983.
Melzack R, Wall P. Pain mechanisms: a new theory. *Science* 1965, 150:171–179.
Merskey H, Bogduk N. *Classification of Chronic Pain: Descriptions of Chronic Pain Syndromes and Definitions of Pain Terms,* 2nd ed. Seattle: IASP Press, 1994.
Mischel W. *Personality and Assessment.* New York: Wiley, 1968.
Mischel W. Sex-typing and socialization. In: Mussen PH (Ed). *Carmichaels' Manual of Child Psychology,* Vol. 2. New York: Wiley, 1970.
Murray AD. Infant crying as an elicitor of parental behavior: an examination of two models. *Psychol Bull* 1979; 86:191–215.
Ohman A. Automaticity and the amygdala: nonconscious responses to emotional faces. *Curr Direct Psychol Sci* 2002; 11:62–66.
Pillai RR, Ho GH, Craig KD, Court C. A comparison of pain ratings and pain cues utilized by nurses and parents. *Abstracts: 10th World Congress on Pain.* Seattle: IASP Press, p 559.
Pilowsky I, Spence ND. Ethnicity and illness behavior. *Psychol Med* 1977; 7:447–452.
Prkachin KM, Craig KD. Influencing non-verbal expressions of pain: signal detection analyses. *Pain* 1985; 21(4):399–409.
Rosmus C, Johnston CC, Chan-Yip A, Yang F. Pain response in Chinese and non-Chinese Canadian infants: is there a difference? *Soc Sci Med* 2000, 51:175–184.
Sargent C. Between death and shame: dimensions of pain in Bariba culture. *Soc Sci Med* 1984; 19:1299–1304.
Stevens B. Pain in infants and children: assessment and management strategies within the context of professional guidelines, standards, and roles. In: Giamberardino M (Ed). *Pain 2002—An Updated Review.* Seattle: IASP Press, 2002.
Stevens BJ, Koren G. Evidence-based pain management for infants. *Curr Opin Pediatr* 1998; 10:203–207.
Tu W. A religiophilosophical perspective on pain. In: Kosterlitz HW, Terenius LY (Eds). *Pain and Society.* Weinheim: Verlag Chemie, 1980.
Tucker CM. Expanding pediatric psychology beyond hospital walls to meet the health care needs of ethnic minority children. *J Pedatr Psychol* 2002; 27(4):315–324.
Tursky B, Sternbach R. Further physiological correlates of ethnic differences in responses to shock. *Psychophysiology* 1967; 4:67–74.
Unruh A. Voices from the past: ancient views of pain in childhood. *Clin J Pain* 1992; 8(3):247–254.
Weisenberg M. Pain and pain control. *Psychol Bull* 1982; 84:1008–1044.
Weisz JR, McCarthy CA, Eastman CL, Chaiyasit W, Suwanlert S. Developmental psychopathology and culture: ten lessons from Thailand. In: Luthar S, Burack J, Cicchetti D, Weisz J (Eds). *Developmental Psychopathology: Perspectives on Adjustment, Risk and Disorder.* Cambridge: Cambridge University Press. 1997.
Willis DJ. Economic, health, and mental health disparities among ethnic minority children and families. *J Pediatr Psychol* 2002; 27(4):309–314.
Zborowski M. *People in Pain.* San Francisco: Jossey Bass, 1969.
Zola IK. Culture and symptoms: an analysis of patients presenting complaints. *Am Sociological Rev* 1966; 31:615–630.

Correspondence to: Kenneth D. Craig, PhD, Department of Psychology, University of British Columbia, 2136 West Mall, Vancouver, BC, Canada V6T 1Z4. Email: kcraig@psych.ubc.ca.

8

Health Center Policies and Accreditation

Ada K. Jacox and Carol D. Spengler

*School of Nursing, University of Virginia, Charlottesville, Virginia, USA;
Clinical Practice Guidelines Program, American Pain Society,
Glenview, Illinois, USA*

In this chapter we will consider several major sociopolitical and economic factors that have influenced the behavior of individual clinicians and health care organizations in the management of pain, especially in infants and children. These factors include the evidence-based practice movement, which is worldwide; the lack of basic and clinical research in pain, especially in infants and children, and a related lack of knowledge of pain management by clinicians; and values that inform resource use. Following this general consideration of factors that influence health center policies, we will consider the state of accreditation in pain management services including the purpose of accreditation, precursors of accreditation, and current pain accreditation programs.

As far as possible, we have tried to adopt an international focus. Accreditation of pain management services is, however, a fairly recent phenomenon even in the more developed countries, and the literature on some aspects is sparse. Similarly, little research has addressed organizational factors that influence pain management, except for some early anthropological studies on social interactions in hospital units where patients were experiencing pain (Institute of Medicine 2002).

POLICY MAKING IS A DYNAMIC PROCESS

In every country, health centers operate within a broad social context of values and national policies that influence policies of the local centers. One example is the recent U.S. adoption of national accreditation standards that will significantly influence pain management in local health care organizations.

A policy is a decision made by a group or individual to guide a particular course of action. Public policy is made by a state, local, or national government. Private sector policies are the decisions made by private organizations such as professional associations and religious groups. Policy is dynamic; it evolves over time in response to changes in the social environment and leadership, and as knowledge advances. Interaction occurs across policy sectors, so that local actions influence national policies and vice versa, and private and public sector policies influence each other. At times, policy sectors or levels of government may disagree over who should make a particular policy. The term "policy agenda" refers to the issues policy makers are considering at a particular time. An issue may rise closer to the top of an agenda due to pressure from various interest groups such as professional associations, following events such as an outbreak of a serious infectious disease, or by many other means. Local health centers are influenced by policies from all of these sectors, and their leaders also make policies that affect their own organizations. As with policy made at levels above the local health center, organizational policies are affected by the values, priorities, and internal politics of the organization.

Health care policies evolve over time as recognition of a need for change gradually coalesces into group action, which leads to the publication of statements of what is desirable. International examples of this process include the analgesic ladder (1990) of the World Health Organization (WHO) and its application to children (World Health Organization 1998), and the 1990 statement of the International Association for the Study of Pain (IASP) regarding desirable characteristics for pain treatment facilities. Over time and with pressure from interested stake holders, a formal regulation or law requiring change in behavior may result. This process is now occurring in the accreditation of pain services. Policies and regulations often evolve in the more developed countries and gradually disperse to other countries wishing to make similar changes.

In the evolution of a social change such as adoption of a formal policy regulating pain management in organizations, changes occurring in related areas may facilitate progress. In this case the significant attention given to hospice and end-of-life care and the general concern with improving the quality of health care both clearly enhance recognition of the need to improve pain management. It is likely that increased scrutiny and improvement of pain management services through regulation will be accompanied not only by greater attention to pain management in institutions, but also by more thorough education of clinicians and increased pain research.

THE EVIDENCE-BASED PRACTICE MOVEMENT

For the past several decades, health care professionals and the public alike have assumed that health care, especially in the developed countries, was heavily based on science. Not until the latter part of the last century did it become abundantly clear that few health care practices are based on scientific evidence. David Sackett, a Canadian physician who practices in Oxford, England, defined evidence-based medicine as "the conscientious, explicit and judicious use of current best evidence in making clinical decisions about the care of individual patients." Sackett and colleagues (1996) emphasize that both external scientific evidence and the clinician's experience and judgment are necessary in making decisions and that neither alone is sufficient. The term "evidence-based practice" has quickly become embedded in our professional language, and resources are being expended to apply it to everyday practice. The current health care literature is replete with discussions of evidence-based practice. Sometimes these discussions are simply the pouring of old wine into new bottles, but often they represent serious and much-needed efforts to evaluate the scientific evidence for use in practice.

An important part of this development is the international attention being given to efforts such as the Cochrane Collaboration, named after Archie Cochrane, a British epidemiologist who in the 1950s and 1960s emphasized the need to conduct research to improve the quality of medical care. The Cochrane Collaboration has set for itself the ambitious task of synthesizing the experimental evidence for medical practice. This collaboration, originating in Oxford, now includes scientists and professionals in more than 70 countries, with more than 50 chapters focused on the evaluation of research in specific fields. Only one chapter is specifically devoted to pain—Pain, Palliative and Support Care (PaPas; www.jr2.ox.ac.uk/cochrane)—but many others include reviews of pain research in specific medical conditions such as arthritis, along with other aspects of the condition.

In the United States, increasing costs of health care and acknowledgment of the widespread variations in clinical practice prompted Congress to establish the Agency for Health Care Policy and Research (AHCPR) in 1989 (now known as the Agency for Health Care Research and Quality, AHRQ). This agency focuses on evaluating the organization, delivery, and cost of health care, all geared toward understanding how to reduce costs and improve quality.

A current AHRQ program supports 13 Evidence-Based Practice Centers, which evaluate and synthesize the research literature in various areas of health and illness. An important part of the agency's original mission was the establishment of clinical practice guidelines, which were defined as systematic statements to assist clinicians and consumers in making decisions about appropriate health care for specific clinical conditions (Institute of Medicine 1992). In this program, multidisciplinary panels came together to synthesize the research evidence and to make recommendations for practice based on scientific evidence and expert judgment, clearly an expression of evidence-based practice. The initial conditions identified were medical diagnoses such as benign prostatic hypertrophy and myocardial infarction. An early meeting of the acting director of the agency with a group of nurse researchers suggested focusing on conditions that cut across diagnoses, rather than only on specific medical conditions. Subsequently, pain, urinary incontinence, and wounds were selected for guideline development. The visibility given to pain by a federal agency helped to put this important topic on the national policy agenda.

The first evidence-based guideline published by AHCPR in 1992 was for acute postoperative pain (Carr et al. 1992). The ninth guideline, published in 1994, was for cancer pain management (Jacox et al. 1994). The panels that developed both guidelines drew upon position statements from the American Pain Society, the American Academy of Pediatrics, the Oncology Nursing Society, and other professional associations. The publication and widespread dissemination of the AHCPR guidelines prompted the Joint Commission on Accreditation of Healthcare Organizations (JCAHO) to reconsider an earlier decision rejecting pain as a focus for development of standards. JCAHO adopted pain standards, which they described as their first evidence-based standards, in 1999 and implemented them in January 2001.

The national and international focus on evidence-based practice manifests in many ways in health centers. Among these are the identification of "best practices," rapid and widespread development of clinical protocols, adaptation of clinical practice guidelines for local use, and use of care maps and algorithms focused on specific clinical problems.

LACK OF RESEARCH ON PAIN AND INADEQUACY OF HEALTH PROFESSIONALS' KNOWLEDGE OF PAIN

Although research addressing pain management in children has increased in recent years, the scientific evidence base for clinical practice is still weak. An important stage in the development of clinical practice guidelines is to summarize the strength of scientific evidence available for various interventions. Table I shows the strength of evidence for various interventions in children and adults for pain related to cancer, sickle cell disease, and arthritis. The American Pain Society adopted the process used in the AHRQ

Table I
Strength and consistency of scientific evidence for selected pain interventions

Intervention	Cancer Pain Adult	Cancer Pain Child	Sickle Cell Pain Adult	Sickle Cell Pain Child	Arthritis Adult	Arthritis Child
Analgesics						
Nonselective NSAIDs	A, B	A, B, D	A, B	A, B, D	B, C	B
Parenteral opioids	A	A, B, D	A	A, B, D	B	D
Relaxation	A	B	A	B	B	C
Surgery	D	D	–	–	B, C†	B
TENS	C	D	C	D	C	D
Use of superficial heat or cold	D	D	D	D	D	D

Note: A = strongest and most consistent scientific evidence; D = weakest scientific evidence (case reports and clinical examples only). Evaluation of evidence on cancer pain is from Jacox et al. (1994), on sickle cell pain from Benjamin et al. (1999), and on arthritis from Simon et al. (2002). NSAIDs = nonsteroidal anti-inflammatory drugs; TENS = transcutaneous electrical nerve stimulation.
†Depends on surgical procedure.

guidelines to develop guidelines for sickle cell pain and arthritis. As is abundantly clear, the science base for adults is weak in some areas, but for children it is nearly nonexistent in most areas.

In a recent article titled "Why aren't more pediatric trials performed," Barett (2002) discusses the widespread off-label and unlicensed use of medications in children. "Off-label and unlicensed use means that a drug is used in situations not covered by the manufacturer's product license or summary of product characteristics. ... [A drug may be] used in a different dose or frequency, in different clinical indications, in different age groups, by another route, or in a formulation not approved for children." Analgesics are one of two classes of drugs most frequently used off-label. A study of pediatric medication use in five European countries (Conroy et al. 2000), for example, found that 67% of children needing medication received off-label drugs and that 39% of all prescriptions written for children were off-label. It is likely that the data are similar in the United States and other countries, given the widespread lack of medication research in children and infants. Pediatric clinicians who wish to use these medications must adapt the dosages and routes of administration without the benefit of guidance from clinical trials in these populations.

Several reasons explain the lack of pediatric pain medication research, including regulatory barriers that have made research in infants and children difficult to conduct, and lack of adequate financial incentives for pharmaceutical companies to manufacture appropriate drugs. National governments in the United Kingdom, several other European countries, and the United

States are making efforts to encourage research in children (Nordenberg 1999; Boardman 2001; European Legion Clinical Trials Directive 2001). In the United States, legislation extending pharmaceutical manufacturers' patent protection for pediatric uses is intended as an incentive for them to develop medications for children. Although these comments have focused primarily on medications, as Table I shows, research on other interventions is also meager. There has been some significant research on pain in children, of course, as is obvious from the presentations at the conference on which this book is based and other conferences. Anand's research on the use of adequate analgesia in surgery for neonates literally changed anesthesia practice in infants overnight (Anand and Hickey 1987). In general, however, the evidence base for pain management in children is weak. As Barett (2002) noted, "The desire to protect individual children from exposure to research risks may have the effect of harming children as a class by inhibiting research into pediatric health and disease."

VALUES THAT INFORM USE OF RESOURCES

Many factors affect health policies related to pain management, including the amount of resources devoted to health care and how the available funds are allocated and used. Nations vary widely in their wealth and in the resources they devote to health care. The allocation of scarce resources for health care and for specific health services is determined by competing social values and norms that change over time. Values influence not only how much should be spent on an area, but how it should be spent, and how the work will be done. Such decisions commonly are made on political and economic grounds; they influence health center policies in important ways.

Payment mechanisms, for example, affect many practice areas, including pain management. Fee-for-service payments can encourage overuse of services, while capitation methods (uniform per capita fees) may promote underuse. For example, several years ago U.S. health insurers stopped direct payment to anesthesiologists to provide certain interventional therapies and instead bundled these services into a capitation payment. The consequence was a drastic reduction in the provision of those services in many health care settings across the country. What is paid for and who receives payment influence the care given.

The use of resources also affects pain management when unnecessary constraints are placed on the delivery of care. The legal regulation of health professionals through licensure, for example, is reserved for the province, state, or nation, depending on the country. Licensure defines the scope of practice within which the licensee has demonstrated the ability to practice safely. What happens in practice is that organizations limit what professionals may do (even though they *can* legally perform certain activities), which can have a major influence on how pain is managed. A current case involving the JCAHO pain standards illustrates how factors other than evidence influence health center policies, even in so-called evidence-based practice standards. Although registered nurses in all 50 of the United States are licensed to make judgments in the administration of medication, a current debate focuses on whether or not they should have authority to use their own judgment in administering medication orders that have a dosage range or that are to be given "as necessary" (p.r.n.).

Preliminary indications suggest that attempts will be made to discourage the use of range orders, or to require a protocol for their interpretation. The Standards FAQ section of JCAHO's Web site (www.jcaho.org), for example, states that "range orders are acceptable only if policies exist which clearly specify how such orders are to be interpreted, and the prescribing physician is aware of the protocol." An example cited by JCAHO is that "an order for one or two tablets should always start out as being given one tablet and orders for every 4 to 6 hours should always start out as being given every 6 hours" (D. Rich, personal communication, March 2002).

Such interpretation of a dose range and similar interpretations that preclude the professional judgment of clinicians who provide care to patients will unnecessarily constrain practice by requiring the "cookbook recipes" that early critics of evidence-based practice feared. Such practice omits the crucial judgment component in evidence-based practice. Just as efforts to protect individual children from exposure to research risks may harm children as a class, attempts to overly and prematurely codify pain management and limit professional judgment may result in a lower quality of patient care. It is well known in the policy world that establishing a policy is only the first step. Ensuring implementation in the way the policy makers intended can be a more difficult step.

When such policies are implemented, whether by a national accrediting agency or by a local health center, they can unnecessarily and negatively affect the quality of pain management. Unfortunately, the division of labor in health care often is heavily based on tradition, rather than on who can legally and safely perform care. To achieve significant improvement in pain management, we need a better research base for both clinical strategies and organizational structure and processes that promote the efficient and effective use of resources.

A final, and more easily solved, local resource problem for infants and children is the failure of institutions to purchase appropriately sized equipment or supplies. At least two U.S organizations (the American College of Emergency Physicians and the American Academy of Pediatrics) have promulgated policies related to the need for emergency departments to have available equipment, supplies, and medications oriented toward infants and children. In this area, as in many others, needs of infants and children can be overlooked when the main focus of the institution is on adult patients.

In summary, values related to resource use, the lack of research on pain management in infants and children, and the emerging emphasis on evidence-based practice all are factors that influence pain management in local health centers. One factor that we have touched on is accreditation of pain services. We now further consider accreditation, its precursors, and specific mechanisms of pain services.

ACCREDITATION OF HEALTH CARE ORGANIZATIONS

Accreditation is a formal process by which a nongovernmental agency acknowledges that a specific health care organization meets applicable and published standards. In contrast, certification is a process by which an authorized governmental or nongovernmental organization recognizes either individuals or organizations as meeting predetermined requirements and criteria. Accreditation applies to organizations, while certification may apply to individuals and to organizations. Accreditation is a voluntary process; institutions choose to apply for accredited status and then agree to abide by the standards of the accrediting organization. It is a means of self-regulation and peer review that is adopted by a particular community, in this case the health care community.

As noted earlier, accreditation does not spring full-blown from the minds of the accreditors. It is a step in an evolutionary process by which practice is changed. An early step in trying to change an organization is for individuals or groups of members to try to bring a perceived problem to the attention of influential persons in the organization. With regard to the problem of widespread unrelieved pain experienced by patients, most health care organizations in the developed countries were in the early stage of this process until the last few years. Many less developed countries are still in this stage. A later step in the process of change is for private or public bodies to develop and disseminate position statements on the subject. Many countries are at this stage today. A still later step is the development of regulatory standards, including accreditation.

Each of these steps or phases in the evolutionary process has some impact on an organization. Persuasive individuals, for example, can have a significant effect on changing practice in a particular department, service, or health care organization. By making authoritative statements, professional associations may influence the behavior of their members and others, but these position statements are not binding on the behavior of individuals or institutions. In contrast, accreditation has a significantly greater influence on an organization's activities because it confers some desired status, such as institutional reputation or eligibility for payment. This situation creates a powerful incentive for care organizations to comply with the accreditation standards. Still another stage of individual and organizational change is passage of a law making a particular practice or set of practices mandatory. This stage is illustrated by state and federal controlled substances laws, which Joranson discusses in this volume. Most stages in this process are influenced by the prior stages. That is, influential and persuasive members of professional associations prompt position statements of desired behavior. Accrediting agencies, in turn, often depend upon authoritative statements of professional associations in establishing accreditation criteria and standards.

Various countries, of course, are at different stages in the process of health care accreditation, and accreditation of pain services is even less well developed. Many countries have fairly rudimentary, if any, accreditation systems. However, Canada, the United States, and some European countries including the United Kingdom have formal accreditation systems, with some focusing specifically on accreditation of pediatric services or services related to children's pain. In health care accreditation programs, as in other types of program, regulatory systems usually are pioneered in the more developed countries, and then adapted by less well-developed countries in ways consistent with their needs and resources.

POSITION STATEMENTS: PRECURSORS OF ACCREDITATION

Although we found no accreditation standards published by international associations, various international groups have addressed the problem of pain through position statements. In 1985, the WHO issued its well-known statement that every nation should give high priority to establishing a cancer pain relief policy. This statement called international attention to the problem. WHO's 1990 statement on the analgesic ladder and its 1998 application to children added detail to the policy. Those statements have influenced pain management in cancer worldwide.

IASP in 1990 published desirable characteristics for pain treatment facilities. Although not an accreditation document, the publication provides authoritative information that could be useful in establishing accreditation standards.

WHO is now focusing on the performance of health systems internationally (World Health Organization 2000). Although we could find no mention of pain management in the performance measures, the statement draws attention to the need to establish international standards for health care.

Numerous national professional organizations, including chapters of IASP, have published position statements on various aspects of the management of the pain. Table II lists examples. They include statements regarding the need to manage pain, use of opioids, end-of-life care, and circumcision standards of care. Many of these statements are likely to influence or evolve into accreditation standards.

PAIN ACCREDITATION PROGRAMS

As noted earlier, most health care accreditation programs have been established in the more developed countries, including some European countries,

Table II
Sample organization policies, standards, and position statements related to aspects of pain management in various countries

Organization	Subject	Type of Position Statement
U.S. National Institutes of Health	Integrated approach to pain management	Consensus development conference statement (1986)
Canadian Pain Society	Use of opioid analgesics for the treatment of chronic noncancer pain	Consensus statement and guideline (1998)
Canadian Paediatric Society and American Academy of Pediatrics	Prevention and management of pain and stress in the neonate	Policy statement (2000)
American College of Emergency Physicians	Use of pediatric sedation and analgesia	Policy statement (2001)
American Academy of Pediatrics	Palliative care for children	Policy (2000)
American Pain Society and American Academy of Pediatrics	Assessment and management of acute pain in infants, children, and adolescents	Policy statement (2001)
British Association of Paediatric Surgeons	Religious circumcision of male children: standards of care	Policy standard (2001)
Association of Pediatric Oncology Nurses	Pain management for the child with cancer at the end of life	Position paper (2001)

the British Commonwealth, and the United States. Only a few countries have fully developed accreditation programs, and only a few of those include accreditation of pain services.

The first pain service accreditation program in the United States was developed by the Commission on Accreditation of Rehabilitative Facilities (CARF) in 1983, with consultation from the American Pain Society. The CARF pain accreditation is part of a general program for accrediting rehabilitation facilities (www.carf.org). The American Academy of Pain Management (AAPM) developed the second accreditation program in 1992 (www.aapainmanagement.org).

JCAHO adopted pain standards in 1999 and fully implemented them in January 2001. In 1999, JCAHO also launched an international accreditation program called the Joint Commission International (JCI). It was developed by a task force representing countries in Western Europe, the Middle East, Latin and Central America, Asia and the Pacific Rim, North America, Central and East Europe, and Africa. JCI is a subsidiary of JCAHO and presently lists 40 JCI-accredited organizations in 11 countries (Table III). JCI implemented pain standards in January 2003. How many countries will include the pain standards is unknown at this time. Table IV presents additional information on the domains and types of settings accredited by CARF, AAPM, JCAHO, and JCI.

The CARF accreditation process evaluates the management of pain in both adults and children. CARF evaluates both organizational and clinical practice domains. AAPM develops both nonclinical standards, such as organizational structures and business practices, and clinical standards related to documentation of assessment and management of pain.

Table III
Number of Joint Commission International (JCI) accredited organizations by country

Country	N	Year
Spain	5	1998, 1999, 2001, 2002
Brazil	4	1999–2002
Kingdom of Saudi Arabia	5	2000–2001
Germany	5	2000–2001, 2002
United Arab Emirates	1	2000
Austria	1	2002
Denmark	7	2002
Ireland	5	2002
Thailand	1	2002
Turkey	2	2002
Italy	4	2002

Table IV
Accrediting organizations that include pain standards for adults and children

Organization	Domains Accredited	Standards Implemented	Types of Settings Accredited
Commission on Accreditation of Rehabilitation Facilities (CARF)	Core values and mission Input from persons served Individual-centered planning, design, and delivery Patient rights Continuity of care Quality and appropriateness of service Leadership, ethics, and advocacy Strategic planning, fiscal management Human resources development Accessibility Health, safety, and transportation Outcomes management and public information	1983	Medical rehabilitation program Adult day services Assisted living Behavioral health Freestanding rehabilitation hospitals Interdisciplinary pain rehabilitation programs (inpatient)
American Academy of Pain Management (AAPM)	Organization purpose and structure Business practices Personnel management Physical maintenance and safety General clinical standard applicable to all pain programs	1992	Physicians' offices Medical groups Hospital departments Rehabilitation programs Pain management programs Dental practices Podiatry practices Oral and maxillofacial surgery offices Classification specific clinical standards

Joint Commission on Accreditation of Healthcare Organizations (JCAHO)	Patient rights and organization ethics Assessment of patients Care of patients Education of patients Continuum of care Improving organizational performance	2001	Hospitals Ambulatory care centers Home care Long-term care Ambulatory surgery centers Behavioral health care
Joint Commission International (JCI)	Governance, leadership, and direction Facility management and safety Staff qualifications and education Management of information Access to care and quality of care Patient and family rights Assessment of patients Care of patients Patient and family education Quality improvement and patient safety	2003	All types of health care settings: Hospitals Ambulatory care clinics

Note: JCAHO and CARF offer freestanding rehabilitation hospitals the option of a collaborative study by both organizations at the same time.

The Australia and New Zealand College of Anaesthetists (ANZCA) established an accreditation program in pain management in 2001, and lists 11 hospitals, including two children's hospitals, with accredited pain management units (www.fpm.anzca.edu.au). These units are accredited for the purpose of sponsoring fellowship programs for the education of health professionals, however, and are not directly comparable to the pain accrediting standards developed by CARF, AAPM, and JCAHO.

JCAHO pain standards are divided into six areas: (1) rights and ethics, which recognize the right of individuals to appropriate assessment and management of pain; (2) assessment of persons with pain; (3) pain management; (4) education of persons with pain; (5) continual care, addressing individuals' management in the discharge planning process; and (6) improving organizational performance (Joint Commission on Accreditation of Healthcare Organizations 2001). As noted earlier, JCAHO's pain standards are based heavily upon position statements of various professional groups and clinical practice guidelines developed by the AHCPR. Since adopting pain standards, CARF, and AAPM, and JCAHO have developed educational resource materials to prepare organizations to use their standards.

ORGANIZATIONAL FACTORS THAT INFLUENCE PAIN MANAGEMENT

When developing evidence-based clinical practice guidelines, we are reminded constantly that evidence-based practice is not practice based only on evidence. Rather, it is the use of evidence combined with the clinician's experience and judgment and the patient's preference that provides the basis for decision making in health care. Similarly, when trying to locate empirical studies of organizational factors that influence the management of pain in children, we found that the literature is sparse. This lack of evidence necessitates using consensus statements by experts as guidelines until research results demonstrate the efficacy of certain organizational approaches; then the recommendations may change. Current suggestions for how organizations can influence pain management rely on the IASP desired characteristics of pain centers, the JCAHO organizational standards related to pain, and the Institute of Medicine (2001) report on the improving quality in health care. The IOM report is one of two publications that discuss problems in the health care system and suggest how the system can move toward performance improvement (Institute of Medicine 1999, 2001). Both IOM books cite numerous studies of mistakes that occur in the administration of analgesics and in children's care across multiple health care settings. The reports focus on the need to build organizational supports for change.

The IOM (2002) report on improving quality in health care organizations describes steps to take in redesigning the health care system, including what must be done in health care organizations. The authors discuss six challenges to be met, all of which are applicable to pain management in local health centers.

Redesigning care processes. Here, the emphasis is on standardizing care as much as possible while also providing for individualization of care as necessary. The report describes the 80/20 principle applicable to most work, in which approximately 80% of the work can be done following standardized plans while the remaining 20% requires more expertise and judgment. The adoption of protocols, guidelines, algorithms, and similar devices reflects this approach, and the authors state that clinical judgment must be used in application of the guidelines.

Making effective use of information technologies. The IOM report acknowledges that the health care industry has been slow to implement sophisticated technologies to improve communication between clinicians and patients and consultation with other clinicians. The report describes ways in which such technology is used in other industries and encourages its increased use in health care.

Managing clinical knowledge and skills. The proliferation of health care knowledge, including the understanding of pain mechanisms and pain management, requires going beyond the conferences and publications that at an earlier time sufficed to keep clinicians up to date. Increased use of technology such as interactive computer programs is needed to rapidly bring new and complex knowledge to the fingertips of clinicians. A concomitant need, of course, is to ensure that the content of these programs is valid and as empirically based as possible.

Developing effective teams. The multidisciplinary team approach has long been used in progressive pain management settings. The IOM report recounts the historical factors that have resulted in an overly rigid division of labor in many health care settings and argues for more rational and effective ways to use the skills of the health care team.

Coordination across patient conditions, services, and settings over time. This issue has plagued the health care system for many years, and as care becomes more complex, it seems to become more fragmented. Better ways to coordinate care are clearly needed.

Incorporating performance and outcome measurements for improvement and accountability. This last "challenge" reflects the increased attention to outcomes that has accompanied the evidence-based practice movement. It acknowledges the need to base clinical and organizational decision-making on empirical data.

These final brief comments are based largely on the IOM's excellent report on the improvement of quality in health care. It is interesting to note that many examples of needed changes are related to pain management and medication administration. Clearly the report is of value to those seeking to improve pain management in their local health centers.

Although the JCAHO pain standards and others may be of relatively recent origin, pain itself is not. It has been a problem largely ignored by the health care system in most countries around the world. The subject of pain finally has been placed on the policy agenda in health care. The information presented in this chapter should be useful to those interested in understanding how health policy and health center policies influence the management of pain in children.

REFERENCES

American Academy of Pediatrics. Palliative care for children. *Pediatrics* 2000a; 106(2):351–357.
American Academy of Pediatrics. Prevention and management of pain and stress in the neonate (policy statement). *Pediatrics* 2000b; 105(92):454–461.
American Academy of Pediatrics. The assessment and management of acute pain in infants, children and adolescents (policy statement). *Pediatrics* 2001; 108(3):793–797.
American College of Emergency Physicians. Essential areas and policies of accreditation, 2001. Available via the Internet: www.pain.accp.org/statement.html. Accessed June 2002.
Anand KJS, Hickey PR. Pain and its effects on the human neonate and fetus. *N Engl J Med* 1987; 317:1321–1329.
Barett J. Why aren't more pediatric trials performed? *Applied Clin Trials* 2002; 36–38, 40, 42, 44.
Benjamin LJ, Dampier CD, Jacox AK, et al. *Guideline for the Management of Acute and Chronic Pain in Sickle Cell Disease.* Glenview, IL: American Pain Society, 1999.
Boardman HS. Pediatric drug development: principles and practice. *Int J Pharm Med* 2001; 15:35–47.
Carr DB, Jacox A, Chapman R, et al. *Acute Pain Management: Operative or Medical Procedures and Trauma.* AHCPR Publication No. 92-0032. Rockville, MD: U.S. Department of Health and Human Services, Agency for Health Care Policy and Research, 1992.
Conroy S, Choonara I, Inpicciatore P, et al. Survey of unlicensed and off-label use in paediatric wards in European countries. *BMJ* 2000; 320:79–82.
Institute of Medicine. Field MJ, Lohr KN (Eds). *Guidelines for Clinical Practice: From Development to Use.* Washington, DC: National Academy Press, 1992.
Institute of Medicine. Kohn LT, Corrigan JM, Donaldson MS (Eds). *To Err is Human: Building a Safer Health System.* Washington, DC: National Academy Press, 1999.
Institute of Medicine. *Crossing the Quality Chasm: A New Health System for the 21st Century.* Washington, DC: National Academy Press, 2001.
Institute of Medicine. *Care Without Coverage: Too Little, Too Late.* Washington, DC: National Academy Press, 2002.

International Association for the Study of Pain. Task Force on Guidelines for Desirable Characteristics for Pain Treatment Facilities. *Desirable Characteristics for Pain Treatment Facilities.* Seattle: IASP, 1990.

Jacox A, Carr DB, Payne R, et al. *Management of Cancer Pain.* AHCPR Publication No. 94-0592. Rockville, MD: U.S. Department of Health and Human Services, Agency for Health Care Policy and Research, 1994.

Joint Commission on Accreditation of Healthcare Organizations. *Pain Assessment and Management: An Organizational Approach.* Joint Commission on Accreditation of Health Care Organizations, 2000.

Joint Commission International. *International Accreditation, Care Continuum Draft Standards.* Available via the Internet: www.jcrinc.com/international.ASP. Accessed June 2002.

Nordenberg, T. Pediatric drug studies: protecting pint-sized patients. *FDA Consumer Magazine* 33(3); 1999:May–June.

Sackett DL, Rosenberg WMC, Gray JAM, Heynes RB, Richardson WS. Evidence-based medicine: what it is and what it is not. *BMJ* 312:71–72.

Simon L, Lipman A, Jacox A, et al. *Guideline for the Management of Pain in Osteoarthritis, Rheumatoid Arthritis and Juvenile Chronic Arthritis.* Glenview, IL: American Pain Society, 2002.

World Health Organization. *The WHO Three-Step Analgesic Ladder.* Geneva: World Health Organization, 1990.

World Health Organization. *Cancer Pain Relief and Palliative Care in Children.* Geneva: World Health Organization, 1998.

World Health Organization. *World Health 2000: Health Systems' Performance.* Geneva: World Health Organization, 2000.

Correspondence to: Ada K. Jacox, PhD, RN, 474 Edge Hill Farm Road, Heathsville, VA 22473, USA. Email: ajacox@painguidelines.org.

9

Availability of Opioid Analgesics for Cancer Pain Relief in Children

David E. Joranson, Aaron M. Gilson, Karen M. Ryan, and Martha A. Maurer

Pain & Policy Studies Group, University of Wisconsin Comprehensive Cancer Center, World Health Organization Collaborating Center for Policy and Communications in Cancer Care, Madison, Wisconsin, USA

Despite current medical knowledge and effective pharmacological and nonpharmacological treatments, inadequate management of cancer pain continues to be a serious health problem throughout the world (World Health Organization 1990). The World Health Organization (WHO) estimates that the number of new cases of cancer will double in the next 20 years (Sikora 1998). Presently, the incidence of cancer-related mortality is greatest in developed countries, but in the next 20 years the burden of cancer is predicted to shift to the developing countries (Murray and Lopez 1996), where most patients receive the diagnosis of cancer when the disease is already in the late stage and they are in pain (World Health Organization 1990).

In 1998, in collaboration with the International Association for the Study of Pain (IASP), WHO published the booklet *Cancer Pain Relief and Palliative Care in Children* (World Health Organization 1998). A follow-up to *Cancer Pain Relief* (World Health Organization 1986), it recommends morphine and other opioids such as fentanyl, hydromorphone, oxycodone, oxymorphone, and methadone for the treatment of moderate to severe cancer pain in children. It offers WHO- and IASP-approved pain assessment and treatment guidelines for health care professionals. It also targets policy makers to address misunderstandings that lead to inadequate relief of pain in children with cancer, in particular the fear of drug addiction and dependence when use of opioids is considered. Indeed, these fears have led to inadequate medical use and availability of opioid analgesics for patients of all ages throughout the world (World Health Organization 1996). A publication by a WHO collaborating center in 2001 provides a progress report, educational resources, and a review of recent research on pain in children (Colleau 2001a). In 2002, WHO provided further emphasis and a definition of palliative care for children in *National Cancer Control Programmes* (World Health Organization 2002).

INADEQUATE AVAILABILITY OF OPIOID ANALGESICS

MORPHINE CONSUMPTION

One indicator of a country's progress toward improving the availability of opioid analgesics is a statistic that describes the annual national consumption of drugs for medical purposes (International Narcotics Control Board 2002a). Morphine consumption is used because this drug is an essential part of the WHO analgesic ladder (World Health Organization 1986, 1996). Of course, morphine consumption alone may not represent a country's ability to effectively treat moderate to severe pain. Other opioids should be taken into account, such as fentanyl, hydromorphone, oxycodone, oxymorphone, and methadone. National opioid consumption statistics vary widely according to medical, economic, and social factors and the capability of the health care system to deliver pain relief. Several cautions should be considered when using opioid consumption data to estimate a country's capacity to provide effective cancer pain management. Opioids are also used for postoperative and chronic nonmalignant pain, and overall consumption data do not indicate the percentage used for cancer pain. Increases in a country's consumption of opioids may not necessarily reflect better pain management; some institutions may have a store of morphine but fail to use it, or more patients may be receiving the drug, but at inadequate doses. Nevertheless, morphine consumption statistics can be a starting point in the process to evaluate a country's capability to effectively manage pain.

Prior to 1986, global consumption of morphine was low and stable. After publication of the WHO analgesic method for relieving cancer pain, global consumption of morphine began to increase; from 1972 to 2000, global morphine consumption increased by 1,243% (see Fig. 1). Figs. 2 and 3 show the increasing global consumption of several other opioids during the same period. Most of the increases in consumption of opioids are accounted for by some, but not all, developed countries, which comprise a small portion of the world's population. Adjusting national morphine consumption for population provides a more realistic picture of patient access to morphine in developing countries. Table I shows the per capita consumption for every

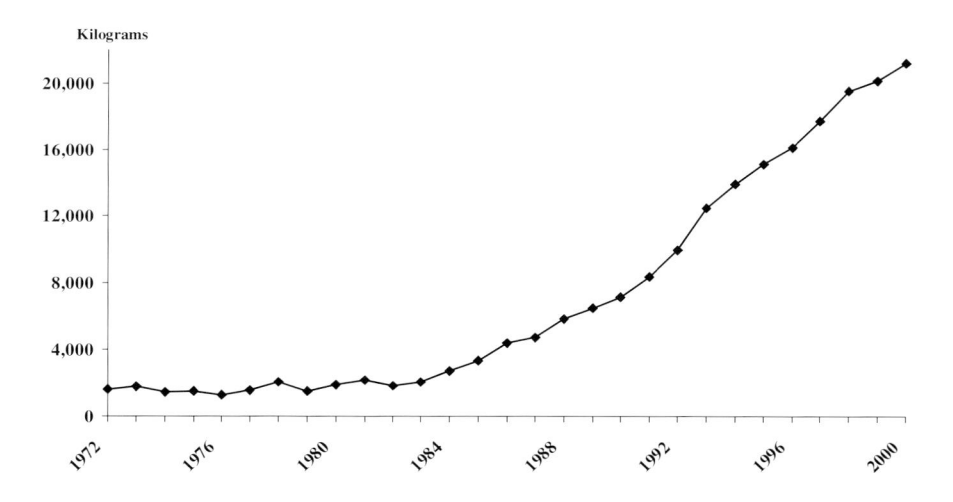

Fig. 1. Global consumption of morphine, 1972–2000. Data from International Narcotics Control Board.

country that reported morphine statistics in 1999. People with cancer—including children—still have very little access to morphine in most countries of the world.

BARRIERS TO OPIOID AVAILABILITY

In 1995, in consultation with WHO, the International Narcotics Control Board (INCB) conducted a survey of all governments to assess the reasons for low availability of opioids. This survey was important because the medical acceptability of using drugs for various indications and patient populations is a matter of national policy, and because it is a government obligation to ensure adequate availability of opioid drugs for medical purposes (International Narcotics Control Board 1996).

Sixty-five governments responded to the INCB survey. Many governments indicated that opioids were not sufficiently available for medical purposes. Furthermore, governments reported that the injectable forms of morphine were more available than the oral form recommended by WHO; injectable morphine was available in 79% of the responding countries, slow-release morphine in 45%, oral immediate-release powder or solution in 40%, and tablets in 29%. Less than half of these governments (48%) reported that hospitals with cancer programs stocked any dosage form of morphine. Fifty-four percent of the responding governments reported shortages of opioids in their hospitals or pharmacies during the last 2 years.

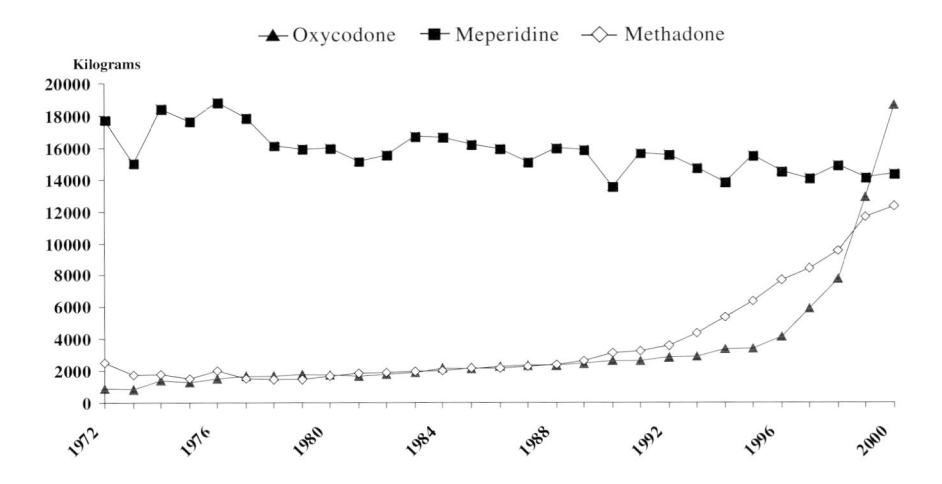

Fig. 2. Global consumption of oxycodone, meperidine, and methadone, 1972–2000. Data from International Narcotics Control Board.

The survey also asked governments to identify the factors that impede adequate availability of opioids. Impediments reported by governments included concerns about addiction (72% of governments); insufficient training of health care professionals (59%); regulatory restrictions regarding manufacture, distribution, prescribing, or dispensing (59%); health professionals' concerns about legal sanctions (47%); and excessively strict regulatory requirements (38%). These national narcotics control authorities appeared to

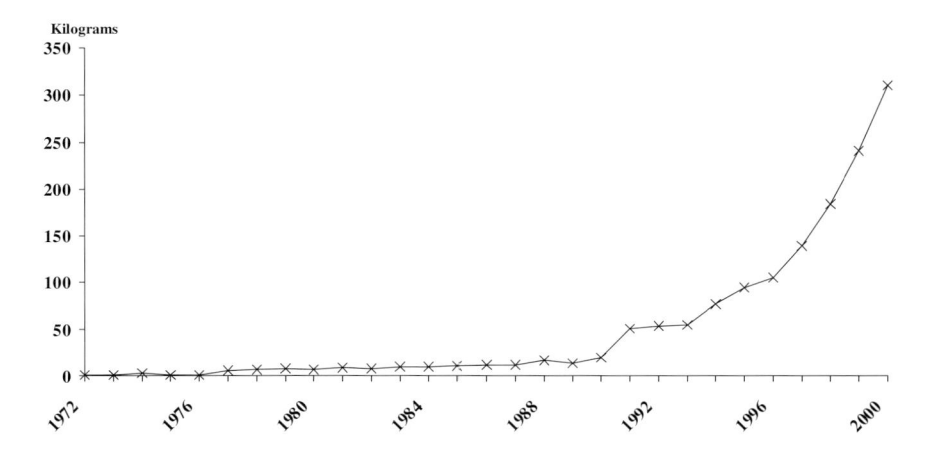

Fig. 3. Global consumption of fentanyl, 1972–2000. Data from International Narcotics Control Board.

be aware of the same barriers that health professionals had identified in several WHO publications (World Health Organization 1990, 1996, 1998).

Based on this survey, the INCB concluded that "while there have been efforts by some governments to ensure the availability of narcotic drugs for medical and scientific purposes, it appears that many others have yet to focus on that obligation" (International Narcotics Control Board 1996). The board reminded governments of their obligation to ensure adequate availability of opioid analgesics, and recommended a number of actions governments should undertake to determine whether national narcotics laws have undue restrictions and make arrangements to ensure adequate availability of opioid drugs to patients. The board recommended that WHO expand its efforts to provide information to the public, health professionals, and policy makers about its recommendations for the relief of cancer pain and the medical use of opioids. It also recommended that organizations such as IASP should teach health professionals and students about the use of opioids and communicate with governments about the availability of opioids for medical purposes (International Narcotics Control Board 1996).

NATIONAL POLICY AND PAIN IN CHILDREN

The INCB's 1995 survey addressed several aspects relating to pediatric pain. Forty-two of the 65 governments (65%) reported that they had issued national policies or guidelines to improve the medical use of opioids; of these policies, 20% related to pain in children. Fifty-two percent of governments reported that they had sponsored, supported, or endorsed an educational program to improve the medical use of opioids, with 19% of these programs addressing the treatment of pain in children.

By 1999, 45 more governments had responded to the questionnaire, bringing the total to 110 (Pain & Policy Studies Group 1999). In updating the survey data regarding pediatric pain, we found that 66 governments (61%) reported that they had issued national policies or guidelines to improve the medical use of opioids, and that of these, 26% said the policies related to pain in children. Forty-eight percent of governments reported that they had sponsored, supported, or endorsed an educational program to improve the medical use of opioids, indicating that 24% of these programs addressed the treatment of pain in children. From these data it appears that there had been an increase in national policies and programs aimed at improving medical use of opioids for relieving pain in children.

Table I
Per capita consumption of morphine (milligrams) in 1999 in 136 different countries

Falkland Islands	74.0000	Hong Kong SAR	3.5837
Denmark	70.7567	Malta	3.3990
Australia	57.0705	South Africa	3.3620
Canada	52.0475	Macedonia	3.2700
Iceland	50.2545	Andorra	3.0933
New Zealand	37.6505	Djibouti	3.0843
Sweden	37.2499	Portugal	2.6719
Austria	36.3185	Cuba	2.5746
France	31.7967	Italy	2.3543
Norway	29.7250	Cyprus	2.2935
United States of America	28.9582	Costa Rica	2.2502
Switzerland	25.7126	Lithuania	2.1614
United Kingdom	19.9868	Bulgaria	2.0328
Kazakhstan	18.3779	Chile	1.9670
Germany	16.8477	Jamaica	1.9531
Ireland	16.5869	Barbados	1.7903
Israel	14.5262	Brazil	1.7769
Belgium	11.3191	Georgia	1.5566
Netherlands	9.9081	Seychelles	1.4750
Slovenia	9.0669	Argentina	1.4729
Luxembourg	8.4149	Belarus	1.3208
Slovakia	7.6669	Colombia	1.2733
New Caledonia	7.6553	Republic of Korea	1.1849
Finland	7.5398	Bahamas	1.1595
Spain	7.2408	Lebanon	1.0343
Hungary	7.1883	Tunisia	1.0121
Japan	6.7843	Singapore	1.0110
Poland	6.5055	Aruba	0.9894
Namibia	5.6814	Latvia	0.9807
Czech Republic	5.4825	Netherlands Antilles	0.9488
Republic of Palau	4.7895	Grenada	0.8602
Estonia	3.9610	Malaysia	0.8440
Cayman Islands	3.8108	Fiji	0.7680

THE IMPERATIVE TO EVALUATE NATIONAL POLICY

In addition to presenting clinical recommendations for the treatment of pediatric cancer pain, the 1998 WHO publication emphasized the importance of adequate governmental and administrative policy, including (a) that governments should institute cancer pain relief programs based on the WHO guidelines for pediatric pain; (b) that drug regulatory systems designed to combat drug abuse should not prevent children with cancer from receiving the drugs necessary for pain relief; (c) that the availability and distribution of oral opioid analgesics should be reviewed and revised to ensure availability to

Table I *(cont.)*

Croatia	0.7398	Mongolia	0.1282
Greece	0.6899	Jordan	0.1223
Saint Vincent/Grenadines	0.6696	Morocco	0.1158
Bahrain	0.6261	China	0.1102
Macao	0.6244	Syrian Arab Republic	0.1059
Albania	0.6200	Nicaragua	0.0972
Oman	0.5557	Zambia	0.0961
Saint Kitts and Nevis	0.5385	India	0.0884
Russian Federation	0.5191	Yugoslavia	0.0715
Armenia	0.5036	Wallis and Futuna Islands	0.0714
Republic of Moldova	0.4306	Kyrgyzstan	0.0711
Panama	0.4279	Iraq	0.0696
Sierra Leone	0.4240	Myanmar	0.0521
Saudi Arabia	0.4169	Uzbekistan	0.0519
United Arab Emirates	0.3824	Rwanda	0.0510
Dominican Republic	0.3434	Dominica	0.0423
Turkey	0.3407	Algeria	0.0392
Cook Islands	0.3158	Honduras	0.0377
Sri Lanka	0.3064	Bolivia	0.0232
Suriname	0.2892	Pakistan	0.0223
Thailand	0.2868	Vanuatu	0.0215
Tonga	0.2857	Nepal	0.0150
Samoa	0.2485	Libyan Arab Jamahiriya	0.0132
Qatar	0.2479	Guatemala	0.0087
Brunei Darussalam	0.2447	Uganda	0.0083
Mauritius	0.2240	Guyana	0.0082
Iran (Islamic Republic of)	0.2025	Cape Verde	0.0072
Paraguay	0.2001	Cambodia	0.0056
Turks and Caicos Islands	0.1875	Indonesia	0.0054
Kuwait	0.1846	Eritrea	0.0051
Peru	0.1741	Niger	0.0048
Egypt	0.1625	Madagascar	0.0045
Antigua and Barbuda	0.1493	Dem. Rep. of the Congo	0.0033
Mexico	0.1437	United Republic of Tanzania	0.0014
Botswana	0.1353	Nigeria	0.0007

Source: International Narcotics Control Board; United Nations (1999). Global mean: 5.934 mg per capita.

cancer patients; and (d) that health professionals should report to the authorities any instances of oral opioids being unavailable for cancer patients.

Indeed, the INCB and the WHO have repeatedly called on national governments to evaluate their health care systems and laws and regulations, and to identify and remove impediments to opioid availability for medical needs (International Narcotics Control Board 1989, 1996; World Health Organization 1990, 1996). Although technical support is available from United Nations drug control authorities to help governments develop policies to prevent abuse and trafficking in illicit drugs (United Nations International Drug Control Programme 1994), there were no criteria to evaluate national drug policy for its ability to ensure availability of opioid analgesics for medical use.

The INCB recommended that the United Nations International Drug Control Programme revise its model national legislation on the control of narcotic drugs to include provisions that ensure the availability of narcotic drugs for medical and scientific purposes (International Narcotics Control Board 1996).

WHO GUIDELINES FOR EVALUATING NATIONAL OPIOIDS POLICY

The first step taken by the WHO to respond to this need was publication of *Cancer Pain Relief with a Guide to Opioid Availability* (World Health Organization 1996). This booklet explained how the international and national drug control system should work to ensure opioid availability for cancer pain relief.

The second step began in 1998 when the Pain & Policy Studies Group at the University of Wisconsin Comprehensive Cancer Center, which has been designated the WHO Collaborating Center for Policy and Communications in Cancer Care (WHOCC), proposed the development of more specific criteria for governments and health professionals to evaluate national policies that govern control of narcotic drugs. The WHOCC believed there was an international consensus about the policy basis for ensuring availability of opioids, and that policy guidelines could help to focus the attention of national governments and health professionals on the need to address regulatory barriers to inadequate pain management. The proposal was accepted by the WHO Office for Essential Drugs and Medicines Policy.

Policy makers must consider several factors when developing policy guidelines. The credibility of the policy basis for guidelines is critically important. The validity of guidelines used for policy analysis depends on the source of authority, as well as the direct relevance to the policies being evaluated (Patton and Sawicki 1993; Weimer and Vining 1999). The first step in developing the guidelines was to identify the key policy principles in the international narcotics control treaties. We identified the principle of "balance" as central to the treaties and therefore to the obligations of national governments to develop and implement national drug control policies. The principle of balance is stated in international conventions (United Nations 1973, 1977), and is further explained in recommendations of United Nations bodies that monitor implementation of the conventions (International Narcotics

Control Board 1996) and in the findings and recommendations of WHO expert bodies. The WHO (2000) summarizes this principle as follows:

> The central principle of "balance" represents a dual imperative of governments to establish a system of control to prevent abuse, trafficking, and diversion of narcotic drugs while, at the same time, ensuring their medical availability. While opioid analgesics are controlled drugs, they are also essential drugs and are absolutely necessary for the relief of pain. Opioids, including those in the therapeutic group of morphine, should be accessible to all patients who need them for relief of pain. Governments must take steps to ensure the adequate availability of opioids for medical and scientific purposes. These steps include empowering medical practitioners to provide opioids in the course of professional practice, allowing them to prescribe, dispense and administer according to the individual medical needs of patients, and ensuring that a sufficient supply of opioids is available to meet medical demand.

The second step was to derive individual criteria (or guidelines) that were consistent with the central principle. A total of 16 guidelines were developed, each one compatible with the principle of balance and the treaties and official WHO and INCB publications. Each guideline expresses an essential policy or administrative principle that should be present in national drug control policy and administration. A narrative accompanies each guideline, containing excerpts from the historic origins of relevant policy and an elaboration of the steps that have been recommended by experts to accomplish the policy objectives expressed in the guidelines.

REVIEW PROCESS

In November 1999, the WHO and the WHOCC sponsored a working group of experts to review and accept the draft guidelines (Pain & Policy Studies Group 2000). The group comprised Tokuo Yoshida (WHO), David E. Joranson (WHOCC), Carmen Selva (U.N. International Narcotics Control Board Secretariat), Liliana De Lima (Pan American Health Organization), Romesh Bhattacharji (Narcotics Commissioner of India), Gu Wei-Ping (State Drug Administration, People's Republic of China), Claudio Blengini (Pain and Palliative Care Specialist, Italy), Philip Emafo (WHO Expert Advisory Panel on Drug Dependence, Nigeria), and Alan Nixon (Palliative Care Specialist, Saudi Arabia). The guidelines, *Achieving Balance in National Opioids Control Policy: Guidelines for Assessment,* were published in 2000 (World Health Organization 2000).

The guidelines emphasize the need to define responsibility at every level of the chain of drug distribution (importer, manufacturer, distributor, hospital, pharmacy, hospice, palliative care program, physician) so that opioid analgesics are available to the patients who need them. The guidelines encourage governmental representatives of narcotics regulation and cancer control to communicate with medical institutions and health professionals working in pain management and palliative care, to exchange information and to identify and make changes in national policies and administration in order to achieve the important public health goal of relieving pain.

In 2002, the INCB endorsed the guidelines, stating: "In the opinion of the Board, the guidelines for the review of national policies contained in that document should always be applied with full respect for the provisions of the 1961 Convention and the corresponding national legislation" (International Narcotics Control Board 2002b).

The guidelines, first published in English, have been translated into French, Spanish and Italian. Internet access is available at www.who.int/medicines/library (English and French), at www.paho.org/spanish (Spanish), and at www.medsch.wisc.edu/painpolicy (English, French, Italian, and Spanish, including monographs and slide presentations relevant to countries in Africa, the Americas, Europe, and Asia).

SUMMARY OF THE GUIDELINES

The content of *Achieving Balance in National Opioids Control Policy* can be grouped into three categories: (1) assessing national policy, (2) estimating annual requirements for opioids, and (3) administering an effective system for distributing opioids to patients.

Assessing national policy. The guidelines explain the rationale and imperative for governments to evaluate their national drug control policy to determine if it is adequate and to take corrective action if needed. The policies of states or provinces within a country should be evaluated as well. National policy should recognize explicitly that opioids are absolutely necessary for medical and scientific purposes, and that the national government has an obligation to ensure adequate availability of opioid analgesics for medical purposes. To fulfill this obligation, governments should designate an administrative authority to implement these responsibilities within the national government.

In order to address exaggerated concerns about addiction, national policies should avoid use of inaccurate terminology that could affect how the medical use of opioids for pain is interpreted; the use of opioids for pain relief should not be confused with drug dependence or "addiction." "Drug dependence" should not be equated with the withdrawal syndrome or tolerance that may occur from prolonged use of opioids for pain management. Instead, "drug dependence," if used in law or regulation, should be defined as compulsive use of a drug that results in impaired functioning and decreased quality of life.

Further, national policy should not impede a physician's ability to make medical prescribing decisions based on individual patient needs, and should avoid restricting the amount or duration of prescriptions or unduly limiting the availability or validity period of prescription forms. Governments should establish a national policy that makes palliative care, pain relief, and availability of opioids priorities in the health care system (World Health Organization 1996). WHO emphasizes the need for governments to include palliative care in their national cancer control programs (Sepúlveda 2000).

Estimating annual requirements for opioids. The guidelines emphasize the need for governments to submit to the INCB realistic estimates of the amounts of each opioid that will be needed in the country during the following year, taking into account unmet needs and the possibility of increasing needs. Governments are encouraged to collaborate with health professionals and medical institutions to learn about the quantity, type, and dosage forms of opioids that are needed. The estimate must be submitted to the INCB in a timely fashion and confirmed by the INCB, so that the government can lawfully import, manufacture, and distribute opioid pain medications. If unforeseen needs arise, governments should submit supplementary estimates to the INCB in order to avoid any interruption in supply of pain medications to patients (Selva 1997). The INCB can confirm supplemental estimates quickly if there is an urgent need to increase the national estimate to permit increased import or manufacture.

Administering the national opioid distribution system. The guidelines emphasize that governments must administer an efficient national system to procure and distribute opioids in a timely fashion to all medical institutions that need them and are properly licensed. Governments should communicate with health professionals to clarify the legal requirements for prescribing, stocking, and dispensing opioids, and to address any fears about legal repercussions for opioid prescribing and dispensing. Governments are encouraged to provide access to opioids for patients throughout their country, including access for patients in hospitals as well as those living at home, while maintaining reasonable controls to prevent diversion.

USING THE GUIDELINES

The guidelines are intended to be used by governments and health professionals in several ways: (1) as an educational tool to learn about the role of national government and its drug control policy with respect to making opioid analgesics available for pain relief, (2) as a policy evaluation tool to identify strengths and weaknesses in national drug control policy, and (3) as a method to formulate new policies or improve existing policies.

For educational purposes, the guidelines should be distributed to the relevant government and nongovernmental organizations in all countries, especially to those individuals and groups who are interested in improving cancer pain relief and palliative care for adults as well as children.

To implement the guidelines, several approaches are suggested. One approach would be for the government to appoint a commission or task force to prepare a study of national policies, using the guidelines and the self-assessment checklist (World Health Organization 2000) as a template to identify barriers and recommendations for change. A task force should include the national competent authority for narcotics control (United Nations 2000); and representatives of organizations dealing with cancer control, HIV/AIDS, essential drugs, and law enforcement; and health professionals including pain clinicians and specialists in pediatric pain and palliative care. In addition, one or more national organizations dedicated to cancer, HIV/AIDS, or pain or palliative care could appoint a commission or task force to conduct a guideline-based study of national policy leading to recommendations and a national strategy meeting. Another approach would be for the competent authority to participate in a workshop or strategy session with health professionals and stake holders to review the WHO checklist and determine the steps needed to implement them in their country. All of these strategies require cooperation between government representatives and health care providers in order for the narcotics control system to work as intended.

Prior to the 2000 guidelines, some governments and health care professionals were cooperating to improve pain management by identifying and addressing unduly restrictive regulation of opioid analgesics: China (Joranson et al. 1995), India (Rajagopal et al. 2001), Italy (Blengini et al. 2003), Japan (Takeda 1993; Japanese Ministry of Health and Welfare 1999), Mexico (Allende and Carvell 1996), the United States (Pain & Policy Studies Group 2000), Malaysia (World Health Organization Western Pacific Regional Office 1999), Germany (Zenz 1993), and France (Brasseur and Larue 1993).

Shortly after the guidelines were published, WHO began sponsoring regional workshops to begin a process to implement them. The WHO, the Pan American Health Organization, and the WHOCC sponsored the first workshop in Quito, Ecuador, in December 2000. Teams of government and health professionals from six Andean countries (Bolivia, Chile, Colombia, Ecuador, Peru, and Venezuela) came together to use the guidelines to evaluate their national policies (Pan American Health Organization 2000; Colleau 2001b).

The second WHO regional workshop was held in Budapest, Hungary, in 2002, where teams from six eastern European countries (Bulgaria, Croatia, Hungary, Lithuania, Poland, and Romania) used the guidelines to develop action plans for improving patient access to opioid analgesics (World Health Organization Regional Office for Europe 2002). Later in 2002, a WHO workshop was held in Gaborone, Botswana, for teams from five African countries (Botswana, Ethiopia, Tanzania, Uganda, and Zimbabwe) to develop palliative care plans for cancer and HIV/AIDS, with a strong component of opioid availability (Joranson and Jorenby 2002). Successful implementation of these action plans will require resources to provide encouragement, technical support, and monitoring in each country.

CONCLUSIONS AND RECOMMENDATIONS

The barriers that impede access to cancer pain management for adults are basically the same for children, although they may be magnified. Lack of knowledge about pain and its treatment, and exaggerated concerns about opioids and fear of dependence and addiction interfere with the use and availability of opioid analgesics, although these drugs are deemed essential for cancer pain management in adults as well as children (World Health Organization 1990, 1998).

Many countries have yet to address their needs for opioid pain medications, as recommended by the INCB and WHO. *Achieving Balance in National Opioids Control Policy* (World Health Organization 2000) provides an authoritative framework for addressing these needs. Health professionals and national health care organizations, including IASP and its national chapters as well as pain and palliative care organizations, could contribute to better understanding of the role of government in opioid availability and the need for cooperation with health professionals. These individuals and organizations can help by (a) disseminating information about the 2000 guidelines to their members through newsletters and journals (Barnard 2002), (b) developing workshops and task forces as vehicles for health professionals and competent authorities to review the guidelines and assess the unmet need for opioids, and (c) supporting the INCB and WHO in their efforts to improve national opioids policy and increase patient access to the drugs that are essential for cancer pain relief. Strong motivation and political leadership will be necessary to expand palliative care, pain relief, and patient access to opioid analgesics (Stjernswärd 1993).

ACKNOWLEDGMENTS

The authors express appreciation to the members of the guidelines review group. We thank the Office for Essential Drugs and Medicines Policy of the WHO for its consistent support, aimed at achieving balance in national opioids control policy. We also express appreciation to Ms. Maria Monterroso for assisting with the review of international policies, and to Ms. Jody Jorenby for assistance in preparation of the manuscript. D.E. Joranson and A.M. Gilson acknowledge support from the Robert Wood Johnson Foundation, Purdue Pharma, and Janssen Pharmaceutica; D.E. Joranson also acknowledges support from Ortho McNeil.

REFERENCES

Allende S, Carvell HC. Mexico: status of cancer pain and palliative care. *J Pain Symptom Manage* 1996; 12(2):121–123.
Barnard D. World Health Organization guidelines for national narcotics control policies. *J Palliat Med* 2002; 5(4):575–577.
Blengini C, Joranson DE, Ryan KM. Italy reforms national policy for cancer pain relief and opioids. *Eur J Cancer Care* 2003; 12(1):28–34.
Brasseur L, Larue F. France: status of cancer pain and palliative care. *J Pain Symptom Manage* 1993; 8(6):412–415.
Colleau SM. Easing the pain of seriously ill children: a progress report. *Cancer Pain Release* 2001a; 14(3):1–8. Available via the Internet: www.whocancerpain.wisc.edu.
Colleau SM. New World Health Organization opioid guidelines put into action. *Cancer Pain Release* 2001b; 14(1).
International Narcotics Control Board. *Report of the International Narcotics Control Board for 1989: Demand for and Supply of Opiates for Medical and Scientific Needs.* Vienna: United Nations, 1989.
International Narcotics Control Board. *Report of the International Narcotics Control Board for 1995: Availability of Opiates for Medical Needs.* New York: United Nations, 1996. Available via the Internet: www.incb.org.
International Narcotics Control Board. *Narcotic Drugs: Estimated World Requirements for 2002—Statistics for 2000.* New York: United Nations, 2002a.
International Narcotics Control Board. *Report of the International Narcotics Control Board for 2001.* New York: United Nations, 2002b. Available via the Internet: www.incb.org.
Japanese Ministry of Health and Welfare. *Report on Administrative Measures against Narcotics and Stimulants Abuse.* Tokyo: Narcotics Division, Pharmaceutical and Medical Safety Bureau, Japanese Ministry of Health, 1999.
Joranson DE, Jorenby JP. *Availability of Opioid Analgesics in Africa and the World.* Madison, WI: University of Wisconsin Pain & Policy Studies Group, 2002.

Joranson DE, Cai Z-J, Gilson AM. Barriers to opioid availability in China. *Chin Bull Drug Depend* 1995; 4(2):88–91.
Murray CJL, Lopez AD. *Global Burden of Disease: A Comprehensive Assessment of Mortality and Disability from Diseases, Injuries, and Risk Factors in 1990 and Projected to 2020.* Cambridge, MA: Harvard University Press, 1996.
Pain & Policy Studies Group. *Raw Data from 45 Government Surveys Received after Publication of the 1996 Report "Availability of Opiates for Medical Needs."* Madison, WI: University of Wisconsin Pain & Policy Studies Group, 1999.
Pain & Policy Studies Group. *Improving Cancer Pain Relief in the World: 1997–1999, a Report on Three Years of Work.* Madison, WI: University of Wisconsin Pain & Policy Studies Group, 2000.
Pan American Health Organization. *Taller de Reguladores: Asegurando Disponibilidad de Analgésicos Opioides para Cuidados Paliativos.* Washington, DC: Pan American Health Organization, 2000.
Patton CV, Sawicki DS (Eds). *Basic Methods of Policy Analysis and Planning,* 2nd ed. Englewood Cliffs, NJ: Prentice Hall, 1993.
Rajagopal MR, Joranson DE, Gilson AM. Medical use, misuse, and diversion of opioids in India. *Lancet* 2001; 358:139–143. Available via the Internet: www.medsch.wisc.edu.
Selva C. International control of opioids for medical use. *Eur J Palliat Care* 1997; 4(6):194–198.
Sepúlveda C. Cancer control programme: WHO Geneva 2000–2001. *Cancer Detect Prev* 2000; 24(Suppl 1):S63.
Sikora K (Ed). *Developing a Global Strategy for Cancer.* Geneva: World Health Organization, 1998.
Stjernswärd J. Palliative medicine—a global perspective. In: Doyle D (Ed). *Oxford Textbook of Palliative Medicine.* Oxford: Oxford University Press, 1993, pp 803–816.
Takeda F. Japan: status of cancer pain and palliative care. *J Pain Symptom Manage* 1993; 8(6):425–426.
United Nations. *Single Convention on Narcotic Drugs, 1961.* Geneva: United Nations, 1973. Available via the Internet: www.incb.org).
United Nations. *Single Convention on Narcotic Drugs, 1961, as Amended by the 1972 Protocol Amending the Single Convention on Narcotic Drugs, 1961.* New York: United Nations, 1977.
United Nations. *Competent National Authorities under the International Drug Control Treaties, 1999.* New York: United Nations, 2000.
United Nations Department of Economic and Social Affairs. *Demographic Yearbook,* 51st ed. New York: United Nations, 2001.
United Nations International Drug Control Programme. *Format and Guidelines for the Preparation of National Drug Control Master Plans.* Vienna: United Nations, 1994.
Weimer DL, Vining AR (Eds). *Policy Analysis: Concepts and Practice,* 3rd ed. Upper Saddle River, NJ: Prentice Hall, 1999.
World Health Organization. *Cancer Pain Relief.* Geneva: World Health Organization, 1986.
World Health Organization. *Cancer Pain Relief and Palliative Care,* Technical Report Series 804. Geneva: World Health Organization, 1990.
World Health Organization. *Cancer Pain Relief: With a Guide to Opioid Availability,* 2nd ed. Geneva: World Health Organization, 1996.
World Health Organization. *Cancer Pain Relief and Palliative Care in Children.* Geneva: World Health Organization, 1998.
World Health Organization. *Achieving Balance in National Opioids Control Policy: Guidelines for Assessment.* Geneva: World Health Organization, 2000. Available via the Internet: www.who.int/medicines/library/qsm.
World Health Organization. *National Cancer Control Programmes: Policies and Managerial Guidelines,* 2nd ed. Geneva: World Health Organization, 2002.

World Health Organization Regional Office for Europe. *Assuring Availability of Opioid Analgesics for Palliative Care*. Copenhagen: World Health Organization Regional Office for Europe, 2002.

World Health Organization Western Pacific Regional Office. *Mission Report: Review of Drug Availability for Cancer Pain Relief*. Manila: World Health Organization Western Pacific Regional Office, 1999.

Zenz M. Germany: status of cancer pain and palliative care. *J Pain Symptom Manage* 1993; 8(6):416–418.

Correspondence to: David E. Joranson, MSSW, Pain & Policy Studies Group, University of Wisconsin Comprehensive Cancer Center, 406 Science Drive, Suite 202, Madison, WI 53711, USA. Tel: 608-263-7662; Fax: 608-263-0259; email: joranson@wisc.edu; Internet: www.medsch.wisc.edu/painpolicy.

Index

Locators in *italic* refer to figures.
Locators followed by t refer to tables.

A

Abdominal pain
  chemotherapy-related, 135
  cognitive-behavioral therapy for, 121
  encouragement of illness behavior, 118
  in families, 113
  school functioning and, 146
  vomiting and, 135
Accreditation
  health care organizations, 183, 190–191
  international programs, 193, 193t
  pain programs, 192–193, 196
  pain standards for adults and children, 194t–195t
Acetaminophen, 139
Achieving Balance in National Opioids Control Policy (WHO), 210–212, 213
Acute pain
  caregiver reaction to, 165–167, *166*
  defined, 99
  family involvement in child care, 104
Adenylyl cyclases, calmodulin-stimulated, 15
Adolescents, 92, 119–120
Adrenocorticotropic hormone (ACTH), 9
A-fibers, 10
Age factors, 64, 90–91
Agency for Health Care Policy and Research, 185–186
Agency for Health Care Research and Quality, 185
American Academy of Pain Management, 193
AMPA (α-amino-3-hydroxy-5-methyl-4-isoxazole propionate), 11
Analgesia and analgesics
  analgesic ladder, cancer pain, 139, 202
  endogenous, 12
  genetics and efficacy of, 58, 61–62
  off-label usage, pediatric, 187
  pre-emptive, for cancer pain, 139
  range orders, 189
  stress and animal models, 60–61
Anesthesia induction, parent presence during, 100–103
Anger, attachment and, 82
Anhidrosis, 58–59
Animal models
  neonatal pain, 3–10
  pain sensitivity, 59–61
  spinal pain mechanisms, 10–13
Anterior cingulate cortex, 13
Anticipation, pain and, 90
Antidepressants, 140
Anxiety, 103, 145
Arousal
  interaction with performance, 26, *26*
  needle sticks and, 27
  ontogenetic adaptation, 47–49
  pain thresholds and, 25
  reactions to novelty and, 44
  regulation of, 24, 31–32
Arthritis, pain interventions in, 187t
Attachment, 81–84
  chronic pain and, 83
  defined, 81–82
  disordered behaviors, 82
  in older children, 83
  painful experiences and, 82–83, 165
  parental separation and pain, 83
  secure vs. insecure, 82, 93–94
Attention, 30–31, 34
Australia and New Zealand College of Anaesthetists, 196

B

Back pain, 59
Balance, in opioids policy making, 208–209
Bayley Behavior Rating Scale, 27
Bayley Scales of Infant Development, 27, *28*
Bee venom, 5
Behavior. *See* Child behavior
Behavioral Style Questionnaire, 84

217

Biofeedback, 121
Bone marrow, aspiration and biopsy, 136
Brain
 development time across species, 4, *5*
 pain-processing structures, 13, *14*
Burns, 103
BXD mice, 68–69

C
CACNA1A gene, 59
Calcitonin gene-related peptide (CGRP), 4
Calcium channels, 59
CAMPIS (Child-Adult Medical Procedure Interaction Scale), 105–106
Cancer pain, 131–150
 assessment of, 137–138
 cancer incidence, 131, 201
 disability from, 143
 epidemiology
  cancer-related, 137
  children vs. adults, 132
  prevalence, 132–134, 144
  procedure-related, 135–137
  treatment-related, 134–135
 family impact of, 144–145
 feeding tubes and, 137
 impact of, 143–146
 long-term effects of, 146
 national policies and opioid analgesia, 205–213
 physical activities and, 143
 psychosocial outcomes, 145–146
 quality of life and, 145
 school functioning and, 143
 self-report of, 137–138
 social activities and, 144
 treatment of, 138–142
  evidence-based interventions, 187t
  inadequacies in, 201–202
  opioid analgesia, 201–214
  palliative, 140
  pharmacological, 139–140
  psychological, 141–142
  psychosocial interventions, 149–150
  sedation for procedures, 135–136
Cancer Pain Relief with a Guide to Opioid Availability (WHO), 208
Cannulation, intravenous, 103
Capitation and pain management, 188
Capsaicin, 5
Carbamazepine, 140
Caregivers
 attachment to, 81–82, 93–94
 child development and, 29–30
 pain response and, 29–30
 reaction to acute pediatric pain, 165–167, *166*
 self-regulatory behaviors and interactions with, 23–24, 31
CARF (Commission on Accreditation of Rehabilitative Facilities), 193
Carpal tunnel syndrome, 59
Carrageenan, 5, 6, 11–12
Catheterization, 103
CBX mice, 68
CCA. *See* Corrected chronological age (CCA)
Cerebral blood flow, regional, 13
CGRP (calcitonin gene-related peptide), 4
Charleston Pediatric Pain Pictures, 83
Chemotherapy, 132, 135
CHEOPS (Children's Hospital of Eastern Ontario Pain Scale), 138
Chest tube insertion, neonatal pain models, 7
Child behavior
 attachment, 82
 etiology of, 35–46
 individual differences in, 159–160
 neonatal pain experiences and, 39, 40, 40t
 parental factors in, 24
 predicting disorders of, 41–43
 temperament and, 39, 39t
 very low gestational age and, 36–39
Child development. *See also* Social development
 arousal regulation and, 24
 caregiver influences on, 29–31
 early pain experience and, 46–47
 plasticity in, 30
 sleep regulation in, 32–33
 temperament and, 34–35
Child Health Questionnaire, 149
Child-Adult Medical Procedure Interaction Scale (CAMPIS), 105–106
Children's Hospital of Eastern Ontario Pain Scale (CHEOPS), 138
Children's Somatization Inventory, 172
Chinese medicine, pain interventions, 169
Chloral hydrate, 135
Chromosome 19p13, 59
Chronic constriction injury, 14
Chronic fatigue syndrome, 73–74
Chronic pain
 in adolescents, 119

assessing impact of, 148–149
attachment behaviors and, 83
cognitive-behavioral therapy, 120–121
defined, 99
family environment and, 115
illness behavior encouragement in, 117–118
impact of, generally, 142–143
impact on family, 119–120, 142
long-term impact of, 147
modeling in, 114
parent training for, 120
parental behavior effects on child, 114–119
physical activities and, 146–147
quality of life and, 147
school functioning and, 143, 146
social activities and, 144
social consequences of, 92–93
Cingulate cortex, anterior, 13
Circumcision, 7
Clinical practice guidelines, 186–187, 196
Clinical trials, pediatric, 186–188
Clonidine, 61
Coaches, parents as, 108–110
Cochrane Collaboration, 185
Codeine, 58
Cognition, 9–10, 27–29
Cognitive assessment
 child behavior etiologies, 35–46
 experimental stress and, 35
 neonatal pain experiences and behaviors, 39
 parent-child interactions in, 24, 37
 premature vs. full-term 3-year-olds, *38*, 38–39
Cognitive-behavioral therapy
 for cancer pain, 141
 family interventions, 120–121
 for painful procedures, 108
Cold pressor task, 86, *86,* 107
Colic, 31–32
Commission on Accreditation of Rehabilitative Facilities (CARF), 193
Communication, social, 164–165
Community, pain and, 162
Compete Freund's adjuvant, 4–5, 11
Conditioned response. *See* Reinforcement
Congenital insensitivity to pain, 58–59, 65
Coordination of health care, 197
Coping
 emotion-focused, 89

mother-child interactions and, 116
pain consequences and, 116–117
pain expression and, 90–91
painful procedures and, 105–106
problem-focused, 89
self-comforting behaviors, 87–88
Corrected chronological age (CCA)
 altered self-regulation and, 33
 experimental stress and, 35
 facial reactivity to pain and, 26, 28
 maternal-child interactions and, 30
 pain reactivity and dampening and, 25
Corticotropin-releasing factor, 9
Crying, 90, 165
Culture
 concept of, 162
 interpretation of, 176–177
 pain interventions and, 169–170
 research methodology and, 177–179
 sensitivity in clinical practice, 176–177
 socially sanctioned pain exposures, 167
 sociocommunications model, *166,* 167
 transformations in, 174–175
 transmission of, 175–176
Cutaneous reflexes, neonatal, 4
CYP2D6 gene, 58
Cytarabine, 135

D

Deep breathing, 141
Dendritic morphogenesis, 2
Dental procedures, 103
Depression, 11, 145
Descending inhibitory systems, neonatal, 4
Despair, 82
Development. *See* Child development; Social development
Diazepam, 135
Diffuse noxious inhibitory controls (DNIC), 12
Distraction, 109, 141
DNA microarrays, 65
DNA sequencing, 57
Dorsal horn cells, 4, 10
Dysmenorrhea, 59
Dyspepsia, 135

E

Electroencephalography (EEG), 33
Emotions, regulation of, 87–89
Endogenous analgesia, 12
Enkephalins, neonatal, 4

Environment, pain and, 159–160
Epibatidine, 61
Ethnicity
    attitudes toward pain, 170–172
    pain and, 161, 171
    research methodology and, 177–179
    sensitivity in clinical practice, 176–177
    sick role and, 170–171
    situational adaptations, 171
    stereotypes and, 176–177
    variation and, 170–174
Evidence-based practice
    growth of, 185–186
    organizational factors in, 196–198
    pain interventions, pediatric, 186–188, 187t
    values affecting, 187t, 188–189
Evolution, social, 164
Experimental pain, 86–87, 107
Extremely low birth-weight (ELBW) infants. *See also* Very low gestational age (VLGA) infants
    child behavior etiologies in, 35–46
    cognitive assessment and, 27
    maternal interactions and child development, 30
    pain thresholds, 25

F
Faces Pain Scale, 138
Facial reactivity to pain, 25–26, 88–89
Familial hemiplegic migraine, 59, 65
Familial Mediterranean fever, 72–73
Family, 99–122. *See also* Parent-child interactions
    chronic pain and, 113–114, 119–121, 147
    encouragement of illness behavior, 117–118
    pain impact on, 144–145, 161
    parents and painful procedures, 100–110
    postoperative pain management and, 110–112
Feeding tubes, 137
Fee-for-service, 188
Fentanyl, 201, *204*
Fibromyalgia
    genetics, 65, 73–74
    heritability of, 59
    juvenile, 73–74, 115
Foot shocks, 6
Formalin, 5–6
Freund's adjuvant, complete, 4–5, 11

Functional Disability Inventory, 149
Functional Status II, 149

G
Gabapentin, 64, 140
Galanin, 4
Gastrointestinal disorders, 115
Gate control theory of pain, 174
Gender, temperament and, 85
Genetics
    age factors in pain sensitivity, 64
    analgesic response, 58, 61–62
    DNA microarray technology, 65
    haplotype analysis, 71
    interindividual variability in pain, 57–61
    mouse strains and pain, 60–61
    pain genes, identification of, 64–71
    pain traits and, 61–64
    pediatric pain and, 71–74
    quantitative trait locus mapping, 65, 67–68
Glutamate, 11
Guided imagery, 141

H
Headache. *See also* Migraine
    biofeedback for, 121
    chronic, 93
    family environment and, 115
    parental behavior and, 119
    school functioning and, 146
Health care policies, 183–198. *See also* Policy making
    accreditation and, 189
    evolution of, 184
    resource utilization, 188–190
Health Utilities Indexes (HUI), 148
Heel stick
    aversion and, 27
    cueing and stress, 49
    neonatal pain models, 6–7
Hereditary sensory neuropathy, type IV, 58–59
Hospitalization, stressors in, 82
Hydromorphone, 201
Hyperalgesia
    capsaicin-induced, 15
    excitatory mechanisms, 10–11
    inflammation-related, 10–11
    needle sticks and, 6, 11
    thermal, 4–5, 14–15
Hypnosis, 141
Hypothalamic-pituitary-adrenal axis, 34

I

Illness behavior. *See* Sick role
Illness Behavior Encouragement Scale (IBES), 87, 117–118
Imagery, guided, 141
Immunizations, 106, 109
Immunoreactivity, Fos-like, 11
Infant pain. *See also* Neonatal pain
  changing views of, 2, 174–175
  ethnicity and, 172
  learning and memory of, 27–29
  long-term effects of, 1
  social aspects of, 165
  underestimation of, 169
Infant stress response, 9–10
Inflammatory pain
  experimental, substances inducing, 5–6
  long-term effects of, 12
  prostaglandin E$_2$ in, 11
  rodent models, 4–6
Information technology, 197
Injections, pain from, 88–89
Institute of Medicine (IOM), 196–198
Insular cortex, 13
Intelligence quotient (IQ), 29–30
International Narcotics Control Board (INCB), 203–205, 207–208, 210
Interpersonal relations, 163–165
Intestinal pain, 135
Invasive procedures. *See also* Painful procedures
  memory of pain and, 28–29
  pain from, 1
  parental presence during, 103
Irritable bowel syndrome, 7, 8
Isolation, social, 94

J

Joint Commission International (JCI), 193, 193t
Joint Commission on Accreditation of Healthcare Organizations (JCAHO)
  international accreditation program, 193, 193t
  pain standards, 189, 193, 196
Juvenile primary fibromyalgia, 73–74, 115
Juvenile rheumatoid arthritis, 115

K

Kainate, 11
Keratoconjunctivitis, 135
Knockout mice, 70–71

L

Language, 89
Learning, 27–29, 85–87
Lifestyle, 167
Long-term depression, 11
Long-term potentiation, 11
Lumbar puncture, 103, 136

M

Marenostrin, 72
Maternal separation, 9–10, 45
MEFV gene, 72
Memorial Symptom Assessment Scale (MSAS), 132, 149
Memory of pain, 27–29
Menstrual pain, 59
Meperidine, *204*
Metabotropic glutamate receptor 1 (mGluR1), 11
Met-enkephalin, neonatal, 4
Methadone, 201, *204*
Mice
  high-analgesia/low-analgesia strains, 66
  high-analgesic-response/low-analgesic-response strains, 66–67
  knockout, 70–71
  as pain sensitivity models, 59–61
  recombinant inbred strains, 68–69
  transgenic, 70
Midazolam, 102, 136
Migraine. *See also* Headache
  biofeedback for, 121
  familial hemiplegic, 59, 65
  genetics, 59
Modeling of pain behaviors, *86*, 86–87, 94, 113–114
Monoaminergic systems, 10
Morphine
  for cancer pain, 140, 201
  genetics and efficacy of, 58, 61
  global consumption of, 202–203, *203*, 206t
Mother-child interactions. *See also* Parent-child interactions
  child development and, 29, 30
  in chronic pain, 116
  cognitive assessment and, 24
  modeling of pain behavior, 86, *86*
  pain response and, 45
  during painful procedures, 106–107
MSAS (Memorial Symptom Assessment Scale), 132, 149
Mucositis, 135
Musculoskeletal pain, 146

Mutagenesis, 70
Mutations, 69–70

N
Needle sticks, 6, 11, 27
Neonatal Facial Coding System, 27
Neonatal pain. *See also* Infant pain
  adult behavior and, 15
  diffuse noxious inhibitory controls, development of, 12
  endogenous analgesic mechanisms, 12
  excitatory mechanisms, 10–12
  facial reactivity to, 25–26
  from invasive procedures, 1
  long-term effects of
    as clinical problem, 2–3
    human data, 46–47
    primate models, 8–10
    rodent models, 3–10
    spinal pain mechanisms, 10–13
    supraspinal processing, 13–15
  modulatory mechanisms, 12–13
  pain threshold in, 2, 25–26
  reflex leg extension and, 25–26
  research needs, 16
  social factors in, 165
Neuropathic pain
  animal models, 8
  chemotherapy-related, 135
  DRG-derived neurotrophins in, 10
  opioids for, 140
Neuroplasticity
  in child development, 30
  glutamate receptors in, 11
  neonatal pain and, 1, 2
Neurosurgery, 140
Neurotransmitters, neonatal, 4
Neutropenia, 135
Newborn pain. *See* Neonatal pain
N-methyl-D-aspartate (NMDA) receptors, 11, 15
Nociceptors, polymodal, 4
Nonsteroidal antiinflammatory drugs (NSAIDs), 139
NTRK1 gene, 59

O
Objective Pain Scale, 138
Observational Scale of Behavioral Distress (OSBD), 138
Oncology, pediatric. *See* Cancer
Ontogenetic adaptation, 47–49
Opioids
  for cancer pain, 139–140, 201–214
  efficacy, individual variability in, 58
  global consumption of, 202, *204*
  guidelines for evaluating national policies, 208–213
    administering distribution system, 211
    estimating annual requirements, 211
    opioid usage, 212–213
    policy assessment, 210–211
  inadequate availability of, 202–205
  intestinal motility and, 135
  national policy and use of, 205–213
  for neuropathic pain, 140
  underutilization of, 201–202
Oucher scale, 138
Outcome measurement, 197–198
Oxycodone, 201, *204*
Oxymorphone, 201

P
Pain. *See also* specific types of pain
  acute. *See* Acute pain
  anticipation of, 90
  chronic. *See* Chronic pain
  definitions of, 163
  experience of, 167–168, 168t
  expression of, 89–92, 168, 169t
  individual variation in, 58–61
  in infants. *See* Infant pain
  interpersonal aspects, 163–165
  memory of, 27–29
  in newborns. *See* Neonatal pain
  procedural. *See* Painful procedures
  prolonged, consequences of, 92–93
  severity, underestimation of, 169
  social aspects, 81–95, 159–180
  supraspinal processing, 13–15, *14*
Pain behavior
  antecedents of, 87
  consequences of, 87
  modeling of, *86,* 86–87, 94, 113–114
  parental influences on, 86
Pain genes, 64–71. *See also* Genetics
  definition, 65
  inbred strain comparison, 67–68
  recombinant inbred mice, 68–69
  selective breeding for, 66–67
  spontaneous mutations, 69
  targeted mutations, 69–71
Pain management
  accreditation and, 190–196, 194t–195t
  challenges for improving, 197–198
  clinical practice guidelines, 186–188
  evidence-based practice, 185–186, 187t
  health care policy and, 184, 188–190

organization factors in, 196–198
position statements, 191–192, 192t
resource utilization and, 188–190
Pain sensitivity
  age factors in, 64
  assay abbreviations, 63t
  behavior problems and, 42
  child behavior and, 44–45
  genetics of, 58, 61–64, *62*
  individual variation, 57–61, 175–176
  neonatal variables and, 40, 40t
  nociceptive assays, genetic correlations, 62–64
  parent ratings of, 39, 39t
  temperament and, 85
Pain threshold
  in extremely low birth-weight infants, 25
  measurement of, 25–26
  in premature infants, 2, 25–26
  reactivity and recovery in, 23
  temperament and, 84
Painful procedures. *See also* Invasive procedures
  in cancer treatment, 132–137
  cognitive-behavioral therapy for, 108
  interventions with parents, 108–110
  negative effects of parent presence, 103–104
  parent behavior and, 88, 88t, 104–108
  parental anxiety during, 103
  parental presence during, 100–104
Parent-child interactions. *See also* Mother-child interactions
  in chronic pain, 114–119
  coaching, 108–110
  in cognitive assessment, 37
  control of distress and, 31, 105–106
  encouragement of illness behavior, 117–118
  pain response and, 45
  painful procedures and. *See* Painful procedures
  parental modeling of pain behavior, 86, 113–114
  postoperative pain management, 110–112
Parenting style, 24, 44
Parents' Postoperative Pain Measure (PPPM), 111–112
Pediatric Cancer Quality of Life Inventory (PCQL-32), 148
Peer interactions, 95
Peptic ulcer disease, 118
Performance, arousal and, 26, *26*

Perinatal experiences, child behavior and, 35–46
Personality Inventory for Children (PIC), 37, 40, 42t–43t, 44–44
PET (positron emission tomography), 13
PGE$_2$ (prostaglandin E$_2$), 11
Phantom limb pain, 134
Physical activity, 143, 146–147
Physiological pain, rodent models, 6–7
Play therapy, 141
Pleiotropy, 61
Poker chip scale, 138
Policy making, 183–198
  accreditation and, 190–191
  agenda in, 184
  change and, 184
  evidence-based practice and, 185–188
  national opioids policy evaluation, 208–213
  payment mechanisms and, 188
  position statements and, 191–192
  public vs. private, 184
  validity of guidelines for, 208
Polymerase chain reaction (PCR), 57
Polymorphism, single nucleotide (SNP), 68
Position statements, 191–192, 192t
Positron emission tomography (PET), 13
Postoperative pain
  in cancer treatment, 134
  cancer-related, 132
  parental management of, 110–112
  undermedication of, 111
Post-traumatic stress disorder, 146
Potentiation, long-term, 11
PPPM (Parents' Postoperative Pain Measure), 111–112
Premature infants. *See also* Neonatal pain
  child behavior etiologies in, 35–46
  external stimulation, adaptation to, 23
  facial reactivity to pain, 25–26
  long-term effects of early pain, 23–50
  ontogenetic adaptation, 47–49
  pain reactivity vs. dampening, 25
  pain thresholds, 2, 23, 25–26
  self-regulation development in, 31
  sensitivity to novel stimuli, 48
  sleep regulation in, 32–33
Preparation, psychological, 141
Primates, as neonatal pain models, 8–10
Procedural pain. *See* Painful procedures
Prolonged pain. *See* Chronic pain
Prostaglandin E$_2$ (PGE$_2$), 11
Protein kinase A, 11

Psychiatric disorders, 118
Public policy, 184
Pyrin, 72

Q
Quality of health care, 189–190, 196–198
Quality of life, 142, 145, 147
Quality of Life Headache-Youth, 149
Quality of Life Pain-Youth, 149
Quantitative trait locus mapping, 65, 67–68
Quisqualic acid, 14

R
Race, concept of, 162–163
Radiation therapy, 132
Rats
　brain development in, 4, 5
　high-autonomy/low-autonomy strains, 67
　as neonatal pain models, 4–8
Reimbursement, health, 188
Reinforcement
　encouragement of illness behavior, 117–118
　memory of pain and, 28–29
　pain behaviors, maintenance of, 87, 94
　pain in premature infants, 47–48
Relaxation, 141
Religion, pain and, 161–162
Research methodology, 177–179
Resource utilization, values and, 188–190
Rheumatoid arthritis, juvenile, 115
Rocking, 87

S
School functioning, 143, 146
Sciatica, 59
Sedation, 135–136
Self-regulation
　altered, 32–34
　biobehavioral reactivity, 34
　control of distress and, 31
　coping and, 33
　development of, 30–32
　of emotions, 87–89
　landmarks in, 31
　parent-child interactions and, 30, 31
　sleep and waking states, 32–33
　temperament and, 34–35
Self-report, 137–138, 168
Separation Anxiety Test, 83
Sex factors in temperament, 85

Sick role
　ethnicity and, 170–171
　parental encouragement of, 117–119
　socio-environmental factors in, 159–163
Sickle cell disease
　evidence-based pain interventions, 187t
　genetics, 65
　school functioning and, 146
　sleep disorders in, 146
Single nucleotide polymorphism, 68
Sleep, 32–33, 146
Small for gestational age, 36
Social activities, pain and, 144
Social development, 81–95. *See also* Child development
　attachment and, 81–84
　learning and, 85–87
　modeling of pain behavior, 86, 86–87
　pain anticipation and, 90
　pain expression, 89–92
　prolonged pain, consequences of, 92–93
　regulation of emotion, 87–89
　temperament, 84–85
Social influences on pain, 159–180
　communication in, 164–165
　concepts in, 161–163
　cultural transmission of, 175–176
　culturally sanctioned pain exposures, 167
　diverse impacts of, 165–170
　evolution in, 164
　exposure of children to danger, 167
　individual variation, 175–176
　interpersonal aspects, 163–165
　interventions and, 169–170
　isolation, 94
　observers' assessment of child pain, 168–169
　pain experience, 167–168, 168t
　pain expression, 168, 169t
　research design considerations, 177–179
　sociocommunications model, 165–167, *166*
　in young children, 165
Socialization. *See* Social development
Sociocommunications, 165–167, *166*
Socioeconomic status, 29–30, 33
Somatization, 145, 172
Somatosensory cortex, primary (S1), 13
Somatostatin, 4
Spinal pain processes, 10–13

Stanford-Binet Behavior Rating Scale, 37, *38,* 38–39, 41, 41t
Stereotypes, 176–177
Steroid hormones, 140
Stress
  cueing and, 49
  experimentally induced, 35
  in premature infants, 48–49
  temperament and, 34
Substance P, 4
Supraspinal pain processing, 13–15, *14*
Surgical pain, animal models, 7
Synaptogenesis, 2

T
Tail-withdrawal test, 62
Team, health care, 197
Teddy bears, 87
Temperament
  coping and, 35
  defined, 34, 84
  effortful control in, 34–35
  gender and, 85
  pain sensitivity and, 39t, 84, 85
  persistence of, 84
  social development and, 84–85
Temporomandibular disorder, 59
TENS (transcutaneous electrical nerve stimulation), 140
Thalamus, ventroposterolateral, 13
Thumb sucking, 87
Touch sensitivity
  behavior problems and, 41
  child behavior and, 44–45
  neonatal variables and, 40, 40t
  parent ratings of, 39, 39t
Transcutaneous electrical nerve stimulation (TENS), 140
Transgenesis, 70
Trauma, children's exposure to, 167
Tricyclic antidepressants, 140
TRKA receptor, 59

U
U50,488 (κ-opioid agonist), 61
United Nations International Drug Control Programme, 208

V
Values, resource utilization and, 188–190
Variation, individual, 58–61, 175–176

Vasoactive intestinal polypeptide, 4
Venipuncture, 103
Very low gestational age (VLGA) infants. *See also* Extremely low birth-weight (ELBW) infants
  child behavior etiologies in, 35–46
  early pain experience, 36–39
  effortful control and, 44
  parent concerns about cognitive development, 45
  prediction of child behavior, 41–44
  reactions to novelty, 44
  stress in, 48
  temperament and child behavior, 39, 39t
Vinca alkaloids, 135
Vincristine, 135
Visceral pain, 7–8
Visual analogue scale (VAS), 138

W
WIN55,212-2 (cannabinoid receptor antagonist), 61
Windup, C-fiber-mediated, 10
Withdrawal, attachment and, 82
Withdrawal latency, 11–12
World Health Organization (WHO)
  analgesic ladder, cancer pain, 139, 202
  call for national opioid policy reviews, 206–208
  Collaborating Center for Policy and Communications in Cancer Care (WHOCC), 208
  guidelines for evaluating national opioids policy
    development of, 208–209
    review process, 209–210
    summary of, 210–211
    use of, 212–213
  Office for Essential Drugs and Medicines Policy, 208
  pediatric cancer pain recommendations, 201–202
  position statements, 192

Progress in Pain Research and Management Series

Pediatric Pain: Biological and Social Context, edited by Patrick J. McGrath and G. Allen Finley, 2003

Opioids and Pain Relief: A Historical Perspective, edited by Marcia L. Meldrum, 2003

Proceedings of the 10th World Congress on Pain, edited by Jonathan O. Dostrovsky, Daniel B. Carr, and Martin Koltzenburg, 2003

Spinal Cord Injury Pain: Assessment, Mechanisms, Management, edited by Robert P. Yezierski and Kim J. Burchiel, 2002

Complex Regional Pain Syndrome, edited by R. Norman Harden, Ralf Baron, and Wilfrid Jänig, 2002

Neuropathic Pain: Pathophysiology and Treatment, edited by Per T. Hansson, Howard L. Fields, Raymond G. Hill, and Paolo Marchettini, 2001

Acute and Procedure Pain in Infants and Children, edited by G. Allen Finley and Patrick J. McGrath, 2001

The Child with Headache: Diagnosis and Treatment, edited by Patricia A. McGrath and Loretta M. Hillier, 2001

Pain Imaging, edited by Kenneth L. Casey and M. Catherine Bushnell, 2000

Sex, Gender, and Pain, edited by Roger B. Fillingim, 2000

Proceedings of the 9th World Congress on Pain, edited by Marshall Devor, Michael C. Rowbotham, and Zsuzsanna Wiesenfeld-Hallin, 2000

Psychological Mechanisms of Pain and Analgesia, by Donald D. Price, 1999

Opioid Sensitivity of Chronic Noncancer Pain, edited by Eija Kalso, Henry J. McQuay, and Zsuzsanna Wiesenfeld-Hallin, 1999

Chronic and Recurrent Pain in Children and Adolescents, edited by Patrick J. McGrath and G. Allen Finley, 1999

Assessment and Treatment of Cancer Pain, edited by Richard Payne, Richard B. Patt, and C. Stratton Hill, 1998

Sickle Cell Pain, by Samir K. Ballas, 1998

Measurement of Pain in Infants and Children, edited by G. Allen Finley and Patrick J. McGrath, 1998

Molecular Neurobiology of Pain, edited by David Borsook, 1997

Proceedings of the 8th World Congress on Pain, edited by Troels S. Jensen, Judith A. Turner, and Zsuzsanna Wiesenfeld-Hallin, 1997

Pain Treatment Centers at a Crossroads: A Practical and Conceptual Reappraisal, edited by Mitchell J.M. Cohen and James N. Campbell, 1996

Reflex Sympathetic Dystrophy: A Reappraisal, edited by Wilfrid Jänig and Michael Stanton-Hicks, 1996

Visceral Pain, edited by Gerald F. Gebhart, 1995

Temporomandibular Disorders and Related Pain Conditions, edited by Barry J. Sessle, Patricia S. Bryant, and Raymond A. Dionne, 1995

Touch, Temperature, and Pain in Health and Disease: Mechanisms and Assessments, edited by Jörgen Boivie, Per Hansson, and Ulf Lindblom, 1994

Proceedings of the 7th World Congress on Pain, edited by Gerald F. Gebhart, Donna L. Hammond, and Troels S. Jensen, 1994

Pharmacological Approaches to the Treatment of Chronic Pain: New Concepts and Critical Issues, edited by Howard L. Fields and John C. Liebeskind, 1994